Empowering Health Decisions

Jerrold S. Greenberg, PhD
Professor Emeritus
School of Public Health
University of Maryland
College Park, Maryland

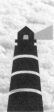

JONES & BARTLETT
LEARNING

World Headquarters
Jones & Bartlett Learning
5 Wall Street
Burlington, MA 01803
978-443-5000
info@jblearning.com
www.jblearning.com

Jones & Bartlett Learning books and products are available through most bookstores and online booksellers. To contact Jones & Bartlett Learning directly, call 800-832-0034, fax 978-443-8000, or visit our website, www.jblearning.com.

Substantial discounts on bulk quantities of Jones & Bartlett Learning publications are available to corporations, professional associations, and other qualified organizations. For details and specific discount information, contact the special sales department at Jones & Bartlett Learning via the above contact information or send an email to specialsales@jblearning.com.

Production Credits
Publisher: William Brottmiller
Editorial Assistant: Sean Coombs
Associate Production Editor: Jill Morton
Developmental Editor: Jennifer Angel
Senior Marketing Manager: Jennifer Stiles
V.P., Manufacturing and Inventory Control: Therese Connell

Composition: Publishers' Design and Production Services, Inc.
Cover Design: Scott Moden
Director, Photo Research and Permissions: Amy Wrynn
Cover Image: © Ilja Mašík/ShutterStock, Inc.
Printing and Binding: Courier Companies
Cover Printing: Courier Companies

To order this product, use ISBN: 978-1-4496-9040-3

Library of Congress Cataloging-in-Publication Data
Greenberg, Jerrold S.
    Empowering health decisions / by Jerrold S. Greenberg.
        p. cm.
    Includes bibliographical references and index.
    ISBN 978-1-4496-1738-7 — ISBN 1-4496-1738-7
1. Health—Decision making. 2. Health behavior. I. Title.
    RA776.9.G75 2013
    613—dc23
                                    2012027218

6048

Printed in the United States of America
17 16 15 14 13   10 9 8 7 6 5 4 3 2 1

Dedication

Empowering Health Decisions is dedicated to my three grandchildren: Garrett, Jonah, and Zoe. It is my hope that their grandfather's book will help them live a healthy and satisfying life full of family, joy, accomplishment, and service to others.

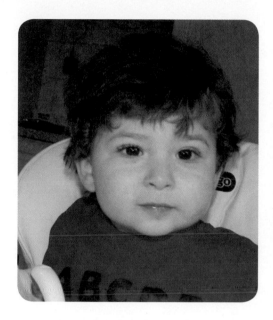

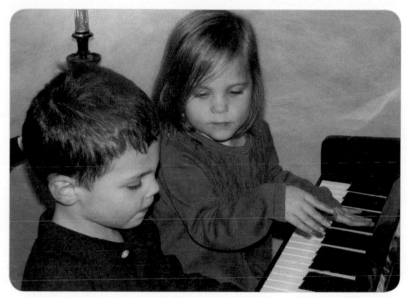

Brief Contents

Contents

Contents

Chapter 3   Improving Your Psychological Health   53

Chapter 4   Managing Stress, Rather Than Letting Stress Manage You   81

Contents

Contents

Preface

Over three decades of teaching, I have been bothered by several troublesome concerns regarding health textbooks for college students. Primary among these concerns is that these texts are inconsistent with what is known about effective health communication. Health communication research advises that important messages not be diluted with other messages of lesser importance. When communication becomes diluted in this manner, the primary message gets lost and learning suffers. In the case of college health texts, readers do not as readily learn which behaviors are health enhancing and which are associated with health risks—even if they do learn the names of anatomical structures or complex physiological processes. This is because college health texts often present a wealth of health information that is not necessary for readers to know in order to make decisions that enhance their health and well-being.

Consequently, when writing *Empowering Health Decisions*, an attempt was made to include only content necessary for college students to make healthy lifestyle decisions. Admittedly, decisions regarding inclusion or exclusion of content cannot be made with total objectivity. That is, there is no way to apply strict and rigid rules and standards to make these determinations. However, valid decisions about what to include and what not to include can still be made. To do so in *Empowering Health Decisions*, content inclusion was guided by the following questions:

- Can a healthy decision be made by the reader without having this information? If yes, then that content was omitted.

- Is this information necessary for the reader to behave healthfully? If yes, then that content was included.

As a check and balance for these decisions, experts in health education and college instructors of health education courses reviewed drafts of this book to ensure that content was not omitted that, in their determination,

needed to be included. The result is confidence that extraneous content is not included and necessary content is.

This process led to a book of fewer pages than the typical college health text, albeit more effective in communicating and highlighting health information necessary for readers to adopt and maintain a healthy lifestyle.

Theory Based

Health behavior change theories and models of decision-making can be quite helpful in aiding students to behave in healthy ways. Yet descriptions of these theories and models are too often presented in a complicated and confusing manner. *Empowering Health Decisions* describes behavior change theories and models of decision-making in a way that readers can easily understand, and applies these theories throughout the text. In an early chapter, several behavior change theories and models of decision-making are described in detail, and examples of how to use these models to make health-enhancing decisions are presented. Subsequently, following chapters refer back to these theories and models, and include an exercise in which students select one scenario to which they wish to apply one of the behavior change theories or decision-making models.

Pedagogical Features

Empowering Health Decisions includes several pedagogical features to enhance student learning. Among these features are:

- *Learning Objectives.* Listed at the beginning of each chapter, learning objectives guide the student and instructor to the major learning components that follow.

- **Health Check Up.** Consists of scales, questionnaires, numerous assessments, and other activities to help students determine how they would behave with regard to the information presented in each chapter.

- **What I Need to Know.** Interesting content, pertinent to making health-enhancing decisions, is highlighted to emphasize its importance.

What I Need to Know

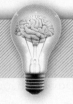

College Students' Health

The American College Health Association regularly collects data on the health of college students. Some of the highlights from those studies are as follows.

Students experienced various health problems during the past 12 months:

Allergies	20%
Asthma	9%
Back pain	13%
Ear infection	7%
Migraine	8%
Strep throat	11%
Sinus infection	18%

Only 33% received Human papillomavirus (HPV) vaccination, 40% flu vaccination, and 55% meningococcal meningitis vaccination.

Only 34% of males performed a testicular self-exam, and 54% of females had a gynecological exam in the past year.

Less than half of college students used sunscreen regularly for sun exposure.

When riding a bicycle, 42% never used a helmet.

Depression was prevalent. Ten percent were diagnosed with depression, and 31% reported difficult functioning as a result of feeling depressed. Depression affected academic performance for 12%, and 61% reported feeling very sad.

Anxiety is also prevalent with 48% feeling overwhelmingly anxious and 18% stating anxiety affected their academic performance.

Alarmingly, 6% of students considered suicide within the past 12 months, and 1% actually attempted suicide.

Sleepiness was problematic as well. Sleepiness interfered with the daytime activities of 16%, and sleep difficulties affected the academic performance of 20%.

Stress also created problems for students. Forty-one percent experienced *more than average stress* and another 10% experienced *tremendous stress*. For 27%, stress interfered with their academic performance.

Alcohol is the most commonly used drug on campuses, with 80% of students using it. In spite of driving and drinking concerns, 27% drove after ingesting alcohol. The last time they partied, 43% drank five or more drinks. Alcohol drinking led to 35% doing something they later regretted. Furthermore, under the influence of alcohol, 17% had unprotected sex, and 17% physically injured themselves.

Students are also sexually active with 50% engaging in sexual intercourse during the past year, but only 51% using a condom or other protective barrier. The result is that 2% of those who had sexual intercourse experienced an unintended pregnancy.

Only 49% of students met the recommended guidelines for moderate-intensity or vigorous-intensity exercise.

DATA FROM: American College Health Association. *American College Health Association–National College Health Assessment II: Reference Group Executive Summary Spring 2010*. Linthicum, MD: American College Health Association, 2010.

■ *Myths and Facts.* Myths and misconceptions specific to each chapter's content are presented. Alongside each myth, the correct information (fact) is discussed. Only the necessary facts and myths that should be dismissed to make health-enhancing decisions are included.

■ *Running Glossary.* Key terms are defined at the bottom of the pages on which they appear to help students better understand each chapter's content.

■ *Applying Behavior Change Theory.* Students are asked to choose a health behavior specific to each chapter's content that they want to modify. They will choose a behavior change theory or decision-making model to modify that behavior, outline the steps to apply that theory or model, and make a judgment regarding how successful they think they would be in modifying that health behavior if they applied the theory or model as described.

Myths *and* Facts
About Behavior Change Theories

MYTH	FACT
Each health behavior change theory is unique.	Many behavior change theories have similar constructs. Social support, self-efficacy, and the influence of the environment are several of these constructs.
All health behavior change theories take a similar approach to affect behavior change.	Some health behavior change theories take very different approaches. For example, stages of change theory suggests different activities for people who fall into different stages. In contrast, the health belief model suggests similar activities for people regardless of their readiness for change. Some theories rely more heavily on the influence of the environment (social learning theory), whereas others are more inner/individual directed (social marketing theory).
Theories that were developed many years ago are outdated and should not be used.	For a theory to be useful, it must be tested over many years, in many different settings, with many different groups of people. If that type of research demonstrates the validity of the theory, then one can be confident it accurately explains health behavior and can be used to modify that behavior. Therefore, theories developed many years ago may actually be more valid and useful than theories developed more recently.

- **My Health Commitment.** A behavioral contract is included in which the student commits to a health behavior change. The reader is asked to apply a decision-making model or behavior change theory to facilitate this change.

- **Summary.** At the end of each chapter, a summary of the content included in that chapter is provided. This summary guides students to the most important knowledge and skills included in that chapter.

- **Internet Resources.** At the end of each chapter, a list of websites that pertain to that chapter's content are listed so students can acquire more information about topics in which they are particularly interested.

- **References.** Included at the end of the chapter, these current citations validate content presented in *Empowering Health Decisions* and provide students with resources for continued health education.

- **Companion Website.** Access to the student companion website (go.jblearning.com/Empowering) is included with every new text. Students can use the interactive glossary, flashcards, crossword puzzles, practice quizzes, web links, and other resources to master the material covered in the text.

My Health Commitment: A Behavioral Contract

I _____ (your name) am committed to better management of stress. To do that, I need to _____ (the behavior you wish to change) because _____ (the reason you need to make this change).

Hint: Make sure the behavior you identify is very specific. You should specify how much and/or how often you are able to measure the outcome. For example, "I will meditate for 30 minutes five times a week."

If I am successful at changing this behavior, I will reward myself by _____ (the reward you will apply). I have decided I will make this behavior change by _____ (date).

Hint: Make sure the reward is something you would not usually give yourself; for example, calling a friend enrolled at another university.

If I do not make this change, I will reevaluate this contract and adjust it so it can be more successful as an aid to achieve my behavior goal. Then I will implement it again.

_____ (your signature)   _____ (today's date)

_____ (witness signature)   _____ (today's date)

Hint: Having a friend or relative witness the contract will encourage you to adhere to it and increase your chances of being successful in changing the behavior.

The Health Decision Portfolio

go.jblearning.com/Empowering

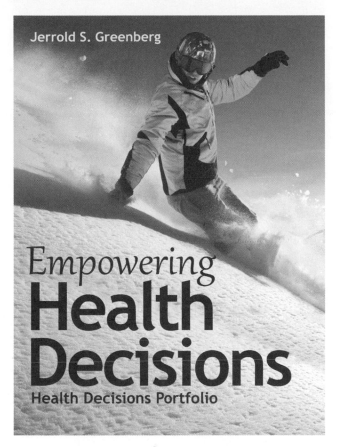

An integral part of *Empowering Health Decisions* is the *Health Decision Portfolio*. Too often, students complete assignments associated with one chapter only to forget about those assignments as they move to another chapter. In this disjointed way, students fail to see the relationship between health-related information. Failing to see how assignments or content from one chapter relate to decisions regarding content from another chapter results in a reductionistic view of health.

The *Health Decision Portfolio* remedies this situation. Readers develop an online *Health Decision Portfolio* that maintains assignments, exercises completed in the book, and material from websites. Then, at the conclusion of the course, the instructor can ask students to tie all of that together in a variety of ways. For example, a term paper could be written on the topic "What I Learned About My Own Health and How to Maintain It." Alternatively, students could be asked to identify gaps in their health knowledge and information after compiling their *Health Decision Portfolios*—gaps they feel impact their abilities to make lifelong health decisions. Once the gaps are recognized, students can identify how they propose to close those gaps. Another option is for students to complete a behavior change contract that refers to future health goals to which they are willing to commit. In other words, the *Health Decision Portfolio* summarizes the course and the student's interaction with the course content. It then challenges students to identify health-related behavior changes they need to make, and decide which strategies they will use to make these changes, to maintain a healthy lifestyle long after the completion of the course.

The goal, then, of *Empowering Health Decisions* is to provide students with the knowledge and skills they need to modify their health behavior, and to be able to do so throughout their lives. If we have succeeded in achieving this goal, the time spent writing this book and the cost of producing it will be well worth the effort. Let us know how we did—both students and instructors. Now, on to better health.

Acknowledgments

The author wishes to thank the following reviewers for their feedback and advice while writing this manuscript:

- Jeanne M. Clerc, EdD, MT(ASCP)SH, Health Sciences Department, Western Illinois University

- Charles "Pete" LeRoy, New Mexico Highlands University

- Elizabeth Lincoln, MD, Sauk Valley Community College

- Dr. Kirsten Lupinski, Albany State University, Department of Health, Physical Education and Recreation

- Dr. Alan Temes, Zero Point Field

The author also wishes to thank Jennifer Angel for her feedback and suggestions while developing this text.

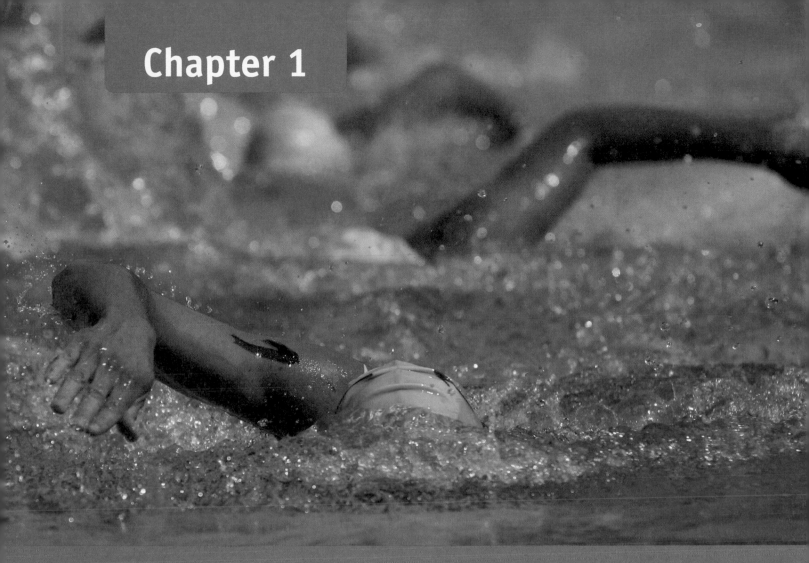

Chapter 1

Health: What It Is, Why You Need It, and How to Get It

 Access Health Check Ups and Health Behavior Change activities on the Companion Website:
go.jblearning.com/Empowering.

Learning Objectives

- Describe the difference between illness, health, and wellness.
- Define mental health, emotional health, social health, physical health, and spiritual health.
- Discuss the factors affecting health and illness.
- Explain the effect of social policy on health and illness.
- Distinguish between factors affecting health that are within your control and those that are beyond your control.

The last time Miguel saw his friend Larissa was 2 years ago in high school. She'd been kind of overweight then. When he ran into her on campus, he noticed she was looking much more fit. While they were catching up, he learned that she had started running and was now up to 50 miles a week. She'd also become a vegetarian and joined a running club around which her social life revolved. However, Miguel also noticed she looked tired and that, beneath all her new-found enthusiasm for running, she seemed unhappy. She admitted that because training takes up so much of her time, her grades have been slipping and she rarely goes to family gatherings or church anymore. Still, she said, she was feeling great.

Larissa believed she was *healthier* than she had ever been. Her doctor told her that her cholesterol level was within the recommended range, her immunological system was more effective resulting in her being ill less often, and her stamina was such that she seldom felt fatigued. Whether, in fact, Larissa was healthy is the focus of this chapter. What is health and how is it related to illness? Can one be healthy and yet not possess wellness? In terms of your lifestyle, are you healthy and functioning at a high level of wellness? As this chapter will show, answers to these questions relate to the quality of your life and whether you lead a life of true satisfaction. We will refer back to Larissa throughout this chapter to make this point.

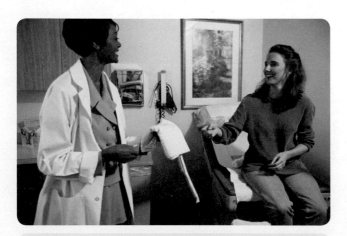

Physicians can help you be physically healthy, but you also have a major role in becoming physically healthy and maintaining physical health.

Know the Meaning of and Differences Between Illness, Health, and Wellness

Illness

If someone told you that your aunt is ill, you would probably assume that she has cancer, heart disease, had an accident, or came down with a common cold. What these conditions have in common is that they are all physical ailments. And yet, people can develop mental impairment, can be emotionally unstable, or be socially isolated. These, too, are illnesses. Illness is defined as one of the components of health not functioning as well as it should. Although we may know this intellectually, we tend not to think of nonphysical ailments when we speak of illness.

That is because we view nonphysical ailments as less serious than physical ailments, and this view is reinforced by the medical and health establishment. Evidence for this conclusion can be seen by health insurance companies only recently being required to cover mental illness in a similar fashion as they have covered physical illness for many years. Is someone with a mental illness less ill than someone with a physical illness? Is someone who angers easily and becomes aggressive (emotional illness) resulting in poor relationships with family members and friends less ill than someone with a physical illness? Is someone who has no friends and feels all alone less ill than someone with a physical illness? No. Illness encompasses much more than merely being physically ill.

Health

Although physical health is important, being healthy entails more than just being physically healthy. Beside physical health, components of **health** include mental health, emotional health, social health, and spiritual health. Some experts include vocational health, environmental health, financial health, and family health in this mix as well.

Physical Health

To achieve **physical health**, you need to have your physiology functioning well. For example, your blood pressure needs to be within normal range, your blood cholesterol needs to be within recommended limits, and you need to have sufficient muscular strength and endurance to meet life's demands. Throughout this book, we show you how to achieve and maintain physical health and ward off physical illness.

Mental Health

Mental health is such a complex concept that there may be no one *official definition* of mental health. Cultural differences, subjective assessments, and competing professional theories all affect how mental health is defined (World Health Organization, 2001). The World Health Organization defines mental health as "a state of well-being in which the individual realizes his or her own abilities, can cope with the normal stresses of life, can work productively and fruitfully, and is able to make a contribution

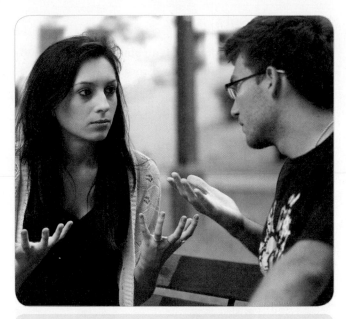

Being emotionally healthy involves learning how to control your emotions and expressing them appropriately.

to his or her community" (World Health Organization, 2005). To be mentally healthy, you also need to perceive events and people in a way that is not dysfunctional but rather realistic. Some mental illnesses, for example, result in the unrealistic belief that others are out to harm you or lead to alternating extremes of sadness and euphoria or to the inability to live life fully because of extreme fear or anxiety. To be mentally healthy is to function as the society or culture defines *normal*.

Health: composed of physical health, mental health, emotional health, social health, and spiritual health.

Physical health: having your physiology functioning well such as blood pressure within normal range, blood cholesterol within recommended limits, and sufficient muscular strength and endurance to meet life's demands.

Mental health: a state of well-being in which the individual realizes his or her own abilities, can cope with the normal stresses of life, can work productively and fruitfully, and is able to make a contribution to his or her community.

Emotional Health

Emotional health is defined as an ability to express emotions and feelings appropriately. Emotionally healthy people can control their emotions when that is the right thing to do and, when they choose to, express their emotions in a manner that does not harm their relationships or interfere with their goals. They are empathetic and understanding of the needs of others and are good listeners. These are skills that can in fact be learned and improved upon throughout life.

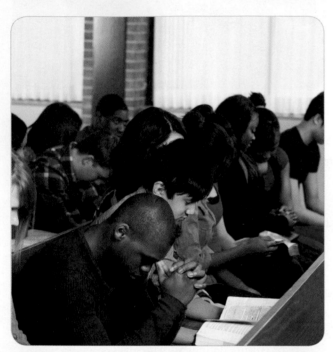

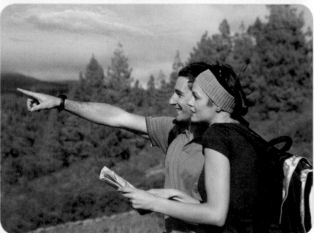

Someone can be spiritual without necessarily being religious. Feeling a connection to nature and to humankind are expressions of spirituality.

Social Health

Socially healthy people interact well with others and their environment. They have satisfying relationships, close friends, and people in whom to confide. **Social health** is characterized by involvement with other people, be that as a member of a club or just hanging out. A number of studies have demonstrated the importance of developing a social support system to maintain overall health. Having others with whom to share your joys and sorrows, from whom to seek advice, to encourage and help you achieve your goals, and even to provide financial support when needed goes a long way in preventing illness and disease.

Spiritual Health

Spirituality encompasses a feeling of connection to the world and others in it, which may or may not be conceptualized as religion. **Religion** is a social entity that involves beliefs, practices, and rituals related to the sacred—sacred defined as mystical or supernatural or God or, in Eastern religious traditions, the ultimate truth or reality. Religions usually speak to life after death and proscribe rules to guide behavior within a support group. Spirituality is more personal than religion in that it is something people define for themselves that is largely free of rules, regulations, and responsibilities typical of religions. Therefore, you can be spiritual but not religious. In that case, you deny a connection with any organized religion

Emotional health: being able to express emotions and feelings appropriately.

Social health: interacting well with others and the environment; having satisfying relationships, close friends, and people in whom to confide.

Spirituality: a feeling of connection to the world and others in it, which may or may not be conceptualized as religion.

Religion: a social entity that involves beliefs, practices, and rituals related to the sacred—sacred defined as mystical or supernatural or God or, in Eastern religious traditions, the ultimate truth or reality.

and define your spirituality in secular and individualistic terms. **Spiritual health** is achieved when you have a clear view of meaning and purpose in life, connections with others (those who came before you and those who will follow) and with nature, peacefulness, and comfort with life choices (Koenig, 2009). Part of being spiritually healthy is being able to forgive (Berry, Worthington, O'Connor, Parrot, and Wade, 2005). Being unforgiving evokes brain activity consistent with stress, anger, and aggression and an increase in blood pressure. It also negatively affects mental health and makes the immunological system less effective. In contrast, adopting a forgiving attitude results in lower levels of anxiety, depression, and stress; fewer illnesses; less back pain; and spiritual well-being.

The Health–Illness Continuum

To understand better the difference between health, illness, and wellness, imagine that health appears on one side of a continuum and death and illness on the other (FIG. 1.1 ▼). Further imagine that this continuum is not made up of a straight line but rather a dotted line with each dot consisting of the five components of health (FIG. 1.2 ▶). The healthier the person, the larger will be each component of health and, therefore, the larger the dot. The implications of this is that someone may be at the illness part of the continuum—for example, a physically challenged man—but have a large health dot because he has a lot of friends, is empathetic and understanding, is a good learner, and has a sense of his or her place in the universe. If he participates in physical challenges, such as training for the Paralympics, the physical health component of his dot may also be quite large in spite of the physical challenges he faces.

Wellness

Whereas health is the total of the components of health, **wellness** refers to the balance between these components.

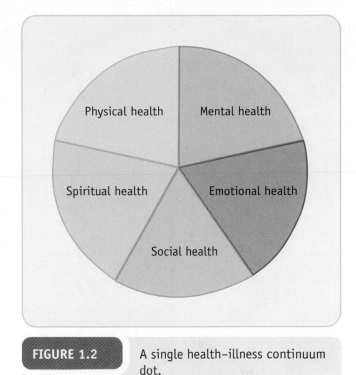

FIGURE 1.2   A single health–illness continuum dot.

Larissa, referred to earlier in the chapter, had improved her physical health tremendously. At the same time, she neglected her mental, emotional, social, and spiritual health. Her health dot would appear as depicted in FIG. 1.3 ▶ . She has an enlarged physical health component but shrunken mental, emotional, social, and spiritual health components. If Larissa's health dot were a tire on a car or bicycle, it would be *out of round* and result in a bumpy ride. Similarly, with her health dot as it is, she can expect a bumpy ride through life. Larissa could pay more attention to all of the components that make up health and thereby achieve high-level wellness. Wellness relates to the level of each of the health sections and, in particular, the balance between them.

| Perfect Health | Health | Illness | Death |

FIGURE 1.1   The health–illness continuum.

Spiritual health: having a clear view of meaning and purpose in life, connections with others and with nature, peacefulness, and comfort with life choices.

Wellness: having the components of health in the recommended amounts and in balance with each other.

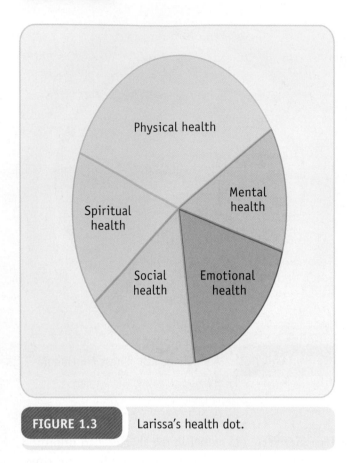

FIGURE 1.3 Larissa's health dot.

High-Level Components of Wellness

Larissa's running is not a problem. The fact that she improved her physical health is to be applauded. However, her neglect of the other health components is indeed problematic and unnecessary. Larissa could have improved her mental health by reading about running; for example, how nutrition relates to faster running, how carbohydrate loading can improve endurance, or how to recover from injuries quickly. She could have improved her emotional health by learning to accept that sometimes she will not run as fast as she would like or by not attempting to prevent faster runners from passing her and getting angry at them and at herself when that happens. Larissa's social health could also have improved if she ran with her friends, shared her passion for running with her family, or organized group running events for friends and family. Lastly, Larissa could have become more spiritually healthy by focusing on the sound of birds or the wind rustling through the leaves or by volunteering 10 hours in her community for every race she ran. One of the criteria for achieving high-level wellness is that all health components are expanded, like a properly inflated tire.

Balance of Components of Health

The second criterion for achieving high-level wellness is that the health components are in balance. Certainly, Larissa failed at that. As discussed earlier, however, that need not have been the case. Expanding all health components in a comparable amount will ensure balance in your life and a smooth ride on your health tire.

Complete Health Check Up 1.1 to determine your level of wellness (see Health Check Up 1.1 on the companion website). Once completed, place Health Check Up 1.1 in your Health Decision Portfolio so you can refer to it when you are motivated to improve your wellness status.

Factors Affecting Health and Illness

There are many factors that affect health and wellness. These factors vary in the degree to which they are within your control. For example, your heredity and genetics are out of your control but may increase or decrease your likelihood of developing an illness or disease or even the number of years you may live. Your immunological system's effectiveness in responding to microorganisms that cause illness and disease is partly inherited but also partly within your control; for example, your diet and sleep habits can affect its performance. Social policies that facilitate or create barriers to healthful behavior are largely out of your control, but being aware of them can help you turn them to your advantage. The factors most in your control are, of course, the lifestyle choices you make that enhance your health or threaten it.

Communicable Diseases

Communicable diseases can be transmitted from person to person or from contaminated objects to those who come in contact with them. This transmission most often

Communicable diseases: diseases that are transmitted from person to person or by contact with infected objects.

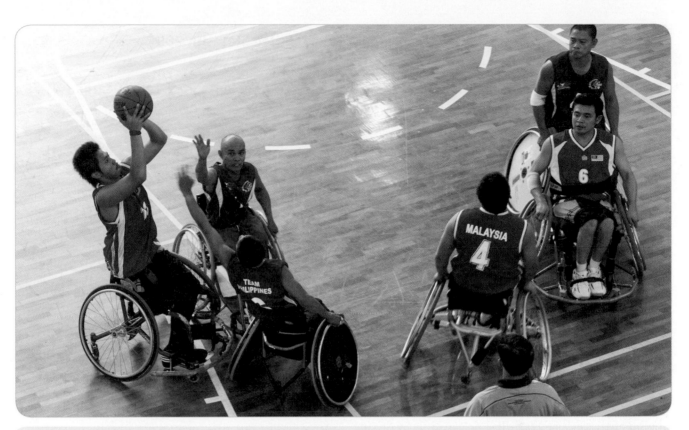

A person may be physically challenged but have other health components functioning well and, therefore, may be classified as healthy.

occurs by breathing contaminated air (e.g., when someone ill sneezes near you), touching something with the disease-causing organism on it (such as equipment at the gym), drinking contaminated water or eating contaminated food, or coming in contact with bodily fluids (such as blood, saliva, or semen) of a contaminated person (Currin, 2007). Examples of communicable diseases are influenza, botulism, sexually transmitted infections, tuberculosis, chicken pox, measles, and strep throat (Rhode Island Department of Health, 2011).

One of the best ways to prevent contraction of a communicable disease is to wash your hands often and thoroughly (Centers for Disease Control and Prevention, 2010). Even better is to avoid contact with disease-causing organisms such as bacteria and viruses. This can take the form of wiping down gym equipment with a disinfectant before working with it, using safer sex methods if sexually active, or avoiding contact with people who have a communicable disease. Another effective method is to get vaccinated against communicable diseases (such as influenza,

measles, chicken pox, malaria, and polio) so your body develops antibodies that can prevent disease even if you come in contact with the disease-causing organism.

Lifestyle Illnesses

Americans are killing themselves. Although that may sound dramatic, it is not far from the truth. In the early 1900s, the leading causes of death were communicable diseases: tuberculosis, pneumonia, influenza, and diarrhea and enteritis. These diseases were caused by viruses or bacteria, and, consequently, health officials could do something to prevent them, and they did. Sanitation, quarantine, and the development of vaccines have eliminated or significantly decreased the prevalence of these diseases. Today, however, the leading causes of death are the result of our unhealthy behaviors. Table 1.1 lists the 10 leading causes of death, the number of deaths for each cause, and the percentage of total death for each cause. Note that the leading

TABLE 1.1 — Ten Leading Causes of Death in the United States in 2007

Cause of Death	Number of Deaths	Percentage of Total Deaths (%)
Heart disease	616,067	25.4
Cancer	562,875	23.2
Stroke	135,952	5.6
Respiratory disease	127,924	5.3
Accidents	123,706	5.1
Alzheimer's disease	74,362	3.1
Diabetes	71,382	2.9
Influenza/pneumonia	52,717	2.2
Kidney disease	46,488	1.9
Septicemia (blood poisoning)	34,828	1.4

REPRODUCED FROM: Centers for Disease Control and Prevention. *Deaths and Mortality*. 2010. Available at: http://www.cdc.gov/nchs/fastats/deaths.htm.

causes of death are **lifestyle diseases**, which are caused by our health behaviors: smoking, eating unhealthy foods, adopting a sedentary lifestyle that lacks the recommended amount of physical activity, behaving carelessly by driving unsafely or not using sun block when in the sun, and so forth. These are all behaviors over which we have control or should have control. To behave in these ways is to shorten our lives and risk our health.

Tobacco Use

One of the unhealthiest behaviors is the use of tobacco. Tobacco use accounts for more than 400,000 deaths, or more than 18% of all deaths, in the United States per year. It is associated with three leading causes of death: cancer, heart disease, and stroke. Although cigarette smoking is the predominant culprit, pipe and cigar smoking, as well as chewing tobacco, are also related to these three leading causes of death. Approximately 20% of Americans are current cigarette smokers, with cigarette smoking most prevalent between the ages of 18 and 34 years and among males. Twenty-five percent of males ages 18–24 and 29% ages 25–34 are current cigarette smokers. Nineteen percent of females ages 18–24 and 20% ages 25–34 are current cigarette smokers (National Center for Health Statistics, 2010, p. 276). Notably, the more educated one is, the less likely that person is to be a smoker. Only 9% of Americans who have a bachelor's degree or higher degree

are current cigarette smokers (National Center for Health Statistics, 2010, p. 278).

Sedentary Lifestyle

Regular exercise or other forms of physical activity such as gardening or dancing improves the health of your heart, circulatory system, and respiratory system. It is for this reason that physical activity can help prevent or postpone heart disease, stroke, and other causes of early disability or death. Regular physical activity is also good for your mental health as it has been shown to help with depression and anxiety. Lastly, it is good for your social health, especially when you exercise with others. Unfortunately, either due to a perceived lack of time or lack of interest, 39% of Americans 18 years of age or older are physically inactive, with just 31% active regularly (National Center for Health Statistics, 2010, p. 299). Those numbers are a little better for college students, but not much. For those with some college education, 29% are physically inactive, with just 38% active regularly—that in spite of the availability of

Lifestyle diseases: diseases caused by health behaviors that place one at risk of developing such conditions as coronary heart disease, stroke, and cancer.

What I Need to Know

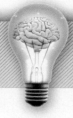

College Students' Health

The American College Health Association regularly collects data on the health of college students. Some of the highlights from those studies are as follows.

Students experienced various health problems during the past 12 months:

Allergies	20%
Asthma	9%
Back pain	13%
Ear infection	7%
Migraine	8%
Strep throat	11%
Sinus infection	18%

Only 33% received Human papillomavirus (HPV) vaccination, 40% flu vaccination, and 55% meningococcal meningitis vaccination.

Only 34% of males performed a testicular self-exam, and 54% of females had a gynecological exam in the past year.

Less than half of college students used sunscreen regularly for sun exposure.

When riding a bicycle, 42% never used a helmet.

Depression was prevalent. Ten percent were diagnosed with depression, and 31% reported difficult functioning as a result of feeling depressed. Depression affected academic performance for 12%, and 61% reported feeling very sad.

Anxiety is also prevalent with 48% feeling overwhelmingly anxious and 18% stating anxiety affected their academic performance.

Alarmingly, 6% of students considered suicide within the past 12 months, and 1% actually attempted suicide.

Sleepiness was problematic as well. Sleepiness interfered with the daytime activities of 16%, and sleep difficulties affected the academic performance of 20%.

Stress also created problems for students. Forty-one percent experienced *more than average stress* and another 10% experienced *tremendous stress*. For 27%, stress interfered with their academic performance.

Alcohol is the most commonly used drug on campuses, with 80% of students using it. In spite of driving and drinking concerns, 27% drove after ingesting alcohol. The last time they partied, 43% drank five or more drinks. Alcohol drinking led to 35% doing something they later regretted. Furthermore, under the influence of alcohol, 17% had unprotected sex, and 17% physically injured themselves.

Students are also sexually active with 50% engaging in sexual intercourse during the past year, but only 51% using a condom or other protective barrier. The result is that 2% of those who had sexual intercourse experienced an unintended pregnancy.

Only 49% of students met the recommended guidelines for moderate-intensity or vigorous-intensity exercise.

Data from: American College Health Association. *American College Health Association–National College Health Assessment II: Reference Group Executive Summary Spring 2010*. Linthicum, MD: American College Health Association, 2010.

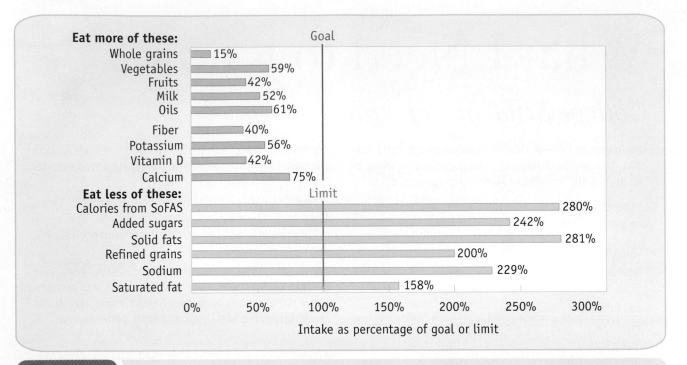

FIGURE 1.4 Dietary intakes in comparison to recommended intake levels or limits. Bars show average intakes for all individuals (ages 1 or 2 years or older) as a percentage of the recommended intake level or limit. SoFAS = Solid fats. Reproduced from: Center for Nutrition Policy and Promotion. *Report of the Dietary Guidelines Advisory Committee on the Dietary Guidelines for Americans, 2010.* Available at: http://www.cnpp.usda.gov./DGAs2010-DGACReport.htm.

exercise facilities on most campuses. Do you take advantage of those facilities or is the portion of your student fees that support these facilities being wasted?

Nutrition

What we eat affects every organ in our bodies. Among other functions, foods provide us energy and the ability to heal, prevent illness and disease, and help us lead a healthy life. Yet, too many of us pay too little attention to the foods we ingest, other than some of us who are trying to maintain or lose weight. As noted in **FIG. 1.4 ▲**, what we eat contains too many fats, added sugars, refined grains, sodium, and saturated fats. We ingest too few whole grains, vegetables, fruits, milk, oils, fiber, potassium, vitamin D, and calcium. And, too many of us are overweight or obese. Consequently, the federal government recommends that Americans limit caloric intake by adopting portion-control strategies. In addition, it is recommended that we eat more vegetables, fruits, and high-fiber whole grains; more fat-free or low-fat milk and milk

products; and more seafood, lean meat, poultry, eggs, soy products, nuts, seeds, and oils. Lastly, it is recommended that Americans eat fewer solid fats and sugars and limit their intake of salt (Center for Nutrition Policy and Promotion, 2010, p. B2-15).

Sexual Behavior

Whereas sex can be pleasurable, it can also result in tragic consequences. Contraction of sexually transmitted infections is always possible, and pregnancies can result from engaging in sexual intercourse—this in spite of adopting **safer sex strategies**. No contraceptive is 100% effective in

> **Safer sex strategies:** behaviors that decrease the chance of someone who is sexually active contracting a sexually transmitted infection or creating pregnancy; included are using a condom, limiting the number of sexual partners, and maintaining a monogamous sexual relationship.

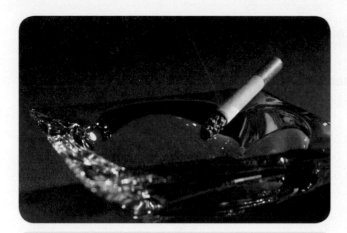

Use of tobacco products is the lifestyle behavior most associated with disability and early death.

preventing pregnancy or sexually transmitted infections. Therefore, the only sure-fire way to not contract a sexually transmitted infection or experience an unintended pregnancy is to be sexually abstinent. For many, however, this is not an acceptable lifestyle. For them, adapting sexual behavior to be safer can limit the chances of experiencing these consequences. Some of these safer sex strategies include using a condom during coitus, being in a sexually monogamous relationship or limiting the number of sexual partners, and refraining from high-risk sexual behaviors such as anal intercourse. And yet, these safer behaviors are too often absent among college students. Numerous researchers have found that "hookups" (oral, vaginal, or anal sex) are common on college campuses. For example, Fielder and Carey (2010b) found that 51% of college students reported hookups before college and 36% during the first semester of college. Unfortunately, they also found that condoms were used in only 69% of hookups involving vaginal sex. One researcher concluded that "even though students were reported to be efficacious in condom usage, they used them inconsistently with their sexual partners" (Gullette and Lyons, 2006). One of the reasons for the lack of condom use is that alcohol is often associated with hookups, interfering with judgments and decisions regarding safer sex behaviors (Fielder and Carey, 2010a,b). In another study, 39% of college students who engaged in vaginal intercourse did not use a condom, and alcohol use was found to precede many of these hookups (Brown and Vanable, 2007). Other researchers have also found a significant relationship among alcohol and hookups and the nonuse of condoms (Higgins, Trussell, Moore, and Davidson, 2010). Furthermore, consumption of alcohol is related to college students having multiple sex partners—another risk factor associated with sex. One researcher found that drug use and drinking were associated with having multiple sex partners and that sexual behavior while intoxicated predicted condom nonuse and multiple sex partners (Caldeira et al., 2009).

Environmental Factors

Our environment also affects our health. What you eat and how that food is grown or raised result in you ingesting healthy or nonhealthy substances. Likewise, if the water you drink and the air you breathe are unclean—that is, contain substances that can cause illness and disease—you are placed at risk. The U.S. Food and Drug Administration, the U.S. Environmental Protection Agency, and other governmental entities establish regulations pertaining to the environment and monitor the adherence to those regulations to limit our risk of illness and disease. However, we sometimes contribute to the pollution of our own environments. For example, we may smoke cigarettes thereby transmitting carcinogens into our bodies and by secondhand smoke into the bodies of others or we may buy products produced by environmentally unfriendly companies, which perpetuates their unhealthy practices. What are you willing to do to contribute to the health of the environment and, as a result, your health?

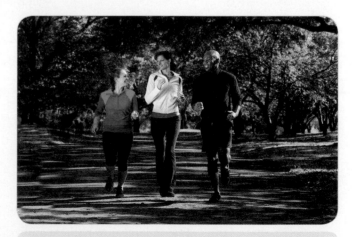

Are you taking advantage of the exercise facilities on your campus to become healthier?

TABLE 1.2	**Poverty by Race, Ethnicity, Family Status, and Age: United States, 2009**

Characteristic	Number	Percentage (%)
Total population in poverty	43,569,000	14.3
Race/Ethnicity		
White	18,530,000	9.4
African American	9,944,000	25.8
Hispanic	12,350,000	25.3
Asian American	1,746,000	12.5
Type of Family		
Married couple	3,409,000	5.8
Female householder (no husband present)	4,441,000	29.9
Male householder (no wife present)	942,000	16.9
Under 18 Years of Age		
Total	15,451,000	20.7
White	9,938,000	17.7
African American	4,033,000	35.7
Hispanic	5,610,000	33.1

REPRODUCED FROM: U.S. Census Bureau. *Current Population Survey, 2009 and 2010 Annual Social and Economic Supplements*. Washington, DC: U.S. Census Bureau, 2010.

Researchers report that the actual causes of death are the result of unhealthy behaviors over which we all have control. Tobacco use accounts for 18% of deaths annually in the United States, and poor diet and physical inactivity account for another 17% of annual U.S. deaths. The next most prevalent cause of death was alcohol consumption (4%) (Mokdad, Marks, Stroup, and Gerberding, 2004).

Social Policy Issues

Imagine living in poverty, lacking health insurance, and being poorly educated. You would guess that these conditions would lead you to be less healthy than those not experiencing these conditions, and you would be right. Social policy has a tremendous effect on health.

Poverty

Before we discuss **poverty**, it is important to realize exactly what that means. The federal government publishes poverty guidelines that are updated yearly. It is these guidelines that provide the definition of poverty for government assistance programs and that are used to compile poverty-related statistics. In 2009, if a family of four had an income of less than $21,954, the federal guidelines defined the family as living in poverty. A family of three with an income of less than $17,098 was defined as living in poverty. The key phrase is *defined as living in poverty*. Certainly, those families with incomes slightly higher than the poverty guidelines are, for all practical purposes, living in poverty even though the federal government does not define them as such. The poverty statistics presented above only represent those people falling within the government's definition, meaning there are many others who are essentially living in poverty but are not included in these statistics.

> **Poverty:** defined by the federal government poverty guidelines based on income: in 2009, if a family of four had an income of less than $21,954, the federal guidelines defined the family as living in poverty.

TABLE 1.3 Percentage of Individuals Who Lacked Health Insurance Coverage for at Least Part of the Past Year or for More Than a Year, by Poverty Status: United States, 2009

Total	Poor	Near Poor	Not Poor
17.5%	30.2%	29.4%	10.7%

REPRODUCED FROM: Centers for Disease Control and Prevention/National Center for Health Statistics, *National Health Interview Survey, 1997–2009, Family Core Component.* Available at: www.cdc.gov/nchs/data/nhis/earlyrelease/insur201006.htm.

TABLE 1.4 Percentage of Americans Who Lacked Health Insurance Coverage for at Least Part of the Past Year or for More Than a Year, by Race/Ethnicity: United States, 2009

Race/Ethnicity	Uninsured for at Least Part of the Year (%)	Uninsured for More Than a Year (%)
Hispanic or Latino	35.3	24.9
Non-Hispanic, white	15.1	7.4
Non-Hispanic, black	22.2	11.4
Non-Hispanic, Asian	17.1	10.8
Non-Hispanic, other races and multiple races	23.3	10.6

REPRODUCED FROM: Centers for Disease Control and Prevention/National Center for Health Statistics, *National Health Interview Survey, 1997 2009, Family Core Component.* Available at: www.cdc.gov/nchs/data/nhis/earlyrelease/insur201006.htm.

In 2009, 43,569,000 (14.3%) of Americans lived in poverty. Table 1.2 shows the poverty status by race, ethnicity, family status, and age (U.S. Census Bureau, 2010). Note that the percentage of African Americans and Hispanics living in poverty (more than 25%) is significantly higher than the percentage of white or Asian Americans living in poverty. Also, the percentage of African-American and Hispanic children under 18 years of age living in poverty (more than 33%) is significantly higher than the percentage of white children living in poverty.

Poverty has a major impact on health. For example, depression is more prevalent among those living in poverty (QuickStats, 2008), and those in poverty are more likely to smoke cigarettes, to be physically inactive and obese, and to sleep less than 6 hours a night (QuickStats, 2010b). Furthermore, they are less likely to have health insurance.

Lack of Health Insurance

Without health insurance, people are less likely to seek medical care. If they do, they often wait too long, making the illness more difficult to treat, or they get care at hospital emergency departments where they are often treated by less experienced health care providers. In the United States in 2009, more than 46 million people did not have health insurance—15.5% of the population (Cohen, Martinez, and Ward, 2010). Table 1.3, Table 1.4, and **FIG. 1.5 ▶** depict the health insurance status of Americans and, specifically, that of minorities and those living in poverty. Because minorities are disproportionately represented among those living in poverty, it is no surprise that they are similarly disproportionately represented among the uninsured. The health reform legislation passed in 2010 seeks to remedy this situation by

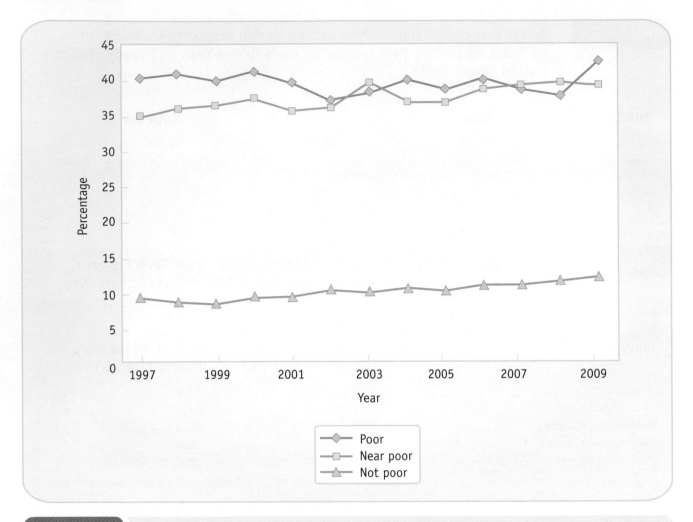

FIGURE 1.5 Percentage uninsured by poverty status for adults aged 18–64 years: United States, 1997–2009. Reproduced from: Centers for Disease Control and Prevention/National Center for Health Statistics, *National Health Interview Survey, 1997–2009, Family Core Component*. Available at: www.cdc.gov/nchs/data/nhis/earlyrelease/insur201006.htm.

increasing health insurance coverage for more Americans. In addition, through the development of national health objectives, the nation is being mobilized to decrease the health disparity between minorities and other Americans. Part of that effort is to increase the health insurance rate among minorities.

Discrimination

African Americans have a higher risk of dying from chronic diseases such as coronary heart disease or hypertension than that of any other ethnic group. Racial discrimination in everyday life explains part of the reason for this situation. In fact, in the past decade, more than 100 studies have been published documenting the harmful effects of racial discrimination on a variety of health measures (Ornish, 2008). For example, in a 6-year study involving 593 women with breast cancer, a relationship was found between the development of cancer and everyday and major discrimination, with women reporting more discrimination having a higher incidence of cancer (Taylor et al., 2007). Women reporting discrimination on the job had a 32% higher incidence of cancer, and those reporting major discrimination had a 48% higher incidence.

What I Need to Know

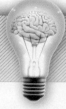

Poverty and Physical Activity

Minority and low-income Americans engage in less physical activity than majority and higher-income Americans. Because of this, and because of other important factors (e.g., less access to health care, less education, and financial constraints), minority and low-income Americans are typically less healthy than others. Several researchers have investigated the reason for this lack of physical activity. We know that there is a relationship between the availability of physical activity–related facilities and exercise behavior. Consequently, researchers have looked at the availability of physical fitness facilities in minority and low-income neighborhoods. When they assessed the presence of parks, sports facilities, fitness clubs, community centers, and walking/bike trails, they found significantly fewer of these in low- and medium-income communities (Eastabrooks, Lee, and Gyuresik, 2003; Powell, Slater, and Chaloupka, 2004). In addition, barriers to physical activity in these neighborhoods included transportation issues, expense, and community safety (Centers for Disease Control and Prevention, 2003). One team of researchers concluded that a "lack of availability of facilities that enable and promote physical activity, may in part, underpin the low levels of activity observed among populations of low socioeconomic status and minority backgrounds" (Powell, Slater, Chaloupka, and Harper, 2006).

In another study (Troxel, Matthews, Bromberger, and Sutton-Tyrrell, 2003), African Americans who reported that they experienced racial discrimination had more blockage of their carotid arteries supplying the brain than those who did not report experience of racial discrimination. Lastly, African-American women who reported having experienced racial discrimination were more likely to develop uterine fibroids than African-American women not reporting such discrimination (Wise et al., 2007). It is hypothesized that discrimination, whether it be racism, sexism, or ageism, has direct and an indirect effects on health. Directly, the stress associated with discrimination can increase blood pressure, heart rate, blood fats, and a host of other physiological variables. Indirectly, discrimination can lead to increased smoking, drinking of alcohol, overeating, physical inactivity, and less social support.

Complete Health Check Up 1.2 to identify the behaviors in which you engage that create risk to your health and wellness (see Health Check Up 1.2 on the companion website). Once completed, place Health Check Up 1.2 in your Health Decision Portfolio.

National Health Objectives

Every 10 years, the U.S. government publishes **national health objectives.** These objectives are developed in coordination with health experts and health-related organizations throughout the country. The intent is to focus health organizations—government agencies, private and public health organizations, businesses, schools and colleges, volunteer organizations, and so forth—on a specific set of achievable goals and objectives they will work toward for the next 10 years. This coordinated endeavor has been found effective enough to pursue national health

National health objectives: objectives developed by the federal government every 10 years targeted at health issues.

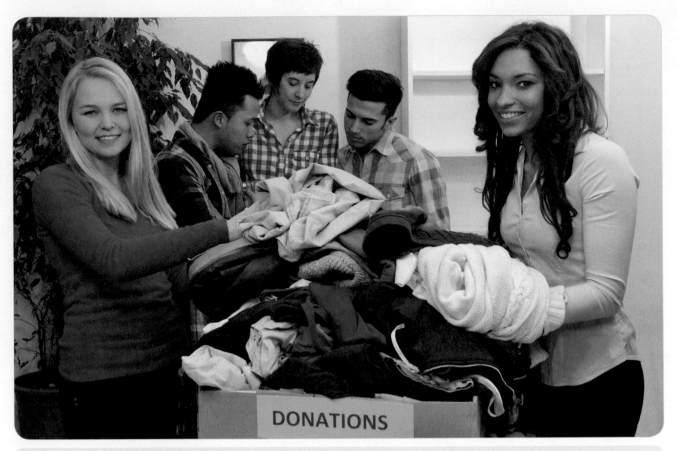

There are many things you can do to become healthy and maintain high-level wellness: you can eat well, you can engage in relaxation techniques, you can volunteer your time, and you can exercise regularly.

objectives ever since 1990. The latest objectives were published in December 2010. In 2020, there will be a determination as to which objectives were achieved and which were not. Adjustments will be made, and a new set of objectives will be developed.

You will encounter many activities designed to achieve these national health objectives. You will see public service announcements in traditional and new media. You will see posters pasted on the sides of buses. You will see ads on the internet. You will hear about local legislators passing laws and regulations to help achieve these objectives. As a responsible citizen, it is up to you to decide which of these objectives you will work toward in your own life. If everyone enhanced their health status by achieving some of the national health objectives, we would be a healthier country. That would obviously be good for the health of the populace, but it would also be good for our country's economy, as national health costs would decline.

What You Can Do to Be Healthy

As we have seen, social policy factors such as poverty, health insurance, and discrimination affect our health. Yet, you need not feel like a victim of these factors even if they seem to be working to diminish your health. In spite of them, there are many things you can do to develop and maintain health and wellness.

Factors Within Your Control

It is clear that numerous behaviors influence health. These behaviors are within your control. You can engage in behaviors that place your health at risk or behaviors that enhance your health. Someone once said: *If you do what you always did, you'll get what you always got.* Likewise with your health-related behavior. If you smoke and continue to do so, you endanger your health. If you engage in unsafe sexual behavior, you risk contracting a sexually

What I Need to Know

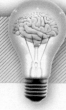

Sample 2020 National Health Objectives

The following is a sample of the 2020 national health objectives pertaining to college-age Americans. A complete listing of the objectives can be found at http://www.healthypeople.gov/2020/default.aspx.

Increase the proportion of adults who engage in aerobic physical activity of at least moderate intensity for at least 150 minutes/week, or 75 minutes/week of vigorous intensity, or an equivalent combination.

Increase the proportion of adults who perform muscle-strengthening activities on 2 or more days of the week.

Increase the proportion of adults with mental health disorders who receive treatment; for example, for depression.

Reduce the proportion of college students engaging in binge drinking during the past 2 weeks, and reduce average annual alcohol consumption.

Reduce chlamydia rates and gonorrhea rates among females aged 15–44 years.

Increase the proportion of Americans who have access to a food retail outlet that sells a variety of foods that are encouraged by the *Dietary Guidelines for Americans*.

Source: U.S. Department of Health and Human Services. Office of Disease Prevention and Health Promotion. Healthy People 2020. Washington, DC. Available at http://www.healthypeople.gov/2020/topicsobjectives2020/default.aspx. Accessed June 25, 2012.

---

transmitted infection or facing an unwanted pregnancy. If you remain physically inactive, you risk heart and circulatory system illness. And, if you overeat or eat unhealthy foods, you risk disability and early death. So which health-related behaviors do you need to eliminate, and which behaviors do you need to adopt? You completed Health Check Up 1.2 earlier, which helped you to identify these behaviors. Now it is time to plan to eliminate unhealthy behaviors and start engaging in healthy ones. Complete Health Check Up 1.3 to strategize ways to overcome barriers to your behaving more healthfully (see Health Check Up 1.3 on the companion website). Once completed, place Health Check Up 1.3 in your Health Decision Portfolio and work to implement those strategies. Recommendations for adoption of healthier behaviors are presented throughout this text. It is up to you, however, to adopt these recommendations and actually become a healthy person possessing high-level wellness.

One important factor in determining your motivation to take control of your health behavior is your **locus of control**. Locus of control is your perception of the control you have over events in your life. If you have an **internal locus of control**, you believe you can do things to improve your life. If you have an **external locus of control**, you believe that how your life turns out is a matter of luck, chance, fate, or will be determined by significant others such as teachers, bosses, and doctors. With an internal locus of control, you are more likely to take charge of behaviors associated with better health because you believe that what you do affects your health. Complete

---

Locus of control: your perception of the control you have over events in your life.

Internal locus of control: the perception that you are in control of most events in your life.

External locus of control: the perception that events in your life are the result of fate, luck, chance, and significant others.

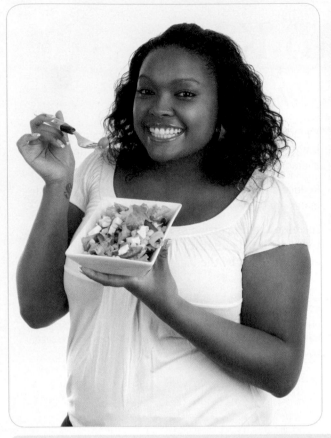

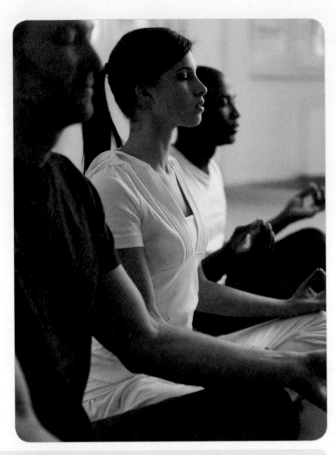

There are many things you can do to become healthy and maintain high-level wellness: you can eat well, you can engage in relaxation techniques, you can volunteer your time, and you can exercise regularly.

Health Check Up 1.4 to identify your locus of control (see Health Check Up 1.4 on the companion website). Once completed, place Health Check Up 1.4 in your Health Decision Portfolio and develop ways to be more in control of events that shape your life.

Complete Health Check Up 1.5 to develop your personal family health history (see Health Check Up 1.5 on the companion website). Once completed, place Health Check Up 1.5 in your Health Decision Portfolio so you can adjust your health behaviors to minimize your risk of development of diseases that are prevalent in your family.

Factors Beyond Your Control

Although heredity and genetics are beyond your control, knowing your family health history can help you adopt

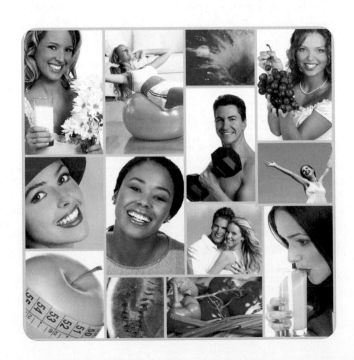

behaviors to minimize your health risks. Similarly, there are several other factors that affect your health but are also seemingly beyond your control. We already discussed some of these: social policy, poverty, availability and cost of health insurance, discrimination, and national health objectives. The operative word here is *seemingly*. As citizens, we have a responsibility to become knowledgeable about these issues and to try to influence them. And, we are not only citizens of our country but of our communities and campuses as well. Lobbying for changes in these factors so as to encourage greater health and wellness is one way we can exert this influence.

Lobbying Key Decision Makers

Key decision makers have a great deal of influence on our health. Among these key decision makers are state and federal legislators and policy makers on campus. The 2010 health insurance reform legislation is but one example of the important role legislators play. Further, your campus health center facilities, staff, level of funding, and outreach programs also have an impact on your health and that of your fellow students. Ways to exert influence on health decisions made by these key decision makers are described in the following sections.

In Government

Legislators are elected and, as such, desire to please those who vote in these elections. Organizing a write-in campaign or visiting your local, state, and federal legislators is one way you can affect their decisions. The more people you get involved with you to advocate for specific health policy, the more influential you will be.

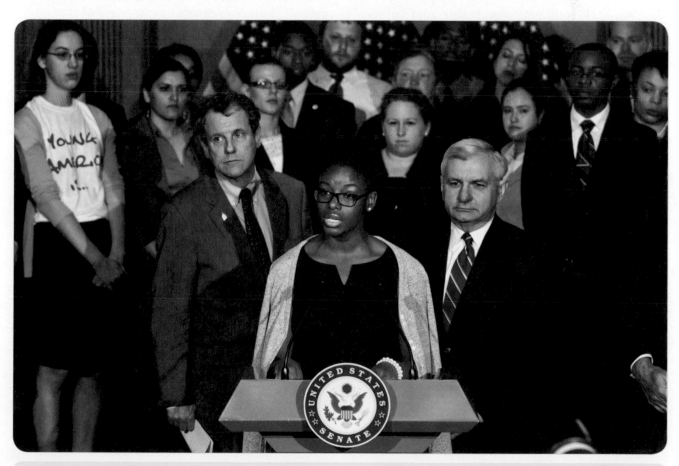

If you join others to lobby for actions to improve your community's health, you are more likely to be effective.

Myths *and* Facts
About Health and Wellness

MYTH	FACT
If I am physically fit, maintain the recommended weight for my height, and do not have any illnesses or diseases, I am healthy.	You may be physically fit and not ill but not be mentally healthy, emotionally healthy, socially healthy, or spiritually healthy. Health has many components, and you need to pay attention to each of these components to be healthy.
If I am physically, mentally, emotionally, socially, and spiritually healthy, I possess high-level wellness.	Even if each of the components of health is classified as healthy, you do not possess high-level wellness unless these components are in balance. If one component is overemphasized to the detriment of others, you do not possess high-level wellness.
There is no reason why everybody should not be physically fit. Even if they can only walk, that can lead to improved fitness.	There are many reasons why people may not be physically fit. Barriers to fitness include a lack of exercise facilities in the neighborhood (such as parks and recreation centers), unsafe neighborhoods with high crime or air pollution, and lack of education about the importance of and ways to become physically fit.
Discrimination is wrong but only marginally related to health and wellness.	Studies have shown that people experiencing discrimination are more likely to develop cancer, blockage of the carotid arteries supplying the brain, uterine fibroids, increased blood pressure, heart rate, and blood fats, and show a greater likelihood of alcohol abuse, overeating, physical inactivity, and social isolation.
Poverty is decreasing in the United States with all racial and ethnic groups benefiting from this decrease.	The latest poverty figures show an increase in the poverty rate, from 13.2% in 2008 to 14.3% in 2009. In 2009, 43.6 million Americans lived in poverty, up from 39.8 million in 2008. The poverty rate increased for all racial and ethnic groups in 2009 with the exception of Asian Americans whose poverty rate remained constant. The poverty rate in 2009 was the highest since 1994.

In Communities

There is an abundance of evidence that residents of communities with high crime and congested traffic and air pollution do not exercise as much for fear of being outside. When we are speaking of low socioeconomic communities, there may be another factor with negative impact: a lack of amenities that promote exercise (such as parks, bike paths, and community recreation centers). In addition, low socioeconomic communities may not have large supermarkets that sell healthy foods thereby requiring residents to travel outside the community for healthy food choices. That necessitates time and travel costs not experienced by residents of wealthier communities. These are but a few examples of the barriers to health and wellness encountered by some of your fellow citizens. It would appear that there is not much any one of us can do to change this state of affairs. However, local leaders can be lobbied to create healthier communities. For example, during budget hearings a group of residents can argue for a bike path to be built, or for leaders to negotiate with a large supermarket chain to open a store in the neighborhood (possibly offering them tax incentives to do so), or for making vans available at no cost to residents to transport those who need medical care to local clinics or hospitals. If you believe you have no control over factors that seem beyond your control, you will actually have no influence. If you refuse to accept this premise, you can be a contributor to the health of the community in which you live.

On Campus

Your campus is a microcosm of the larger community. You might attend school at a university or college that is health-friendly in that fitness classes are offered, health services are available, bike and walking paths abound, and the cafeteria and vending machines offer healthy food choices. In contrast, your campus may offer few or none of these. You need not accept that situation. Over the years, students have exerted a great deal of influence over campus policy. Witness the take-back-the-night marches that led to better lighting, escort patrols, and locked dormitories. Or, student concern about alcohol abuse on campus that led to alcohol-free parties and other activities for students not interested in drinking. Or, the lobbying activities of gay students that resulted in many campuses organizing gay clubs on campus and specifically regulating against sexual orientation discrimination. There is strength in numbers, so when organizing to make your campus a healthier place, recruit others.

Complete Health Check Up 1.6 to start thinking about ways your campus can encourage health and wellness (see Health Check Up 1.6 on the companion website). Once completed, place Health Check Up 1.6 in your Health Decision Portfolio. You might then organize other students to help you advocate for some of these campus health and wellness policies and actions.

Applying Behavior Theory

How can you use behavior change theory to become healthy and develop high-level wellness? Complete the Applying Behavior Change Theory for this chapter on the companion website. Once completed, place it in your Health Decision Portfolio.

SUMMARY

To encourage you to make healthy decisions, this chapter presented information concerning health and wellness and the factors that influence them. To help you become healthy and well and to maintain health and wellness, a summary of this chapter is provided.

■ Health has multiple components and includes physical, mental, emotional, social, and spiritual health. You can be healthy in one of these components but not in others.

■ Wellness denotes a balance in the components of health so that no one component of health is emphasized at the expense of other components.

■ Spirituality encompasses a feeling of connection to the world and others in it, which may or may not be conceptualized as religion. Religion is a social entity that involves beliefs, practices, and rituals related to the sacred—sacred defined as mystical or supernatural or God or, in Eastern religious traditions, the ultimate truth or reality.

■ The leading causes of death—heart disease, stroke, and cancer—are in large part a result of lifestyle choices. Among the behaviors that result in these conditions are tobacco use, physical inactivity, poor nutrition, unsafe sexual behaviors, and several environmental factors.

■ Social policy affects health and wellness. Among these social policies are the lack of availability of physical activity facilities in low socioeconomic and minority communities, poverty, lack of health insurance, and discrimination.

■ Every 10 years, the U.S. government publishes national health objectives. The intent is to focus health organizations—government agencies, private and public health organizations, businesses, schools and colleges, volunteer organizations, and so forth—on a specific set of achievable goals and objectives they will work toward for the next 10 years.

■ There are many actions you can take to develop and maintain your health and wellness. Some of these are obviously within your control such as refraining from the use of tobacco products, eating nutritionally, exercising regularly, and engaging in safer sex if sexually active. Some factors that seem beyond your control can be affected by lobbying government legislators, local community leaders, or policy makers on campus.

REFERENCES

Berry, J. W., Worthington, E. L., O'Connor, L. E., Parrot, L., and Wade, N. G. Forgiveness, vengeful rumination, and affective traits. *Journal of Personality* 73 (2005): 1–43.

Brown, J. L. and Vanable, P. A. Alcohol use, partner type, and risky sexual behavior among college students: Findings from an event-level study. *Addictive Behaviors* 32 (2007): 2940–2952.

Caldeira, K. M., Arria, A. M., O'Grady, K. E., Zarate, E. M., Vincent, K. B., and Wish, E. D. Prospective associations between alcohol and drug consumption and risky sex among female college students. *Journal of Alcohol and Drug Education* 53 (2009): nihpa115858.

Center for Nutrition Policy and Promotion. *Report of the Dietary Guidelines Advisory Committee on the Dietary Guidelines for Americans, 2010*. 2010. Available at: http://www.cnpp.usda.gov/DGAs2010-DGACReport.htm.

Centers for Disease Control and Prevention. *Wash Your Hands*. 2010. Available at: http://www.cdc.gov/Features/HandWashing/.

Centers for Disease Control and Prevention. Physical activity levels among children aged 9–13 years. *Morbidity and Mortality Weekly Report* 52 (2003): 785–788.

Cohen, R. A., Martinez, M. E., and Ward, B. W. *Health Insurance Coverage: Early Release of Estimates From the National Health Interview Survey, 2009*. Hyattsville, MD: National Center for Health Statistics, June 2010. Available at: http://www.cdc.gov/nchs/nhis.htm.

Currin, L. *Communicable Disease*. Portland, OR: Oregon Department of Education, 2007.

Eastabrooks, P. A., Lee, R. E., and Gyuresik, N. C. Resources for physical activity participation: Does availability and accessibility differ by neighborhood socioeconomic status? *Annals of Behavioral Medicine* 25 (2003): 100–104.

Fielder, R. L. and Carey, M. P. Predictors and consequences of sexual "hookups" among college students: A short-term prospective study. *Archives of Sexual Behavior* 39 (2010a): 1105–1119.

Fielder, R. L. and Carey, M. P. Prevalence and characteristics of sexual hookups among first-semester female college students. *Journal of Sex and Marital Therapy* 36 (2010b): 346–359.

Gullette, D. L. and Lyons, M. A. Sensation seeking, self-esteem, and unprotected sex in college students. *Journal of the Association of Nurses in AIDS Care* 17 (2006): 23–31.

Higgins, J. A, Trussell, J., Moore, N. B., and Davidson, J. K. Young adult sexual health: Current and prior sexual behaviours among non-Hispanic white US college students. *Sexual Health* 7 (2010): 35–43.

Koenig, H. G. Research on Religion, Spirituality, and Mental Health: A Review. *Canadian Journal of Psychiatry* 54 (2009): 283–291.

Mokdad, A. H., Marks, J. S., Stroup, D. F., and Gerberding, J. L. Actual causes of death in the United States, 2000. *Journal of the American Medical Association* 291 (2004): 1238–1245.

National Center for Health Statistics. *Health, United States, 2009: With Special Feature on Medical Technology*. Hyattsville, MD: National Center for Health Statistics, 2010.

Ornish, D. The toxic power of racism: Recent studies document the harmful effects of discrimination on our health. *Newsweek*, March 25, 2008. Available at: http://www.newsweek.com/2008/03/24/the-toxic-power-of-racism.html.

Powell, L. M., Slater, S., and Chaloupka, F. J. The relationship between community activity settings and race, ethnicity, and socioeconomic status. *Evidence Based Preventive Medicine* 1 (2004): 135–144.

Powell, L. M., Slater, S., Chaloupka, F. J., and Harper, D. Availability of physical activity—Related facilities and neighborhood demographic and socioeconomic characteristics: A national study. *American Journal of Public Health* 96 (2006): 1676–1680.

QuickStats. Percentage of persons aged ≥12 years with depression, by race/ethnicity and poverty status—National Health and Nutrition Examination Survey, United States, 2005–2006. *MMWR Weekly* 57 (2008): 1082.

QuickStats. Prevalence of selected unhealthy behavior-related characteristics among adults aged ≥18 years, by poverty status—National Health Interview Survey, United States, 2005–2007. *MMWR Weekly* 59 (2010b): 689.

Rhode Island Department of Health. *Communicable Disease List*. 2011. Available at: http://www.health.ri.gov/disease/communicable/diseaselist.php.

Taylor, T. R., Williams, C. D., Makambi, K. H., Mouton, C., Harrell, J. P., Cozier, Y., Palmer, J. R., Rosenberg,

L., and Adams-Campbell, L. L. Racial discrimination and breast cancer incidence in US Black women: The Black Women's Health Study. *American Journal of Epidemiology* 166 (2007): 46–54.

Troxel, W. M., Matthews, K. A., Bromberger, J. T., and Sutton-Tyrrell, K. Chronic stress burden, discrimination, and subclinical carotid artery disease in African American and Caucasian women. *Health Psychology* 22 (2003): 300–309.

U.S. Census Bureau. *Current Population Survey, 2009 and 2010 Annual Social and Economic Supplements*. Washington, DC: U.S. Census Bureau, 2010.

Wise, L. A., Palmer, J. R., Cozier, Y. C., Hunt, M. O., Stewart, E. A., and Rosenberg, L. Perceived racial discrimination and risk of uterine leiomyomata. *Epidemiology* 18 (2007): 747–757.

World Health Organization. *World Health Report 2001. Mental Health: New Understanding, New Hope*. Geneva: World Health Organization, 2001.

World Health Organization. *Promoting Mental Health: Concepts, Emerging Evidence, Practice: A Report of the World Health Organization*. Geneva: World Health Organization, 2005.

INTERNET RESOURCES

Mayo Clinic
   http://www.mayoclinic.com
National Institutes of Health
   http://health.nih.gov
The Henry J. Kaiser Family Foundation
   http://www.kff.org

The National Women's Health Information Center
   http://www.womenshealth.gov
About.com. Men's Health
   http://menshealth.about.com

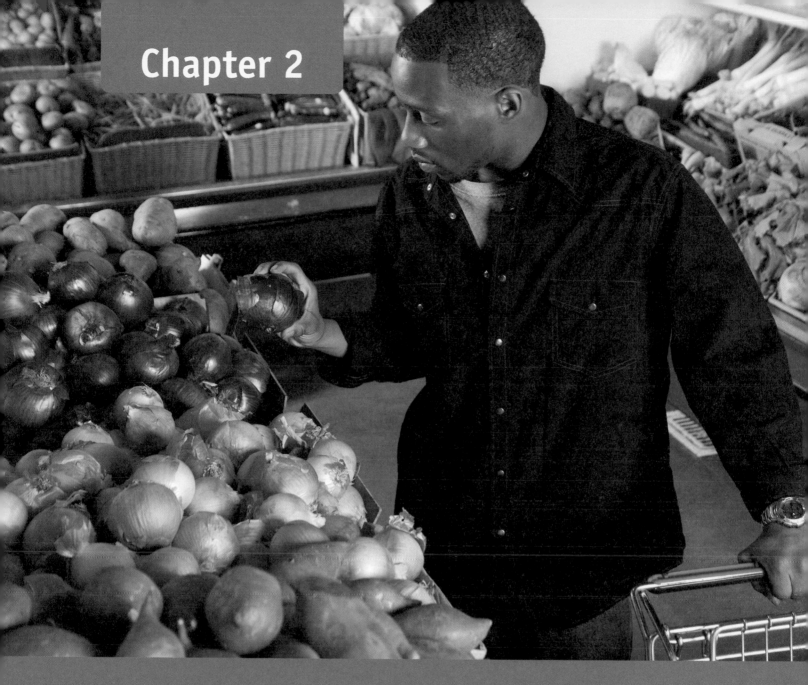

Assuming Responsibility for Your Health

 Access Health Check Ups and Health Behavior Change activities on the Companion Website:
go.jblearning.com/Empowering.

Think of a behavior *you do* that you wish you did not do. Maybe you snack on junk foods, or smoke cigarettes, or your social life revolves around drinking. Write that behavior on a sheet of paper.

Next, think of a behavior *you do not do* that you wish you did do. Perhaps you do not work out regularly, or wear a bike helmet, or use relaxation techniques. Write that down on the same sheet of paper as well. Refer to these behaviors as you read this chapter. Try to apply what you learn so you can change these behaviors and become healthier.

All of us can list several behaviors in both of these categories. At first, it may seem impossible to change them. But, with a greater understanding of why we engage in these behaviors and with strategies for controlling them, we can change how we behave and, consequently, become healthier. This chapter will give you the tools you need to make positive changes in your life.

Understand Why You Behave as You Do

There are many reasons why you decide how to behave. Notice the phrasing of that last sentence. It implies that your behavior is due to choices, decisions, that you make. Too often we *disown* our behavioral decisions. That is, we do not take responsibility for these choices but, instead, blame these decisions on others or the situation. When we say, "It's a habit, I just can't change it," we are not taking responsibility for that decision. We are *disowning* our behavior. Or, when we say, "I was brought up that way, no

one in my family expresses their feelings," we are blaming our families for a behavior we can in fact control. We are *disowning* that behavior.

Your health-related decisions, whether you disown them or not, are affected by your habits, your motivations, your values, your perception of the risks involved, the influences of your culture and family, and environmental and social policy.

Your Habits

People who live near railroad tracks or an airport become desensitized to the noise after a while. They experience the noise so often, they almost do not hear it any longer. Likewise, people who have muscle tension—perhaps their shoulders are always raised—do not even recognize that tense state after a while. They become desensitized to it. Likewise, you engage in health behaviors that, after a while, you just accept as the normal state. For example, there are certain foods you are in the habit of eating. Or, there are certain ways of communicating with others that you have used for so long that they are now habitual. The longer you use certain behaviors, the more of a habit they become, and the more difficult they are to change. You listed two behaviors at the opening of this chapter. Do either qualify as habits?

Your Motivations

You are not irrational, yet you engage in unhealthy behaviors in spite of knowing they are unhealthy. And, you do not adopt certain healthy behaviors that you clearly know are healthy. What's going on here?

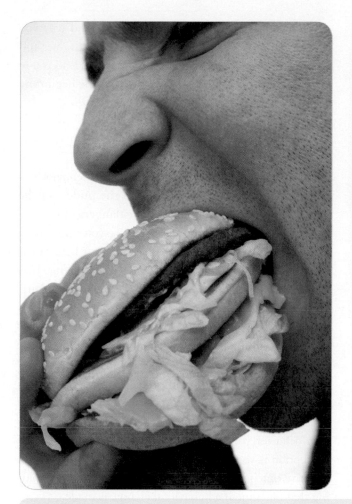
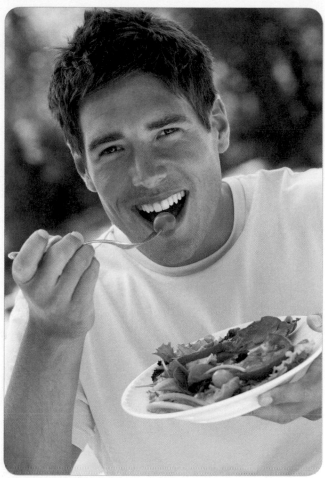

Unhealthy behaviors are ones you want to give up, whereas healthy behaviors are ones you want to strategize to engage in.

Among the factors influencing these decisions is your motivation. For example, you may make health behavior decisions to look good among your peers. People of all ages experience peer pressure. Just think of how similar hair styles, choice of clothing, and recreational activities are among teenagers, retirees, or people from certain cultures. Often, this peer pressure encourages us to behave in healthy ways; such as when we exercise because our friends exercise. At other times, however, it influences us in unhealthy ways, such as when we eat foods high in unsaturated fats at fast food restaurants to spend time with friends.

Another motivational influence on your health behavior may be the desire for immediate pleasure. Let's use dieting

as an example. Dieting to lose weight takes persistence. Because it takes time to reach your desired weight, the reward for dieting is delayed, whereas eating tasty foods, even though high in calories, provides immediate reward. No waiting here! Such is the case with many health behaviors. The reward for choosing to engage in those behaviors is often perceived as occurring some time in the future. So, some people argue, life is too short to not enjoy every day. They might say, "If I like drinking alcohol, or smoking cigarettes, or eating fried foods, why shouldn't I?" On the flip side, other people might argue that a sign of maturity is the ability to postpone immediate pleasure for long-term gain. Although exercising may cause you to sweat and your muscles to ache, for example, in the long run it will increase both the length and quality of your life.

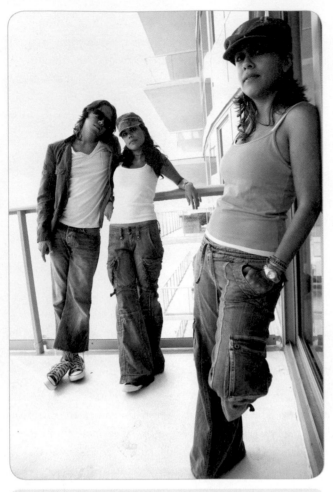

People of all ages are motivated to fit in with their peers.

Your Values

A value is something in which you believe strongly. It is also something upon which you act. If you claim to hold a value, your actions are consistent with it. For example, if you say you value transportation safety, you regularly wear a seat belt when traveling by car, wear a bicycle helmet when biking, and obey traffic laws. More generally, if you value health, you behave in ways to enhance and protect your health. The problem arises when you have two values that compete with one another. For example, you may value safety but also value freedom and spontaneity. In cases of conflict, you have to decide which is more valuable to you; that is, which value carries more weight. If it is safety, you will always take the time to cross streets at the crosswalks. If it is spontaneity, you may jaywalk when it is convenient or when it saves you time, even though

this poses a risk to your safety. To understand why you behave as you do, you need to understand your values and the priorities you place on them. What values lead you to engage in the two behaviors you listed at the beginning of this chapter?

Your Risk Perception

Your **risk perception** affects your health behavior decisions. Assume you usually cross in the middle of the street. If you are educated about the dangers of this behavior—the risk of being hit by a car—you might then use the crosswalk. Still, just being told your behavior is risky might not be enough for you decide to change that behavior. You would have to believe the negative outcome is significant enough to avoid. Certainly, getting hit by a car qualifies. You would also have to believe the negative outcome is likely to occur if you do not change your behavior. Perhaps you believe that if you look both ways before crossing, it is highly improbable you will be hit by a car. In that case, you would not be motivated to use the crosswalk. Lastly, you would have to believe if you change your behavior, you are likely to avoid the risk. So, your risk perception is your view of the likelihood of a significant negative outcome occurring and the likelihood of avoiding that outcome if a behavioral change is made.

Your Culture and Family

Among the healthiest people in the United States are Seventh-day Adventists, which is because they believe the body is a temple and to defile it is sacrilegious. As a result, Seventh-day Adventists refrain from using tobacco and alcohol products, exercise regularly, and eat nutritionally. Religion is just one example of how culture affects health behavior decisions. Ethnicity also affects these decisions. For example, white girls report more concern about their weight than African-American girls. As a result, the prevalence of eating disorders is higher among white girls. First-generation Hispanic immigrants are more likely to breastfeed their newborns than later-generation

Risk perception: the likelihood of a negative outcome as a result of a health behavior.

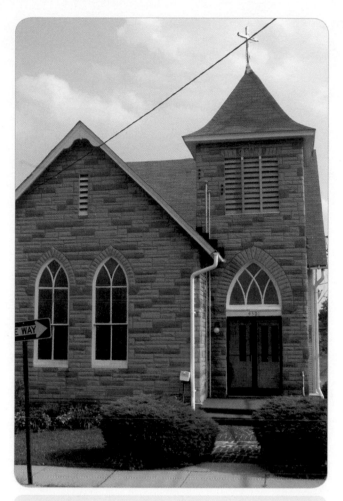

Some religious and cultural groups encourage healthy behaviors and discourage unhealthy ones. As a result, those who belong to these groups tend to be healthier.

exams, you are likely to do that as an adult. Likewise, if a parent or older sibling smokes cigarettes, you are more apt to smoke cigarettes. To achieve better health, you will want to identify the healthy behaviors family members model for you and mimic those behaviors. At the same time, identify unhealthy behaviors in which family members engage, and purposefully refrain from them.

Environmental and Social Policy

If your college cafeteria offers only foods high in saturated fats, you would be hard pressed to limit your fat intake. Likewise, if there is a lot of crime in your neighborhood or a lot of traffic creating unhealthy air, you may decide it is unhealthy to exercise outdoors. In contrast, if there are jogging paths or if there is a health club in your neighborhood, it would be easy to be physically fit. Your environment creates both barriers and opportunities to adopting a healthy lifestyle.

Social policy can have the same effect. Every 10 years, the federal government publishes national health objectives. These objectives guide federal and local expenditures. For example, if breast cancer prevention and early detection are objectives, the government spends money on public service campaigns, health screenings, and education about preventing breast cancer. By bringing this issue to public awareness and providing inexpensive or free screening, the government affects people's health behaviors—women are more likely to obtain breast screenings and mammograms.

Consider another example: the debate about whether to make emergency contraception available without a doctor's prescription. One point of view was that doctors should be consulted before drugs are used. Another proposal was for pharmacists to dispense emergency contraception. It is not difficult to see how this policy decision affects the health behavior of women of childbearing age, especially young women. As environmental factors affect your health behavior, so do social policy factors.

Hispanics. Socioeconomic class is another factor that has a significant affect on health behavior. Poorer Americans have poorer health and riskier health behaviors than their wealthier counterparts. You are a part of a cultural group; whether it is a religious group, a socioeconomic class, an ethnic or racial group, a gender, or an immigrant group. That cultural group affects how you view health and health behavior. It also affects your values.

As cultural groups affect your health decisions, so does you family. Families that value health model healthy behavior that their children often adopt. If family members drive safely, you are more likely to grow up driving safely. If family members obtain regular medical screenings and

What are the factors influencing your health behavior decisions? Complete Health Check Up 2.1 to find out (see Health Check Up 2.1 on the companion website). Once completed, place Health Check Up 2.1 in your Health Decision Portfolio.

Critically Evaluate Health Information

Everyone wants to be healthy. And, everyone wants to know what they can do to become healthy. Multiple sources of health information are offered to the public, not all of equal merit. Your challenge as a health consumer is to recognize the information that is valid and the information that is not.

Sources of Health Information

Pick up any newspaper or magazine and you will find advertisements or articles about health products or behaviors. Watch television for a while and you will see ads for drugs and fitness products. Surf the internet and you will find numerous health-related websites. Carry on a conversation with family members and friends and before long a health-related topic comes up. In the following sections, you will find a discussion of these sources of health information and tools you can use to evaluate them critically.

Advertising

By their very nature, advertisements serve companies, not consumers. That is, someone is trying to get you to buy a product or service. Sometimes, the use of the product advertised will improve your health. Other times, it is a waste of money or, worse yet, harmful to your health. A good rule of thumb is to view ads with a critical eye. Challenge the advertiser to *prove it*! Expect references to studies—conducted by objective third parties—that demonstrate the effectiveness of the product. When drug manufacturers reference studies conducted by scientists they employ or studies funded by their companies, be suspicious.

If the claims for the product seem too good to be true, they probably are. A quick weight-loss diet might work, but you can expect to soon gain back the weight you lost. A vitamin pill might supplement your diet, but you may already be getting enough of that vitamin in the foods you eat. Ads may present narratives by people who swear that glucosamine and chondroitin supplements have healed their knees and prevented knee surgery, but studies have found these supplements to work only on those with severe arthritis. Be suspicious!

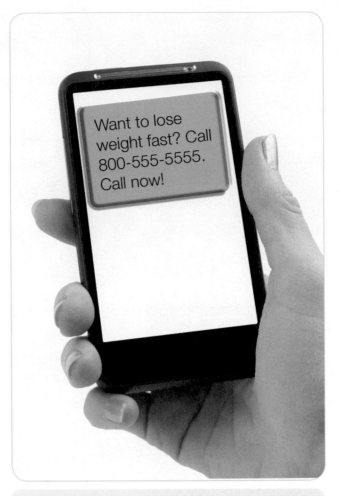

It is important to verify the validity of claims made in advertisements for health-related products.

Read the small print. When a toothpaste is advertised as preventing tooth decay, the small print often qualifies that effect as occurring when a recommended dental health regimen is followed: daily brushing and flossing, regular dental checkups, and eating a nutritious diet. When a fitness device is advertised to "melt inches off of your waist," the small print often qualifies that this result was observed only when use of the device was accompanied by a daily program of other fitness activities and/or a diet of very limited calories. Be suspicious!

It is wise to access government websites to verify health claims of advertised products. Public, respected, and trustworthy professional organizations—such as the American Heart Association, the American Cancer Society, or the American Diabetes Association—are additional sources you can consult to verify health claims.

What I Need to Know

Evaluating Health Information on the Internet

There is a lot of information on the internet that is useful. In contrast, there is a lot of information that is designed to get you to buy certain products or that contains outdated information or statistics. To evaluate health information on the internet, ask the following questions:

1. Who runs the site?

   Any reputable website should make it easy for you to learn who is responsible for the site and the information included on it.

2. Who pays for the site?

   The source of funding for the website can affect what content is presented, how the content is presented, and what the owners want to accomplish on the site. Websites ending in ".gov" are federal government sponsored, ".edu" indicates educational institutions, ".org" is often used by noncommercial organizations, and ".com" denotes commercial organizations.

3. What is the purpose of the site?

   The purpose of the website is related to who runs and pays for it. Many websites have a link entitled "About Us" or "About This Site" that clearly states the purpose of the site and that can help you evaluate the trustworthiness of the information on the site.

4. What is the original source of the information on the website?

   Many health and medical websites post information collected from other websites or sources. If the person or organization in charge of the site did not write the material, the original source should be clearly identified.

5. How is information on the website documented?

   In addition to identifying the original source of the material, the site should identify the evidence on which the material is based. Medical facts and figures should have references (such as citations of articles in medical journals). Also, opinion or ad-vice should be clearly distinguished from information that is *evidence-based* (i.e., based on research results).

6. How is information reviewed before it is posted on the website?

   Health-related websites should give information about the medical credentials of the authors and editors who prepare or review the material on the website. Information about the editorial board and its members should be available on the website. Is there an editorial board in the first place? Do members of the editorial board—who should be people with excellent professional and scientific qualifications—review material before it is posted?

7. How current is the information?

   Websites should be reviewed and updated on a regular basis. It is particularly important that medical information be current. The date when the most recent update or review occurred should be clearly posted. Even if the information has not changed, you want to know whether the site owners have reviewed it recently to ensure it is still valid.

8. How does the site choose links to other sites?

   Reliable websites usually have a policy about how they establish links to other sites. Some medical websites take a conservative approach and do not link to any other sites. Others only link to sites that have met specific criteria. Still other websites link to any site that asks, or pays, for a link.

9. What information about users does the site collect, and why?

   Websites routinely track the path you take through their sites to determine what pages are being used. Some health-related websites ask that you *subscribe* or *become a member*. In some cases, this may be done so they can collect a user fee or select relevant information for the user. However, in all cases, the subscription or membership will allow personal information about you to be collected by the website owners. Any website

(Continues)

asking you for personal information should explain exactly what the site will and will not do with that information. Many commercial websites collect *aggregate* data—information about you that does not personally identify you, grouped with data from many other visitors. The aggregate data might be sold to other companies interested in finding out general characteristics of people who report a certain condition or disease; for example, their gender, socioeconomic class, and location. Be aware that in some cases, personally identifiable data—such as zip code or birth date—may be passed along. You should be certain to understand any privacy policy or similar language on the site and not sign up for anything you do not fully understand.

10. How does the site manage interactions with users?

There should always be a way for you to contact the website owners if you have problems, feedback, and questions. If the site hosts a chat room or other online discussion areas, it should tell you about the terms of using the service. Is the service moderated? If so, by whom, and why? It is always a good idea to spend time reading the discussion without joining in; to feel comfortable with the environment before becoming a participant.

Reproduced from: National Center for Complementary and Alternative Medicine. *Evaluating Web-Based Health Resources*. 2010. Available at: http://www.nccam.nih.gov/health/webresources; National Cancer Institute. *How to Evaluate Health Information on the Internet: Questions and Answers*. 2006. Available at: http://www.cancer.gov/cancertopics/factsheet/Information/internet.

The Internet

Health information is readily available on the internet. All you need do is sit at your computer and type in key words to access any of a number of health-related websites. As a result, many people depend on websites to learn about health issues and to obtain advice regarding their health behavior. This interest in health is to be welcomed. However, depending on the internet as a source of health information is accompanied by several risks. Is the information accurate? Is it current? Is the website owner/manager trying to get you to buy a product? Knowing what you can rely on, and what you cannot, is imperative if you are going to use the internet as a source of health information. The accompanying What I Need to Know box describes how you can evaluate health information on the internet. The Medical Library Association lists the "Top Ten Most Useful Consumer Health Websites" (Medical Library Association, 2006):

- National Cancer Institute: http://www.cancer.gov
- Centers for Disease Control and Prevention: http://www.cdc.gov/
- American Academy of Family Physicians: http://familydoctor.org
- Healthfinder: htpp://www.healthfinder.gov
- University of California San Francisco AIDS Research Institute: http://hivinsite.ucsf.edu
- Mayo Clinic: http://www.mayoclinic.com
- Medem (a project of the leading medical societies): http://medem.com
- Medline Plus: http://medlineplus.gov
- NOAH (New York Online Access to Health): http://www.noah-health.org

Your Family and Friends

Family and friends offer you advice regarding your health. They do so with the best of intentions. They care for you and want you to be healthy. That is why the advice they offer should not be ignored. Yet, they may or may not be offering valid advice. Misconceptions about health

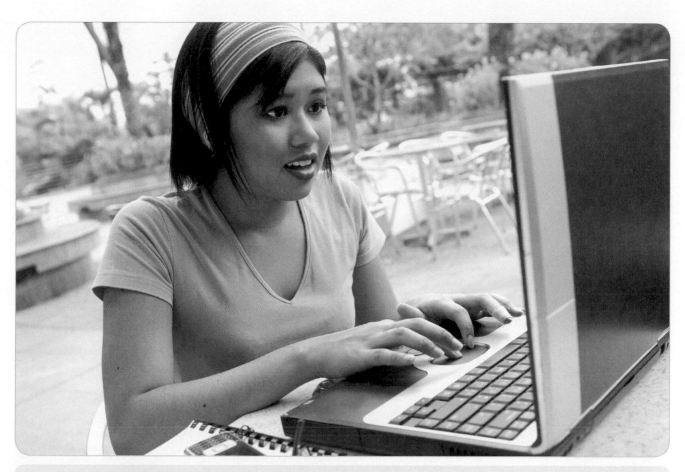

Just because information appears on the internet does not mean that the information is accurate. There are specific ways recommended to validate information found on the internet.

abound. Perhaps family members or friends have been influenced by ads, or television programs, or by the testimonies of people they know who swear by certain products or behaviors. As with all sources of health information, you should verify the accuracy of what family and friends recommend. Are there studies to verify their suggestions? Are their suggestions consistent with the recommendations of health experts? Do government agencies, professional health organizations, or your medical care provider concur with their recommendations? You might also ask an expert on your campus for advice regarding these recommendations. Your health is too important to risk by following health advice of uncertain validity.

Newspaper and Magazine Articles

Your local newspaper publishes articles on health topics. So does your campus newspaper. Articles may report findings from the latest health-related research, columns may offer health advice on dieting or exercise, and health-related websites may be recommended to the reader. Many of these articles and columns offer valuable advice that, if followed, would improve your health. However, as with other sources of health information, these should be read with a critical eye. Newspapers are limited in the amount of space they allow for articles and columns. Consequently, authors must be as brief and concise as possible. The *whole story* may not be told. For example, it may be reported that young drivers are more likely to be involved in traffic accidents. However, the article in the professional journal reporting those findings might describe various limitations in interpreting the results. Perhaps researchers only studied accidents on rural roads, or among youth who had been drinking, or accidents occurring after midnight. Perhaps the important factor in the accidents was not so much the driver's age but rather

35

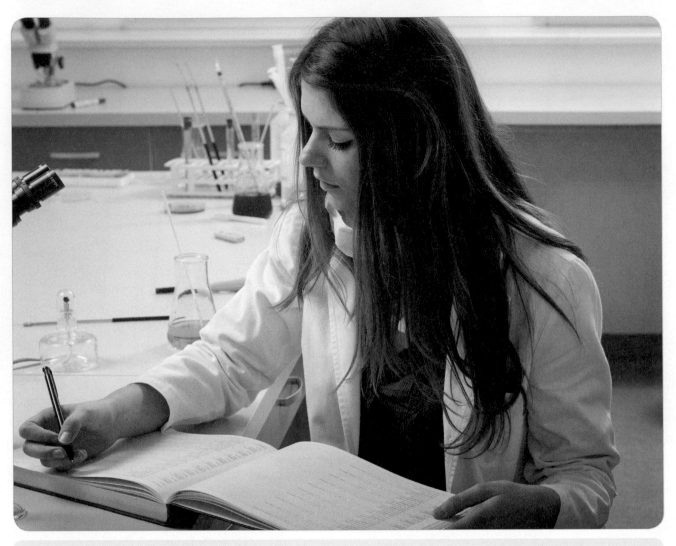

Certain types of research studies result in greater confidence in their results. Among the most valid of these studies is the double-blind, randomized, controlled clinical trial.

the road conditions, alcohol, or some other reason. Whenever possible, the original source of the health information should be read. Do not rely on the interpretation of the newspaper or magazine writer or editor.

Maybe the association being reported is so small as to be meaningless. It may attract readers' attention to have an article entitled "Substance X Causes Cancer!" but often the association is so unsubstantial it should be disregarded. We discuss statistical significance, clinical significance, relative risk, retrospective studies, and prospective studies later in this chapter. That discussion will help prepare you to evaluate health information appearing in newspapers and magazines.

How can you evaluate health information to make better health behavior decisions? Complete Health Check Up 2.2 to find out (see Health Check Up 2.2 on the companion website). Once completed, place Health Check Up 2.2 in your Health Decision Portfolio.

Understand the Different Levels of Medical Evidence

As we have seen, health information and recommendations vary in validity. That is why it is important to base your health behavior decisions on medical evidence. Your confidence in information derived from medical studies should vary based on the type of study. Some types of studies produce more valid findings than others. The types of studies presented in the following sections are listed in order of least to most valid medical evidence.

Case Report

A **case report** is a detailed report of the diagnosis, treatment, and follow-up of an individual patient or research subject (National Cancer Institute, 2006). Case reports also contain some demographic information about the patient (e.g., age, gender, and ethnic origin). A **case series** is the combined reports of several patients with like diagnoses, treatments, or follow-ups. Case reports are the least valid studies because individual patients may differ greatly from the majority of people with the same diagnosis. These types of studies are often called *anecdotal*. Case series are somewhat more valid because they look at patterns across a group and can be valuable if they lead to hypotheses that can be studied in more controlled experiments. Still, data from case series are among the least valid when deciding on your health behavior.

Observational Study

Sometimes researchers want to sit back and see what medical conditions occur without any intervention. These are called **observational studies**. The Framingham Heart Study is an example of an observational study. Started in 1948, this study followed 5,000 adults in Framingham, Massachusetts, to determine what factors were associated with the development of coronary heart disease. If large numbers of people are studied and the right variables elected, observational studies can discover very important health information. On the basis of the Framingham study, for instance, Americans were advised to exercise, lessen their cholesterol intake, and stop smoking if they wanted to prevent coronary heart disease (or at least postpone it until they were of old age).

Case-Controlled Study

A **case-controlled study** compares two groups of people: those with the disease or condition under study, called *cases*, and a very similar group of people who do not have the disease or condition, called *controls* (National Cancer Institute, 2006). Researchers study the medical and lifestyle histories of the people in each group to learn what factors may be associated with the disease or condition. For example, one group may have been exposed to a particular substance that the other was not. Case-controlled studies are also called *retrospective studies*, in that they study people who already have the condition or disease.

Cohort Study

A **cohort study** compares a particular outcome, such as lung cancer, in groups of individuals (cohorts) who are alike in many ways but differ by a certain characteristic; for example, female nurses who smoke compared with those who do not smoke (National Cancer Institute, 2006). One of the challenges to the validity of these studies occurs if the researchers know which people compose the cohort. That may result in the findings being affected by *researcher bias*, which occurs when researchers have a preconceived notion of the results and interpret the study's findings consistent with this view.

Case report: a type of study that provides a detailed report of the diagnosis, treatment, and follow-up of an individual patient or research subject.

Case series: a type of study that provides a detailed report of the diagnosis, treatment, and follow-up of several patients or research subjects.

Observational studies: studies in which researchers observe the medical conditions that occur in association with particular behaviors without interfering with those behaviors.

Case-controlled study: a type of study that compares two groups of people, one with the disease or condition and another group that does not have the disease or condition.

Cohort study: a type of study that compares an outcome in groups of people who are mostly alike but differ on selected characteristics.

Different Types of Clinical Trials

Controlled clinical trials are studies in which one group of participants is given an experimental drug or treatment, whereas another group, called the control, is given either a standard treatment for the disease or a placebo (National Institutes of Health, 2008). A placebo is a medication or treatment that should have no effect on people's health but, because people believe it is a real remedy, they report feeling better. Then the results are compared.

In a specific type of controlled clinical trial called a **double-blind study**, neither the participating individuals nor the researchers know which participants are receiving which treatment. Double-blind studies produce more valid results because the expectations of the researchers and the subjects about the experimental outcome cannot affect the results.

Among the types of research studies producing the most valid findings is the **randomized clinical trial**. A randomized clinical trial is a study in which the participants are assigned by chance to separate groups that compare different treatments; neither the researchers nor the participants can choose which group. Using chance to assign people to groups means the groups will be similar and that the treatments they receive can be compared objectively.

The most valid data derive from studies in which the subjects in a *controlled clinical trial* are *randomized* into treatment groups, and neither researchers nor subjects know to which treatment group subjects are assigned (*double blind*). This is called a **double-blind, randomized, controlled clinical trial**.

Statistical versus Clinical Significance

Statistical significance refers to how likely it is that a study's results are due to chance. If the results are statistically significant at an 0.05 level, there is only a 5% possibility those results are due to chance. For example, if smokers are studied and it is found that they develop lung cancer to a greater extent than nonsmokers and that finding is significant at the 0.05 level, we can be 95% confident that the difference is due to smoking and not to chance.

How can you use this information to be healthier? When you are deciding whether to engage in a health behavior—for example, exercising—you can read studies that have found *statistically significant* differences between those who engage in that behavior and those who do not. That will give you confidence that these differences are a result of that behavior and that you can expect these benefits, too, if you decide to engage in that health behavior.

One word of caution, however: The way the statistics work, it is difficult to find statistical significance when studies are conducted with relatively few subjects. Conversely, when studies are conducted with a large group of subjects, it is relatively easy to have findings that are statistically significant. That is why it is important to differentiate between statistical significance and clinical significance. **Clinical significance** refers to whether the results have a real or meaningful effect on people's health.

Research pertaining to intracytoplasmic injection is a good example of the difference between statistical significance and clinical significance. Intracytoplasmic injection is a

Controlled clinical trial: a type of study in which an experimental group is given a treatment or engages in a health behavior and a control group is not given that treatment or does not engage in that behavior.

Double-blind study: a type of study in which neither the researchers nor the subjects know who receives the treatment and who does not.

Randomized clinical trial: a study in which subjects are assigned to different groups by chance rather than purposefully.

Double-blind, randomized, controlled clinical trial: a controlled clinical trial in which subjects are assigned randomly to treatment groups and neither researchers nor subjects know to which group subjects are assigned.

Statistical significance: the likelihood that a study's findings are a result of chance.

Clinical significance: the clinical meaningfulness of the results of a study; that is, whether the results actually impact health in a real or meaningful way.

Relative risk: how much a particular risk factor influences the risk of a particular outcome in a prospective study.

What I Need to Know

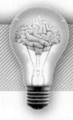

Evaluating Statistics

A cardiologist needed his office furniture reupholstered. When he looked at the furniture, however, he noticed that only the arms and front edge of the seats were worn out. That got him to think about his patients. Perhaps, he wondered, people who sit *on the edge of their seats holding tightly to the arms*—that is, those who are *stressed out*—are more apt to develop coronary heart disease. When he studied his patients with heart disease he indeed found that more of them reported experiencing stress than people who did not have heart disease. So stress leads to coronary heart disease, right? Well, maybe. What this study found was an *association* or *correlation* between stress and coronary heart disease, not a *cause-and-effect relationship*. Yes, it is possible that stress led to coronary heart disease, but it is just as possible that having heart disease led to stress. This highlights the difference between retrospective and prospective studies. *Retrospective studies* investigate people with a condition (e.g., coronary heart disease) and identify variables associated with that condition (e.g., stress). They do not determine causality. *Prospective studies* investigate people who do not have a condition (e.g., people without coronary heart disease), test them on the variable of interest (e.g., stress), and follow them over a period of time to determine if those who have that variable develop the condition. In a classic study, the cardiologist mentioned above studied healthy people, tested their stress levels, and then followed them for more than 20 years. When he found that the people who had more stress developed heart disease to a greater extent than the people who had less stress, he was able to hypothesize that stress preceded and, therefore, led to coronary heart disease.

Someone once said, "Figures don't lie, but liars figure." It's all in how the data are presented. To interpret statistics more accurately, the following should be considered:

Are the statistics describing a cause-and-effect relationship or merely an association or correlation between variables?

Are the findings statistically significant?

Are the findings clinically significant? That is, do the differences reported really make a difference in people's health?

If relative risk is reported, is it greater than 2? **Relative risk** is how much a particular risk factor (such as cigarette smoking) influences the risk of a particular outcome (such as death by age 70) in a prospective study. A relative risk of 2 means a person has a twofold increased risk of having the outcome compared with a person without the risk factor. The higher the relative risk, the more confidence in the association between the risk factor and the outcome. A relative risk of less than 2 is not meaningful. Some epidemiologists even recommend regarding associations with a relative risk of less than 4 as suspect.

Were enough people studied for the findings to be credible?

Were the people studied representative of the general population? Or were they too unique for the findings to be generalized to others? Were the subjects drawn from a wide geographic area? Were they of varied ages, ethnicities, races, cultures, socioeconomic status, and education levels? If the study's subjects were different from you on important variables, you should not be confident the findings pertain to you.

Reproduced from: Friedman, M. and Rosenman, R. *Type A Behavior and Your Heart*. New York: Alfred A. Knopf, 1974; Statistical Assessment Service. *What is the Difference between Absolute and Relative Risk?* Undated. Available at: http://stats.org/faq_risk.htm.

reproductive assistance technology that involves taking a sperm and injecting it into an egg (ovum) to facilitate conception. Studies have found statistically significant differences in the embryos produced. They are four times more likely to have an extra chromosome or a missing chromosome—conditions that lead to various birth defects. At first glance, this would seem to disqualify this technique. After all, would you choose a technique that has a four times greater chance that your child will have a birth defect? And yet, a more careful look at this risk is warranted before the technique is discarded. Studies show that 0.25% (a quarter of 1%) of all births result in an extra or missing chromosome. If intra-cytoplasmic injection results in a four times greater risk, that means that 1% of the resulting births would be affected. In other words, 99% of the babies would be fine. You can see that it is important to look at the clinical significance rather than relying solely on statistical significance that is so small it has no real meaning.

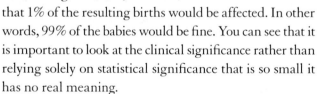

The use of systematic decision making is more likely to result in effective decisions than haphazardly deciding the issue.

How to Make Effective Decisions

If you make decisions haphazardly, you may not make good decisions. When it concerns your health, you do not want to take that chance. Fortunately, you do not have to. There are several ways you can organize the decision-making process to make it more likely your decisions will be the right ones for you. Two of these methods are discussed in the following sections.

Using Systematic Decision Making

Sometimes you have a lot of information about the situation for which a decision is needed, and there are many possible routes you could take. To use **systematic decision making**, generate a number of possible decisions, evaluate each, choose one, and try another decision if the first one was not the best.

Perceive and Define the Problem

Many problems requiring a decision are only minimally understood before a decision is made. This is not the case when using systematic decision making. For example, say you drink too much alcohol. You may decide to drink less. To use systematic decision making, you would have to understand more about this situation. When do you drink? Where? With whom? For what purpose? Explore the situation and attempt to understand it as well as you can.

> **Systematic decision making:** a method of making decisions that involves perceiving and defining the problem, brainstorming and evaluating ideas, and acting on an idea and reacting to the effects.

Brainstorm and Evaluate Ideas

Once you have a handle on the situation, ideas are generated to remedy it. This is done in a brainstorming fashion. List many ideas without judgment; that is, do not reject writing down an idea just because your first impression of it may be bad. If the problem is drinking, the list might look something like this:

- Hang out less with Steve.

- Give up going to the bar with friends on the weekend.

- Go to the gym if I am feeling restless and might drink.

- Play video games rather than go to parties at which alcohol is available.

Once you have a complete list of ideas, go over the list and evaluate each in turn. Given the specifics of the problem or situation, which decision is most likely to be effective?

Act and React

Now implement the decision you selected. Pay attention to what aspects of that decision are working as expected and what aspects are not. Adjust as necessary. Perhaps the decision does not work at all. In that case, try one of the other brainstormed ideas. Repeat the process until you are satisfied with your decision.

You can use systematic decision making to make a health-related decision by completing Health Check Up 2.3 (see Health Check Up 2.3 on the companion website). Once completed, place Health Check Up 2.3 in your Health Decision Portfolio.

Using Force Field Analysis

For any problem or health decision, there are always factors that encourage the desired outcome and factors that interfere with that outcome. When using **force field analysis**, you define the problem well enough to understand the forces that encourage and the forces that oppose the desired action. Then, you identify strategies you can use to maximize the encouraging forces and minimize the opposing forces. Next, you use those strategies and evaluate the results to determine if any adjustments are necessary to increase your likelihood of success.

Minimize Forces Working to Oppose Change

Let's assume you are sedentary but decide you want to exercise more. What forces are pushing you away from exercising regularly? Perhaps you have a lot of schoolwork that occupies your time. Perhaps you do not have exercise clothes. Maybe your friends do not exercise.

How can you minimize these barriers to your exercising? You might not want to devote less time to your schoolwork but might be able to free up time in other ways. For example, you might decide to limit your television viewing. Buying exercise clothing would also encourage you to exercise because, once you did so, you would not want to waste that investment. And, finding a friend or classmate also interested in exercising might provide enough social support to encourage you to exercise.

Maximize Forces Working in Favor of Change

Now you need to identify forces pulling you toward exercising regularly and strategize ways to maximize those forces. Perhaps you have gained a few pounds and want to lose them. Or, your family, being concerned with your health, has been pestering you to exercise regularly. Maybe you have had a checkup and found that your serum cholesterol is too high.

How can you maximize these factors that encourage you to exercise? You could set your alarm clock 30 minutes earlier every morning to make time for the gym. You could download some more up-tempo songs to listen to while you walk or jog. You might buy an article of clothing that would fit if you lose weight by exercising. Recognizing your family's concerns, you might communicate with them when you exercise, thereby receiving encouragement and reinforcement for that behavior. And, you might arrange for periodic blood tests to monitor changes in your serum cholesterol after beginning an exercise

> **Force field analysis:** a method of adopting desired behavior by maximizing forces that encourage the behavior and minimizing forces that oppose the behavior.

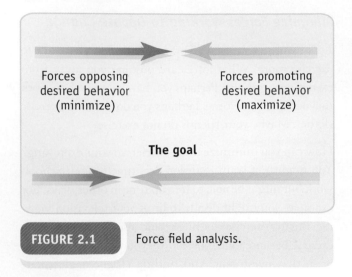

Forces opposing
desired behavior
(minimize)

Forces promoting
desired behavior
(maximize)

The goal

FIGURE 2.1   Force field analysis.

program. When it drops to healthier levels, you will see the benefits of exercising and be more likely to continue that behavior (**FIG. 2.1 ▲**).

You can use force field analysis to make a health-related decision by completing Health Check Up 2.4 (see Health Check Up 2.4 on the companion website). Once completed, place Health Check Up 2.4 in your Health Decision Portfolio.

Understand and Apply Health Behavior Change Theories

Do you want to eat more nutritionally or not get so stressed out? Well, have we got a deal for you! There are several theories you can use to take charge of those health behaviors. At first glance, you may think that study of health behavior change theories is merely an academic exercise. However, you can actually use behavior change theories to take control of your health behaviors and become healthier. This section is designed to help you do just that.

Why Theories Are Useful

"A theory is a set of interrelated concepts, definitions, and propositions that present a *systematic* view of events or situations by specifying relationships among variables in order to *explain* and *predict* the events or situations" (Kerlinger and Lee, 2000). In other words, theories can

be used to determine why people do or do not engage in a health behavior (Glanz, Rimer, and Viswanath, 2008). And, once they know why, people can modify those reasons (also called *constructs*) to encourage healthier behavior. Health behavior change theories, therefore, serve two general purposes: They *explain* why behaviors are adopted, and they provide ways to *modify* those behaviors (**FIG. 2.2 ▶**). We discuss each of these in the following sections.

Explain Behavior

Health behavior change theories include constructs that explain why people choose a health-related behavior. For example, why do people smoke cigarettes? Certainly they know cigarette smoking is related to lung cancer, heart disease, and stroke. This is common knowledge. It must be something else that explains that behavior. Perceptions of the severity and likelihood of contracting these diseases, confidence in the ability to give up smoking, and values are among the constructs in several theories that explain why people smoke or behave in other ways they know to be unhealthy. In fact, knowledge is a *necessary* but *insufficient* condition for people to behave healthfully. You might need to know the reasons for flossing your teeth daily and how to floss correctly, but just knowing that will not ensure that you actually floss each day. Other factors are involved, and health behavior theories identify these factors.

Modify Behavior

Once the factors affecting your behavior are identified, you can manipulate them to change that behavior. For example, if you know you drink alcohol to maintain friendships that provide you social support, you can arrange to acquire that support in other, healthier, ways. Perhaps you decide to join a campus club; or get active in your church, synagogue, or mosque; or organize an intramural sports team. Likewise, if you know that certain barriers interfere with behaving healthfully, you can plan to overcome those barriers. For example, if finances prevent you from going to the doctor for regular health screenings, you can strategize around that barrier by locating a health clinic that offers free screenings. Maybe your campus health center also provides free health services. The point is that once

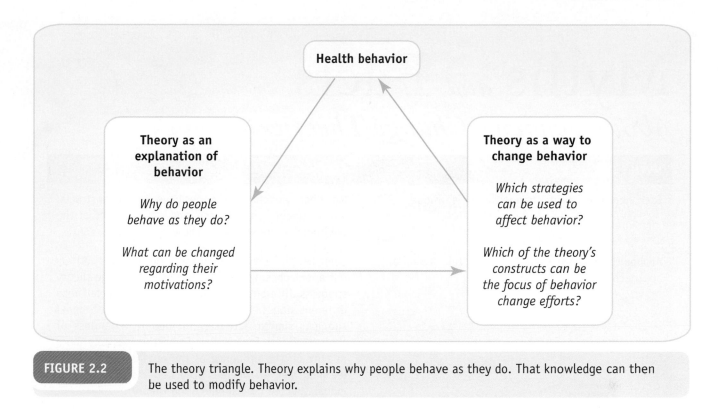

Health behavior

Theory as an explanation of behavior

Why do people behave as they do?

What can be changed regarding their motivations?

Theory as a way to change behavior

Which strategies can be used to affect behavior?

Which of the theory's constructs can be the focus of behavior change efforts?

FIGURE 2.2 The theory triangle. Theory explains why people behave as they do. That knowledge can then be used to modify behavior.

you can explain the factors influencing your health behavior, you can change those factors and, thereby, change your behavior.

Theories You Can Use

Which behavior change theories can you use to take control of your health behavior? Several of these theories are examined in the following sections. Each theory's constructs and applications are discussed, and an example is provided to show how you might use that theory to change your own health behaviors.

Stages of Change Theory

Do you eat a nutritionally sound and healthy diet? Perhaps you may know the reasons you should eat nutritious foods but have never gotten around to doing it regularly. Maybe you have even made a plan to visit the salad bar as part of your routine but have never implemented that plan or, at least, not for long. **Stages of change theory** recognizes that people are at different stages in terms of their health behavior (Table 2.1). Furthermore, this theory suggests different strategies to change health behavior

depending on a person's stage of readiness. People who are thinking about eating better, for example, but have not begun doing it yet need different strategies to help them than those who have started eating healthy meals daily but need help *maintaining* their new habit.

Concepts and Application

Different strategies and applications are developed for people at different stages to encourage them to move to the next higher stage. For example, if you never thought about eating a balanced diet (precontemplation), helping you to develop a plan to do so is useless. Rather, you need to learn about the relationship between diet and health so you start to think about eating more nutritionally (contemplation). Once you contemplate eating more nutritionally, strategies are needed to help you make a plan to do so (decision/determination or preparation). Table 2.1 lists

Stages of change theory: a health behavior change theory that considers people to be at different stages of readiness for change.

Myths *and* Facts
About Behavior Change Theories

MYTH	FACT
Each health behavior change theory is unique.	Many behavior change theories have similar constructs. Social support, self-efficacy, and the influence of the environment are several of these constructs.
All health behavior change theories take a similar approach to affect behavior change.	Some health behavior change theories take very different approaches. For example, stages of change theory suggests different activities for people who fall into different stages. In contrast, the health belief model suggests similar activities for people regardless of their readiness for change. Some theories rely more heavily on the influence of the environment (social learning theory), whereas others are more inner/individual directed (social marketing theory).
Theories that were developed many years ago are outdated and should not be used.	For a theory to be useful, it must be tested over many years, in many different settings, with many different groups of people. If that type of research demonstrates the validity of the theory, then one can be confident it accurately explains health behavior and can be used to modify that behavior. Therefore, theories developed many years ago may actually be more valid and useful than theories developed more recently.

several applications you can use to move to the next stage of readiness.

Example of Stages of Change Theory in Use

Cindy has no idea she should be practicing a method of relaxation to manage stress. She never heard of such a thing. She is at the *precontemplation stage*. Her friend Tonya, however, took a stress management course last semester and learned how to manage stress. Concerned about her friend, Tonya shares what she learned with Cindy. Now knowing the reasons she should incorporate a relation technique into her daily routine, Cindy finds herself in the *contemplation stage*. She is thinking about meditating. Because she knows stages of change theory, she seeks encouragement from her family. She also asks Tonya to help her devise a plan to meditate daily. Cindy is now at the *decision/determination stage*: She decides to meditate at 10 a.m. when her roommate is in class and the room is quiet. Her goal is to meditate at least 3 days the first week and, afterward, 5 days a week. She implements her plan (*action stage*), and after a week she evaluates her progress. Cindy realizes that meditating at 10 a.m. does not work because there is a lot of noise from other residents in her dorm. She changes the time to 2 p.m. She also believes that she needs more encouragement and social support,

TABLE 2.1	Stages of Change Theory: Concepts and Applications

Theory Constructs	Applications
Precontemplation Unaware of problematic health behavior; has not thought about change.	Read about health behavior's relationship to health. Increase awareness of need for change. Learn of risks and benefits of health behavior.
Contemplation Thinking about change, in the near future.	Speak with friends and family about thinking of changing health behavior. Ask them to motivate/encourage you to make specific plans to change health behavior.
Decision/Determination (Preparation) Making a plan to change.	Develop concrete action plans to change health behavior, setting gradual goals.
Action Implementation of specific action plans to change health behavior.	Try the new behavior. If problems arise, get assistance and social support from experts (e.g., health specialists or fitness trainers).
Maintenance Continuation of desirable health behavior, or repeating periodic recommended step(s).	Use reminders (e.g., notes on the bathroom mirror). Find alternative behaviors to add variety that accomplish the same goal.

REPRODUCED FROM: Glanz, Karen and Rimer, Barbara K. *Theory at a Glance: A Guide for Health Promotion Practice*. Washington, DC: National Cancer Institute, Department of Health and Human Services, 2009 (NIH Publication No. 05-3896), http://www.cancer.gov.

so she suggests to Tonya that they each keep a journal describing their meditation experiences and to share their journals with each other once a week. Soon, Cindy is meditating daily, but every once in a while she forgets to make the time to meditate. Using stages of change theory, she writes herself reminders to meditate and leaves them on her bathroom mirror. This helps her avoid relapsing into not meditating. She is now in the *maintenance stage*.

You can use stages of change theory to make a health-related decision by completing Health Check Up 2.5 (see Health Check Up 2.5 on the companion website). Once completed, place Health Check Up 2.5 in your Health Decision Portfolio.

Health Belief Model

Another way of conceptualizing health behavior decisions is the **health belief model**. You have a final examination and you are trying to decide whether to study for it or, instead, party with your friends. If you do not study for the exam, you will likely fail the course. If that means

you will flunk out of school, you probably would study to avoid that serious consequence. However, if you are a graduating senior, you have a 3.98 grade point average, and this course is not needed to graduate, you still might not study, even though you recognize the likely outcome is that you will fail the course. In this case, the consequence is not considered serious enough to encourage studying.

The above example presents two of the constructs of the health belief model, *perceived susceptibility* and *perceived severity*. Other constructs include *perceived benefits* of the behavior, *perception of barriers* to engaging in the behavior, *confidence* in your ability to perform the behavior successfully, and *cues to action* that encourage the behavior.

> **Health belief model:** a health behavior change theory that includes the constructs of perceived susceptibility, perceived seriousness, perceived benefit, perceived barriers, cues to action, and self-efficacy.

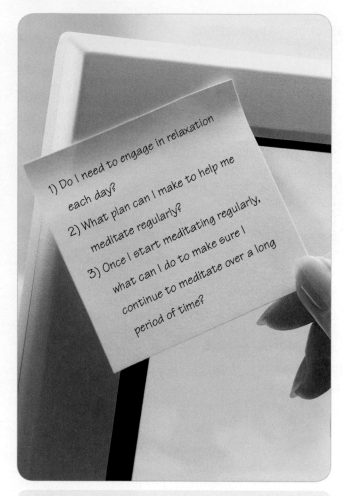

Stages of change theory involves several steps starting from learning of a need for change through adopting and maintaining that change.

1) Do I need to engage in relaxation each day?

2) What plan can I make to help me meditate regularly?

3) Once I start meditating regularly, what can I do to make sure I continue to meditate over a long period of time?

Concepts and Application

The health belief model states that people will decide to adopt a healthy behavior if they:

1. Believe they are at risk to a serious condition if they do not (*perceived susceptibility* and *perceived severity*).

2. Believe that the behavior can prevent this condition (*perceived benefit*).

3. Believe that the cost (in terms of money, time, and effort) of behaving in this way is not too great (*perceived barriers*).

4. Believe that the behavior can be engaged in successfully (*self-efficacy*).

Lastly, the health belief model recognizes that *cues to action*—such as magnets on refrigerators or phone calls—make it more likely the behavior will be adopted. Table 2.2 describes the components of the health belief model.

Example of Health Belief Model in Use

Imagine you have a friend named Carlos who loves to ride his bike on campus. Although his sister encourages him to wear a helmet when biking, Carlos hates the feeling of the strap under his chin, and he thinks he looks *uncool* biking with a helmet. Should he wear a helmet or not? Carlos decides to make this decision systematically using the health belief model that he learned about in his health course.

Carlos decides to find out how *susceptible* he is to a *serious* condition if he bikes without a helmet. He researches the number of bicycle accidents and finds them to occur frequently. Furthermore, he learns that head trauma occurring in a bicycle accident can result in paralysis or even death (*perceived severity*). Reading on, he learns that bicycle helmets are effective in preventing head trauma (*perceived benefit*) and that the costs (*perceived barriers*) are minimal compared to the benefits of wearing a helmet—he can get a helmet for free from the county health department, and the tight chin strap is a small price to pay for his safety. So Carlos decides to wear a helmet when biking. To remind himself to do so (*cues to action*), he stores his helmet by locking it up with his bike, so he is reminded to wear it whenever he uses his bike. He feels confident he can wear his helmet (*self-efficacy*) because he observes other guys on campus wearing theirs.

You can use the health belief model to make a health-related decision by completing Health Check Up 2.6 (see Health Check Up 2.6 on the companion website). Once completed, place Health Check Up 2.6 in your Health Decision Portfolio.

Social Learning Theory

Say you want to be physically fit but the college gym is located far away from your dorm and classes. You recognize

TABLE 2.2	Health Belief Model: Concepts and Applications

Theory Constructs	Applications
Perceived Susceptibility One's opinion of chances of getting the condition/illness/disease.	Read about the risks and benefits of the health behavior to determine how susceptible you are to the consequences of that behavior.
Perceived Severity One's opinion of how serious is the condition/illness/disease.	Study the seriousness of the consequences of the behavior. Do internet searches or speak with a health specialist.
Perceived Benefits One's opinion of the effectiveness of the health behavior to reduce risk or seriousness of impact.	Learn about the benefits of engaging in the behavior by reading, internet searches, or taking a workshop or course.
Perceived Barriers One's opinion of the tangible and psychological costs of engaging in the health behavior.	Identify and reduce barriers by brainstorming solutions. Get assistance from your instructor or a friend who has overcome these obstacles.
Cues to Action Strategies to activate "readiness" to engage in the health behavior.	Provide how-to information; promote awareness; reminders. Send yourself a postcard reminder to engage in the behavior. Place a reminder note on your pillow or with your schoolbooks.
Self-Efficacy Confidence in one's ability to engage in the health behavior.	Try the behavior. Observe others engaging in the behavior. Model your behavior on their behavior.

REPRODUCED FROM: Glanz, Karen and Rimer, Barbara K. *Theory at a Glance: A Guide for Health Promotion Practice*. Washington, DC: Department of Health and Human Services, 1997 (NIH Publication No. 97-3896).

being fit is not going to be easy. One of the basic constructs of **social learning theory** acknowledges the relationship between the environment and the individual. This is called *reciprocal determinism*: an interaction between individuals and their environment in which each affects the other. Several constructs of social learning theory are similar to those you just learned about for other health behavior change theories, whereas others are different.

Concepts and Application

In addition to reciprocal determinism, social learning theory includes *expectations* regarding the likely outcome of engaging in the behavior (similar to *perceived benefit* in the health belief model) and *self-efficacy*, which derives from *observational learning* (seeing others perform the behavior). *Behavioral capability*, the knowledge and skills needed to perform the behavior, is another construct

of social learning theory. Lastly, social learning theory includes *reinforcement* to increase the recurrence of the health-related behavior. Table 2.3 describes the components of social learning theory.

Example of Social Learning Theory in Use

Imagine the following scenario: Your campus is concerned about the prevalence of alcohol abuse and the accidents and fights it leads to. Administrators decide to use social learning theory to respond to this issue. They

> **Social learning theory:** a health behavior change theory that includes the constructs of reciprocal determinism, behavioral capability, expectations, self-efficacy, observational learning, and reinforcement.

TABLE 2.3 **Social Learning Theory: Concepts and Applications**

Theory Constructs	Applications
Reciprocal Determinism Behavior changes result from interaction between person and environment; change is bidirectional.	Change the environment, if warranted. For example, have only healthy foods where you live or take a class in a building in which there is a gymnasium or a walking path nearby.
Behavioral Capability Knowledge and skills to influence health behavior.	Arrange for education or training necessary to engage in health behavior. Take a course or workshop or read a book providing this information.
Expectations Beliefs about likely results of health behavior.	Make a list of the likely results of engaging in health behavior.
Self-Efficacy Confidence in the ability to engage in health behavior and persist in action.	Approach behavior change in small steps. Observe others who are like you engaging in the behavior.
Observational Learning Beliefs based on observing others like oneself engaging in health behavior and noting the results.	Note family, friends, and others' experiences and physical changes as a result of engaging in health behavior. Identify role models to emulate.
Reinforcement Responses to a person's health behavior that increases or decreases the chances of recurrence.	Arrange for incentives, rewards, praise from friends or family for engaging in the behavior. Provide self-reward such as saving money that would have been spent on tobacco or alcohol and buying something with that money.

REPRODUCED FROM: Glanz, Karen and Rimer, Barbara K. *Theory at a Glance: A Guide for Health Promotion Practice*. Washington, DC: Department of Health and Human Services, 1997 (NIH Publication No. 97-3896).

designate a large room in the student union for alcohol-free events and organize parties, film showings, and speeches by guest celebrities in that room (*reciprocal determinism*). They also advertise these events by placing posters in dorms and dining facilities. These posters show the benefits of responsible drinking and/or abstaining from drinking alcohol altogether. As such, administrators are creating a campus environment that is more conducive to resolving the alcohol problem (*reciprocal determinism*). To tackle this problem further, administrators encourage peer leaders—students trained to educate other students—to share knowledge about the effects of alcohol (*expectations*) and teach students to resist pressure to drink (*behavioral capacity*). These tactics help students gain confidence in their ability to resist drinking, even when their friends urge them to do so (*self-efficacy*). This confidence is reinforced when they hear the peer leaders—students like themselves—discuss their ability to

abstain from alcohol consumption (*observational learning* and *reinforcement*). Campus administrators also arrange for students who sign pledges to refrain from drinking alcohol to receive T-shirts on which appear "I Am Alcohol-Free." Visitors to the alcohol-free room also receive these T-shirts (*reinforcement*).

You can use social learning theory to make a health-related decision by completing Health Check Up 2.7 (see Health Check Up 2.7 on the companion website). Once completed, place Health Check Up 2.7 in your Health Decision Portfolio.

How Decision Making and Behavior Change Theory Are Used in This Text

Decision making is the overriding theme of this text. In determining what topics to include in this text, the foremost consideration is whether it helps you make a health behavior decision. The goal is to provide you with the opportunity to lead a healthy life. To accomplish this goal, decision-making strategies are woven throughout this text as described in the following sections.

Decision Making and the Use of Behavior Change Theory Is Applied at the End of Each Chapter

In the online companion website, you should complete an "Applying Behavior Change Theory" activity provided for each chapter. This activity requires you to identify a health behavior discussed in that chapter that you would like to change. Once you select that behavior, you are instructed to select a health behavior change theory and apply theory to make that behavior change. As a result, by the time you finish reading this text, you will have identified at least 11 health behaviors you want to change and developed strategies for making those changes.

Informing the Health Decision Portfolio

As you apply behavior change strategies, you are encouraged to organize those strategies in a Health Decision Portfolio (see the companion website). This includes the Health Check Ups for each chapter and the descriptions of your use of health behavior change theories in the Applying Behavior Change Theory features. Once you organize your strategies in this way, it will be more likely that you will follow up on one or more behavior change goals. The result will be a healthier you, and your quality of life will be enhanced.

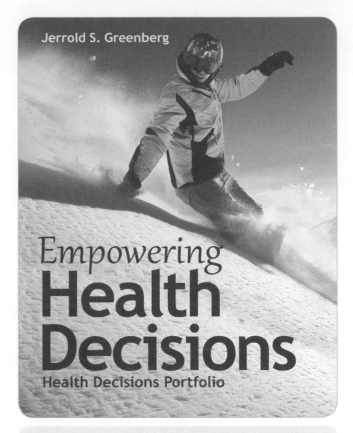

Jerrold S. Greenberg

Empowering Health Decisions
Health Decisions Portfolio

Throughout the course of reading this book, place Health Check Ups and other assignments in your Health Decision Portfolio (see the companion website). Then, at the conclusion of the course, you can better determine which health behaviors you want to change and how you will go about changing them.

SUMMARY

To facilitate your being able to make healthy decisions to improve your physical health, social health, emotional health, mental health, and spiritual health, a summary of this chapter is provided.

- You decide to engage in health-related behaviors for a variety of reasons. Knowledge of the consequences of these behaviors is only one of those reasons. In addition, your health decisions are a function of your habits, motivations, values, risk perception, culture and family, and environmental and social policy.

- There are many sources of health information, some more valid than others. Among these are advertisements, the internet, family and friends, and newspaper and magazine articles. All health information should be critically evaluated for its validity and significance.

- Medical evidence is derived from research. Different types of research studies provide different levels of validity and confidence in the study results. Among the different types of studies are case reports, observational studies, case-controlled studies, cohort studies, controlled clinical trials, double-blind studies, and randomized clinical trials. The most valid data derive from double-blind, randomized, controlled clinical trials.

- Although the results of a medical study may be statistically significant, they may not be clinically significant. Clinical significance refers to the real and/or meaningful effects on the health of study subjects.

- There are several methods of effective decision making. One of these is systematic decision making, which involves perceiving and defining the problem, brainstorming and evaluating ideas, acting on an idea, and reacting to the results of that action.

- Another method of effective decision making is force field analysis. Force field analysis identifies and maximizes the forces that favor adoption of the behavior and identifies and minimizes the forces that oppose adoption.

- Behavior change theories explain why people behave as they do and provide guidance for modifying behavior by intervening in its causes. Among behavior change theories are stages of change theory, the health belief model, and social learning theory.

- Stages of change theory poses that people are at different stages of readiness for change. These stages are precontemplation, contemplation, decision/determination, action, and maintenance.

- The health belief model states that behavior is a function of perceived susceptibility, perceived severity, perceived benefits, perceived barriers, cues to action, and self-efficacy.

- Social learning theory states that behavior is a function of reciprocal determinism, behavioral capability, expectations, self-efficacy, observational learning, and reinforcement.

REFERENCES

Friedman, M. and Rosenman, R. *Type A Behavior and Your Heart*. New York: Alfred A. Knopf, 1974.

Glanz, K., Rimer, B. K., and Viswanath, K. (Editors). *Health Behavior and Health Education: Theory, Practice, and Research*. San Francisco: Jossey-Bass, 2008.

Kerlinger, F. N. and Lee, H. B. *Foundations of Behavioral Research*, 4th ed. Fort Worth, TX: Harcourt College Publishers, 2000.

Medical Library Association. *A User's Guide to Finding and Evaluating Health Information on the Web*. 2006. Available at: http://www.mlanet.org/resources/userguide.html.

National Cancer Institute. *Dictionary of Cancer Terms*. 2006. Available at: http://www.cancer.gov/dictionary/.

National Center for Complementary and Alternative Medicine. *Evaluating Web-Based Health Resources*. 2010. Available at: http://www.nccam.nih.gov/health/webresources.

National Institutes of Health. Glossary of clinical trial terms. 2008. Available at: http://www.clinicaltrials.gov/ct/info/glossary.

Statistical Assessment Service. *What Is the Difference between Absolute and Relative Risk?* Undated. Available at: http://stats.org/faq_risk.htm.

INTERNET RESOURCES

U.S. Food and Drug Administration
How to Evaluate Health Information on the Internet
http://www.fda.gov/Drugs/ResourcesForYou/
Consumers/BuyingUsingMedicineSafely/
BuyingMedicinesOvertheInternet/ucm202863.htm

Jim Grizzell
Behavior Change Theories and Models
http://www.csupomona.edu/~jvgrizzell/best_
practices/bctheory.html

Norman W. Edmund
*Decision Making: A Guide to Creative Decision Making
and Critical Thinking*
http://www.decisionmaking.org/decisionmaking-
booklet.pdf

Free Management Library
Decision Making
http://managementhelp.org/prsn_prd/decision.htm

CancerGuide
The Significance of Statistical Significance
http://cancerguide.org/significance.html

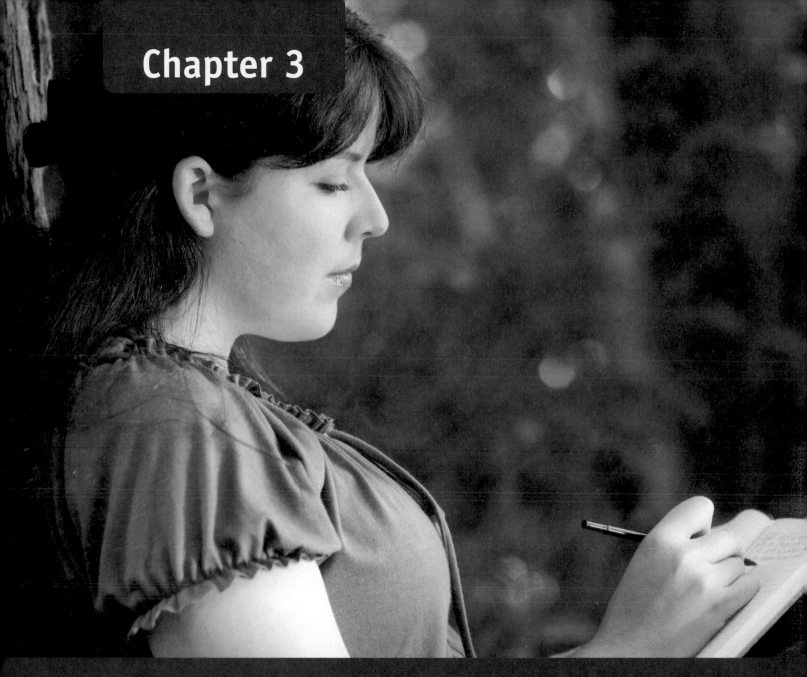

Chapter 3

Improving Your Psychological Health

 Access Health Check Ups and Health Behavior Change activities on the Companion Website:
go.jblearning.com/Empowering.

Learning Objectives

■ Explain the difference between psychological health and mental illness.

■ List the benefits of being psychologically healthy.

■ Summarize symptoms and self-help strategies for common psychological health problems.

■ Describe how to interact with others in a psychologically healthy way.

■ Discuss the signs of mental illness and treatments available.

■ Describe how to recognize and help a suicidal person.

Imagine someone tells you that your favorite relative has become unhealthy. What crosses your mind? Cancer? Heart disease? The flu, a sprained ankle, an ulcer? Some other physical condition? You probably do not think of some psychological ailment, such as depression or panic attacks. Although we know *intellectually* that health is multifaceted, psychological health issues may not come to mind when we learn that someone is in poor health. Yet the health of the body is dependent on the health of the mind. This chapter helps you make psychologically healthy decisions, with the added benefit of also improving the health of your body.

Understand the Difference Between Psychological Health and Mental Illness

Although it seems obvious that there is a significant difference between *psychological health* and *mental illness*, this difference is misunderstood by many people. **Mental illness** refers to alterations in thinking, emotions, or behaviors that produce distress and impaired functioning. It is often a result of biological changes in the brain. Psychological health is marked *not* merely by an absence of mental illness. That is, if you are not depressed, nor suicidal, nor have hallucinations or delusions, it is true you might not be mentally ill. Yet, you may also not be psychologically healthy. Perhaps you have low self-esteem, or are excessively shy in social situations, or have difficulty managing anxious feelings. **Psychological health** is the

ability to express, think, and behave appropriately relative to your emotions.

Psychological Health

In this chapter, you will learn how to be psychologically healthy by first recognizing symptoms of low self-esteem, depression, anxiety, shyness, panic disorder, loneliness, and an inability to resolve conflicts and communicate well with others. Once recognizing which of these challenges to psychological health affect you, suggested remedies are presented so you can respond effectively to these challenges.

Mental Illness

Mental illnesses are quite common. An estimated 30.8 million American adults, or 14.8% of the adult population, experience at least one diagnosable mental illness as defined by the American Psychiatric Association's *Diagnostic and Statistical Manual of Mental Disorders, Fourth Edition* (Grant et al., 2004). When mental illnesses do

---

Mental illness: alterations in thinking, emotions, or behaviors that produce distress and impaired functioning.

Psychological health: the ability to express, think, and behave appropriately relative to one's emotions.

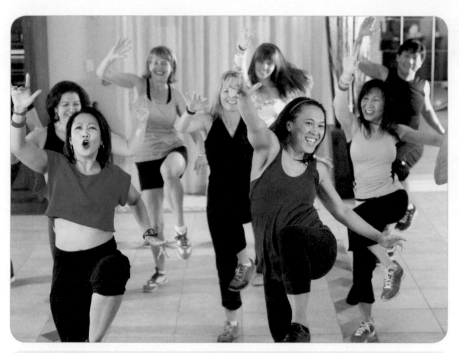

When you are psychologically healthy, you feel better and relate to other people more effectively.

occur, they require the intervention of trained clinicians who may prescribe medications and recommend other therapies depending on the specific illness. How to recognize symptoms of common mental illnesses and then make decisions about treatment are discussed later in this chapter.

Know the Advantages of Being Psychologically Healthy

Knowing the advantages of psychological health will help convince you to engage in activities that improve this aspect of your health. When you are psychologically healthy, you feel better—emotionally and physically—and you interact more effectively with others.

Emotional Benefits

Part of being psychologically healthy is the ability to express emotions appropriately; for example, stating that you are angry rather than acting aggressively, expressing disagreement without insulting other people, and withholding emotions when that is the best strategy. When you are able to express emotions appropriately, you feel more self-assured, more competent, and more effective in managing challenges. In short, you feel better about yourself and your life situation.

Physical Benefits

If you can manage your emotions, you are not only psychologically healthier but also physically healthier. **Psychoneuroimmunology** is a field of science that studies the relationship between the health of the mind and body. This relationship can be understood by considering allergies. Assume your immunological system can manage 100 grains of pollen before an allergic reaction is triggered. It is known that during periods of high emotion, the body's immune system produces fewer pollen-fighting substances. Consequently, it might take only 80 grains of pollen for an allergic reaction to occur. The mind's state of high emotion has lowered the body's production of pollen-fighting substances allowing an allergic reaction.

Social Benefits

You are a social being. Without relatives, friends, colleagues, and others with whom to interact, your life would not be satisfying. When you are psychologically healthy and can manage your emotions, these relationships improve. You communicate better and you resolve conflict more effectively. When these relationships are solid, you are also more likely to obtain the social support you need to get through life's ups and downs.

Psychoneuroimmunology: a field of science that studies the relationship between the health of the mind and the health of the body.

TABLE 3.1	**Percentage of United States College Students Reporting Psychological Health Challenges Within the Past Year**		
Challenge	**Male (%)**	**Female (%)**	**Total (%)**
Felt hopeless	38.7	48.6	45.1
Felt overwhelmed	77.0	91.4	86.3
Felt exhausted	72.7	86.5	81.6
Felt very lonely	50.0	61.3	57.3
Felt very sad	51.3	66.3	61.1
Felt so depressed it was difficult to function	26.9	33.3	31.1
Seriously considered suicide	6.3	6.4	6.4
Attempted suicide	1.1	0.9	1.1
Diagnosed with anxiety	7.2	13.9	11.6
Felt overwhelming anxiety	40.5	56.0	50.6
Diagnosed with depression	7.4	12.4	10.7
Sleep difficulties	23.0	26.6	25.4
Felt tremendous stress	8.1	11.4	10.3

DATA FROM: American College Health Association. *American College Health Association–National College Health Assessment II: Spring 2011 Reference Group Executive Summary*. Hanover, MD: American College Health Association, 2011. Available at: http://www.acha-ncha.org/docs/ACHA-NCHA-II_ReferenceGroup_ExecutiveSummary_Spring2011.pdf.

Understand Challenges to Psychological Health

Some people are just lucky. Or, at least it seems that way. They appear always to be happy, feel good about themselves, perceive situations as challenges rather than threats, have many friends, and communicate well with other people. In other words, they are psychologically healthy. But many of us are not as fortunate. Psychological health does not come as easily to us. The good news is that if you do work at it, you can improve your psychological health. If you face a psychological health problem, know that you are not alone. Many college students face challenges to their psychological health (Table 3.1). This section will help you recognize symptoms of common problems, give you tools to improve many of them, and also alert you to symptoms that require professional help.

> **Self-esteem:** how high a regard or opinion one has of oneself.

Low Self-Esteem

Self-esteem refers to how high a regard or opinion you have of yourself. If you have a good deal of confidence in yourself and your talents, you probably have a high self-esteem. If you think you are inferior to most other people (not as smart, or as good looking, or as well liked), then you probably have a low self-esteem.

Recognizing Symptoms of Low Self-Esteem

Low self-esteem is characterized by a lack of trust in your opinions, letting others make important decisions, following and conforming to others, lacking self-confidence and self-assurance, and believing you are not worthy of being treated respectfully. Some of these characteristics may be present in someone with low self-esteem. People who have low self-esteem are usually shy and socially withdrawn and may hesitate to offer opinions in an attempt to hide their perceived inferiority. Although self-esteem develops over many years and is sometimes difficult to improve, there are effective ways to strengthen it.

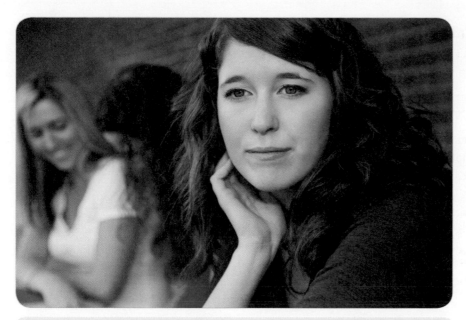

One sign of low self-esteem is shyness resulting from a lack of confidence in one's abilities, ideas, or opinions.

Improving What You Think of Yourself

You have both positive and negative traits. We all do. If you focus on the negative ones, you will feel badly about yourself and have low self-esteem. You will constantly be thinking of what is wrong with yourself and why you developed that way. If, instead, you focus on your positive characteristics, you will be more likely to hold yourself in high regard. Health Check Up 3.1 helps you to organize these positive aspects by identifying your talents, physical traits, social characteristics, and past accomplishments that make you proud (see Health Check Up 3.1 on the companion website). Asking friends and relatives to list your strengths can further help validate your strong points. After completing Health Check Up 3.1, place it in your Health Decision Portfolio.

Depression

Depression may be described as feeling sad, blue, unhappy, miserable, or down in the dumps. Most of us feel this way at one time or another for short periods. It is when these feelings are chronic and persistent that there is a diagnosable problem. **Clinical depression** is a mood disorder in which feelings of sadness, loss, anger, or frustration interfere with everyday life for a long period of time (PubMed

Health, 2010). Clinical depression affects the body, mood, thoughts, behavior, and physical health. Almost 21 million American adults suffer from depression (National Institute of Mental Health, 2010c), and, as noted in Table 3.2, more than 10% of college students have been diagnosed with clinical depression. Fortunately, depression is one of the most treatable of the mental disorders.

Recognizing Symptoms of Depression

Depression may be described as feeling sad, blue, unhappy, miserable, or down in the dumps. Most of us feel this way at one time or another for short periods. Clinical depression, however, interferes with everyday life for a long period of time (PubMed Health, 2010). People who are clinically depressed can be recognized by physical, social, and work/school signs and symptoms.

Physical Signs

Physical signs of depression include low energy, fatigue, a sloppy appearance, sleeping problems, loss of appetite, unexplained weight loss or gain, digestive problems, excessive crying, and difficulty concentrating or making decisions.

Social Signs

Social signs of depression include loss of interest or pleasure in usual activities, withdrawal from others, problems with drugs or alcohol, compulsive spending, antisocial or rude behavior, and irritability.

Clinical depression: a mood disorder in which feelings of sadness, loss, anger, or frustration interfere with everyday life for a long period of time.

TABLE 3.2 **Percentage of United States College Students Experiencing Depression**

Experience	Male (%)	Female (%)	Total (%)
Ever diagnosed with depression	7	12	11
Diagnosed but not treated	1	2	2
Diagnosed and treated with medication	2	4	3
Diagnosed and treated with psychotherapy	2	2	2
Diagnosed and treated with medication and psychotherapy	2	4	3

REPRODUCED FROM: American College Health Association. *American College Health Association–National College Health Assessment II: Reference Group Data Report Spring 2011*. Hanover, MD: American College Health Association, 2011. Available at: http://www.acha-ncha.org/docs/ACHA-NCHA-II_ReferenceGroup_DataReport_Spring2011.pdf.

Work/School Signs

Signs of depression at work or school include decreased productivity, poor performance, morale problems, lack of cooperation, excessive worry, frequent accidents, absenteeism, chronic aches and pains or health changes that seem to have no cause, and frequent complaints of being tired.

Health Check Up 3.2 helps you identify signs and symptoms of depression you may experience (see Health Check Up 3.2 on the companion website). After completing Health Check Up 3.2, place it in your Health Decision Portfolio.

Depression is a serious condition for which help should be sought. Good places to obtain such help are campus health centers.

What to Do When Feeling Clinically Depressed

A number of studies suggest that depression is a factor in at least 30% of suicides (Balázs et al., 2006; National Institute of Mental Health, 2010a). Therefore, it is important that if you have signs of depression, you seek treatment immediately. If you suspect a friend of being clinically depressed, you should speak with a health care provider (someone at your campus health center) or your friend's physician to get your friend into treatment. You may feel awkward about invading your friend's privacy in this manner, but think how you would feel if you did nothing and your friend committed suicide. Treatment consists of antidepressant medication and psychotherapy. The combination of the two can be very effective in alleviating symptoms of depression.

Anxiety

Everyone feels anxious or nervous at one time or another. Even famous people who have to speak or sing in front of an audience experience stage fright. You have probably felt it too, such as when you have to speak in front of the class. This form of nervousness is often popularly referred to as *anxiety*. Occasional anxiety is not a psychological problem, but chronic anxiety can be. Anxiety disorders affect approximately 40 million American adults, about 18% of the population, in a given year (Kessler, Chiu, Demler, and Walters, 2005). Unlike the relatively mild and brief fear of speaking in front of an audience, anxiety disorders last at least 6 months and can get worse if left untreated.

Recognizing Symptoms of Anxiety

Anxiety has three components: (1) an *unrealistic fear*, (2) *physiological arousal* (high blood pressure, heart racing), and (3) *behavior* that either avoids the anxiety-provoking stimulus or escapes from it if it is encountered. People who have test anxiety, for example, are fearful of taking tests and failing (*unrealistic fear*); perspire, have increased muscle tension, and have more cholesterol in their blood (*physiological arousal*); and either cut class the day of the test or turn the test in as quickly as possible to alleviate their fear (*behavior*). Behavioral symptoms of anxiety include excessive worry, an inability to relax, being startled easily, difficulty concentrating, and trouble sleeping. Physical symptoms include fatigue, headaches, muscle tension and aches, difficulty swallowing, trembling, twitching, irritability, sweating, nausea, lightheadedness, and feeling out of breath.

Managing Anxiety

There are several self-help techniques you can use to manage mild anxiety:

- **Environmental planning**: You can adjust your environment so it causes less anxiety. For example, if you experience anxiety when going to the dentist, you can bring a friend with you or bring music and earbuds so you can drown out the sound of the drill.

- **Self-talk**: You can say things to yourself to be less anxious. For example, if you are anxious about taking tests, you can say to yourself, "What's the worst thing that can happen? Failing? That's not good, but there are plenty of worse things that could happen to me. And, most likely the worst thing—failing—will not happen, so anything short of that can't be so bad."

- **Thought stopping**: Every time you have the anxious thought, stop to recognize what is happening and

resign yourself to think of something else. You might even place a rubber band around your wrist and every time you have the anxious thought, snap the rubber band to extinguish that thought.

- **Systematic desensitization**: Imagine you are anxious about flying in an airplane. Systematic desensitization takes you from a safe position (being home and not thinking about a trip) all the way to imagining or doing the anxiety-provoking stimulus (flying in an airplane) in small steps. If you are in a safe position and only take a small step toward the anxiety-provoking stimulus, you should not feel anxious. By taking a series of small steps, you can make it through the event without it causing you anxiety.

The first step in systematic desensitization is developing a *fear hierarchy*—a list of at least 10 steps that start from a safe position and progress until you are experiencing the situation that originally evoked your anxiety. The accompanying What I Need to Know box presents an example of a fear hierarchy. Imagine the first step on the fear hierarchy until you can do so for 30 seconds without experiencing physiological arousal. Then calm yourself by thinking of a place you find extremely relaxing. Proceed through each step in this way. Systematic desensitization may take weeks or

Anxiety: an unrealistic fear accompanied by physiological arousal and avoidance or withdrawal behavior.

Environmental planning: an anxiety-management technique that involves adjusting the surroundings to cause less anxiety.

Self-talk: an anxiety-management technique that involves making reassuring statements to oneself to feel less anxious.

Thought stopping: an anxiety-management technique that involves recognizing when anxious thoughts occur and purposefully thinking about something else.

Systematic desensitization: an anxiety-management technique that involves working from a non-anxiety-provoking situation gradually toward doing the anxiety-provoking stimulus.

What I Need to Know

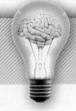

A Fear Hierarchy for Flying in an Airplane

The first step when using systematic desensitization is to develop a fear hierarchy. An example of a fear hierarchy appears below.

Step 1:	Deciding where to travel
Step 2:	Booking my reservation on the internet
Step 3:	Packing a suitcase for the trip
Step 4:	Traveling to the airport
Step 5:	Checking my luggage in at the airport
Step 6:	Sitting in the waiting area prior to boarding
Step 7:	Boarding the plane
Step 8:	Looking out the window as the plane taxis down the runway
Step 9:	Feeling the plane leave the ground
Step 10:	Flying above the clouds

months depending on the nature and degree of your anxiety. It is used by clinical psychologists but can also be useful as a self-help technique.

Complete Health Check Up 3.3 to determine whether you can use these anxiety-management techniques successfully (see Health Check Up 3.3 on the companion website). After completing Health Check Up 3.3, place it in your Health Decision Portfolio.

Chronic Anxiety

Chronic (long-lasting) anxiety can be treated with medications, psychotherapy, or both. Medications include antidepressants, selective serotonin reuptake inhibitors (SSRIs) such as Prozac or Zoloft, tricyclics, monoamine oxidase inhibitors (MAOIs), anti-anxiety drugs such as Xanax, and beta-blockers such as Inderal. One of the most effective forms of psychotherapy is **cognitive behavior therapy** (CBT). CBT helps people change their thoughts that support their unrealistic fear; this therapy often lasts about 12 weeks. CBT starts with therapists helping patients identify the anxiety-provoking behaviors. Then, patients are taught to focus on the behaviors that contribute

to the problem. New skills are taught and practiced that patients can use in real-world situations. For example, patients who become anxious in crowds may be taught how to control their breathing and thought patterns to feel less anxious.

Shyness

Shyness is being afraid of people, especially people who for some reason are emotionally threatening, such as strangers, authority figures, and potential romantic partners. Shy people may avoid social interactions and lack social skills. When shyness becomes severe, it is sometimes referred to as **social phobia**.

Cognitive behavior therapy: a psychological treatment that helps people change the thoughts that support their unrealistic fear.

Shyness: being afraid of people, especially people who for some reason are emotionally threatening.

Social phobia: a severe form of shyness.

Recognizing Symptoms of Shyness

Shyness and social phobia share many symptoms (Henderson and Zimbardo, 2001): heightened arousal in social situations (increased heart rate, perspiring, blushing), social skill deficits (limited eye contact), avoidance of social interactions, and fear of negative evaluations (Chavira, Stein, and Malcarne, 2002). Still, shy people report less socially avoidant behavior than those with social phobia, and their symptoms are often temporary. Forty to fifty percent of people experience some level of shyness, and at least 90% of college students report being shy at some point in their lives (Chavira, Stein, and Malcarne, 2002). One of the unfortunate symptoms of shyness is the delay or avoidance of seeking help. A study of college students found that even when help is readily available, shy students refrain from seeking it because this would require them to initiate a social interaction (Horsch, 2006).

Complete Health Check Up 3.4 to determine how shy you are (see Health Check Up 3.4 on the companion website). After completing Health Check Up 3.4, place it in your Health Decision Portfolio.

Managing Feelings of Shyness

Severe shyness, or social phobia, can be treated with medication and CBT, including systematic desensitization. For less severe shyness, the American Psychological Association (APA) recommends that family and friends help loved ones manage their shyness and suggest ways to do that (APA Help Center, 2010). You can also apply the APA recommendations to manage your own shyness by asking a friend or relative to help you.

- Maintain appropriate expectations while communicating empathy for the shy person's painful emotions.

- Encourage the shy person to tell you about daily experiences and how he or she feels about them.

- Acknowledge the conflict between the need to belong and fears of rejection.

- Role play challenging situations with the shy person.

- Help the shy individual set specific, manageable behavioral goals, and agree upon reasonable means to attain them.

- Help challenge the frequent negative thoughts about self and others, and help the shy person develop constructive alternatives.

- Avoid negative labels and intense pressures for social performance.

- Remember that shyness and social anxiety are common and universal experiences at all ages for most people.

Loneliness

Some people enjoy being alone, whereas other people feel lonely if they are not constantly surrounded by others. *Aloneness* is not the same as *loneliness*. Of course, other than for hermits—people who really prefer to be alone—persistent aloneness will eventually lead to loneliness. **Loneliness** is a psychological condition characterized by a deep sense of social isolation, emptiness, and worthlessness. Those experiencing loneliness find themselves feeling socially isolated (lonely) and uncertain that they can confide in, depend on, or trust others.

Recognizing Symptoms of Loneliness

Loneliness has been described as a strong sense of emptiness, isolation, unimportance, worthlessness, and an aching desire for someone to confide in. Chronic loneliness is a major health risk factor. The stress associated with loneliness can result in damaged arteries, high blood pressure, and conditions such as heart disease, hypertension, obesity, and stroke (Hawkley, Masi, Berry, and Cacioppo, 2006). A study conducted by the Center for Cognitive and Social Neuroscience at the University of Chicago found that loneliness can add 30 points to blood pressure in adults (Wikipedia, 2012). Loneliness also has a negative impact on learning and memory and can interfere with sleep patterns, thus affecting the ability to function in everyday life. Depression and suicidal thoughts can also be signs of loneliness.

> **Loneliness:** a psychological condition characterized by a deep sense of social isolation, emptiness, and worthlessness.

What I Need to Know

Racial Discrimination and Psychological Health

Racial discrimination plays a significant role in the health of Americans. "The evidence is especially clear . . . self-reported everyday discrimination is consistently associated with poorer mental health across multiple racial and ethnic groups (Whites, Latinos, African Americans) and for both women and men." Among the mental health conditions that racial discrimination most affects are depression and low self-esteem. In fact, as racial discrimination continues over a person's lifetime, these conditions may worsen.

Recognizing that discrimination has such a widespread influence on health, the 2010 national health objectives sought to address the issue. However, racial discrimination requires more than just a federal government response. Each of us needs to recognize that when we act in a prejudiced manner, we are affecting the health of others, subjecting them to depression and other mental and physical illnesses. Enrolling in a course that discusses discrimination will help you identify prejudices about which you were previously unaware, as would candid discussions with dorm mates or classmates of different races and ethnicities. Likewise, if you are the object of discrimination, you should recognize the potential implications on your health and work to buffer any ill effects; for example, by viewing the discriminator as humorous, silly, or ignorant.

ADAPTED FROM: Williams, D. R., Neighbors, H. W., and Jackson, J. S. Racial/ethnic discrimination and health: Findings from community studies. *American Journal of Public Health* 93 (2003): 200–208; Schulz, A. J., Gravlee, C. C., Williams, D. R., Israel, B. A., Mentz, G., and Rowe, Z. Discrimination, symptoms of depression, and self-rated health among African American women in Detroit: Results from a longitudinal analysis. *American Journal of Public Health* 96 (2006): 1265–1270; O'Brien, L. T. System-justifying beliefs and psychological well-being: The roles of group status and identity. *Personality and Social Psychological Bulletin* 31 (2005): 1718–1729.

Remedies for Loneliness

If you feel lonely, consider joining a club on campus where you will find others with whom to interact. Campuses have many choices of groups to join: peer counseling programs, student government, social clubs (such as a biking club, sorority or fraternity), or intramural sports teams. Or, you could volunteer to work with students who tutor, visit the elderly, or offer their time at places like the Ronald McDonald House or homeless shelters. Alternatively, you could get a pet if your living arrangements and budget allow. Pets can be wonderful companions and, aside from helping to alleviate feelings of loneliness, have been shown to produce many health benefits for their owners (e.g., lower heart rate and blood pressure). In fact, one study found that just petting a dog lowers the blood pressure in the pet owner and the dog (McLaughlin, 2008).

Panic Disorder

"For me, a panic attack is almost a violent experience. I feel disconnected from reality. I feel like I'm losing control in a very extreme way. My heart pounds really hard, I feel like I can't get my breath, and there's an overwhelming feeling that things are crashing in on me. . . . In between attacks, there is this dread and anxiety that it's going to happen again" (National Institute of Mental Health, 2009). What this person was describing is called a panic disorder. There are approximately 6 million American adults who experience panic attacks in any given year. Panic attacks can disable people if they end up avoiding places where they had a previous attack. For example, if a person's panic attack occurs in an elevator, he or she may develop a fear of elevators so strong that it affects a future job decision about working in a high-rise building. Panic attacks are a symptom of a psychological condition called panic disorder.

Recognizing Symptoms of Panic Disorder

Panic disorder is characterized by sudden attacks of terror accompanied by a pounding heart, perspiration, weakness, faintness, or dizziness. During an attack, people may

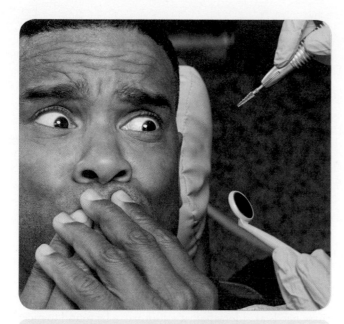

Panic attacks can occur in a crowd or during medical exams resulting in difficulty breathing and feelings of faintness.

become blushed or chilled, their hands may tingle or feel numb, and they may experience nausea, chest pain, or difficulty breathing. There is a fear of impending doom and loss of control.

What to Do if Experiencing Panic Disorder

If you or someone you know experiences panic disorder, help from a mental health professional should be sought. A good place to start is your campus health center. Panic disorder can be treated in a similar fashion as anxiety. Medications may be prescribed to keep the anxiety under control so that psychotherapy can be effective. CBT can help by changing thinking patterns that support irrational fears and by teaching strategies to use during anxiety-provoking situations.

Posttraumatic Stress Disorder

If you ever experienced a horrific car accident, sexual assault, or been the victim of a violent crime, you may have trouble overcoming the fear associated with that traumatic event. Maybe you avoid driving a car, or do not develop love relationships, or refuse to shop at night for fear of being a victim again. In that case, you may be

experiencing posttraumatic stress disorder. **Posttraumatic stress disorder** (PTSD) is a condition that can develop in people who have experienced a traumatic event—an event that was extremely distressing either psychologically, physically, or both. Such trauma may include a threat to one's life, or serious injury, or being subjected to a horrific event, in which intense fear and helplessness are experienced.

Recognizing Symptoms of PTSD

Symptoms of PTSD include:

1. Feelings of intense fear and helplessness.

2. Recurrent flashbacks, repeated memories and emotions, dreams, nightmares, illusions, or hallucinations related to traumatic events.

3. Chronic and recurring condition associated with increased risk of developing secondary disorders, such as depression (American Psychiatric Association, 1994; Ballenger et al., 2000).

PTSD is often experienced by soldiers who serve in war; in particular, among those with combat experience such as being shot at, handling dead bodies, knowing someone who was killed, and killing enemy combatants. An increase in these combat experiences is accompanied by a greater prevalence of PTSD. For example, a study of soldiers and marines serving in Iraq and Afghanistan found the prevalence of PTSD increased with the number of firefights during deployment—4.5% for no firefights, 9.3% for one to two firefights, 12.7% for three to five firefights, and 19.3% for more than five firefights. Rates for

Panic disorder: a psychological disorder characterized by panic attacks: sudden feelings of terror accompanied by a pounding heart, perspiration, weakness, faintness, or dizziness.

Posttraumatic stress disorder: a condition that develops in some people who have experienced a traumatic or extreme psychological or physical event resulting in recurrent fears, flashbacks, and nightmares.

those who had been deployed to Afghanistan were 4.5%, 8.2%, 8.3%, and 18.9%, respectively. Among soldiers serving in Vietnam, 15% experienced PTSD. Ten percent of soldiers serving in the first Gulf War developed PTSD (Hoge et al., 2004).

PTSD is more prevalent than many of us realize. Epidemiologists report that most people will experience a qualifying traumatic event and that up to 25% of them will develop PTSD (Hidalgo and Davidson, 2000; Nutt, 2000). Some experts believe PTSD is as prevalent as any other mental disorder, but that it is underreported because only a minority of people obtain treatment (Kessler, 2000).

Not everyone who experiences trauma develops post-traumatic stress disorder. A history of mental illness in oneself or one's family increases the likelihood of developing PTSD. Being prone to anxiety attacks or depression also increases this likelihood. Among the characteristics of those who have successfully managed PTSD are that they have supportive relationships with family and friends, they do not dwell on the trauma, they have personal faith, religion, or hope, and they have a sense of humor—in other words, their social and spiritual health are strong.

Treatment for PTSD

The most effective treatment for PTSD is called exposure therapy, which is like systematic desensitization, in that the patient confronts the fear in small steps until the threat is diminished. Consultation with a mental health specialist is an important step in overcoming PTSD.

Interact with Others in a Psychologically Healthy Way

Part of being psychologically healthy is the ability to interact with other people in a healthy way. That includes being able to resolve conflict, being assertive, and communicating effectively.

Resolve Conflicts

Suppose Steve wants to invite several friends over to party, but his roommate David wants to use the room to study for an important exam. Steve argues that he pays for half the room and should be able to use it as wanted and that if David wants to study, he should just leave. David argues that he is in school to learn, not party, that he also pays for half the room, and that the library closes at midnight, so he will have nowhere quiet to go. This is a lose–lose scenario: neither roommate wins. If the friends come over to party, David will mope around. If the friends are uninvited, Steve will be resentful.

Conflicts are usually argued over *wants*, although they are really about *needs*. Steve thinks: I *want* to use the room, but, more importantly, I *need* to feel that other people enjoy my company. David thinks: I *want* to use the room, but I *need* to get good grades so I can get into graduate school and meet my life's goal of being a doctor. Once these needs are identified, a solution can be found to meet both sides. Furthermore, recognizing these needs will help Steve and David prevent other conflicts or allow for them to be more easily resolved.

Techniques for Preventing and Defusing Conflict

To resolve conflicts so that both people win—that is, to meet both sets of needs—use RESPECT. **RESPECT** is a conflict-resolution technique in which you:

- **R**ecognize that there is a difference of opinion.

- **E**liminate any thoughts from your mind about what you want. You will come back to this later.

- **S**can and *listen* to what the other person is communicating in words and feelings.

- **P**araphrase the *words* the other person states, as well as the *feelings* you think the other person is experiencing.

- **E**xpress what you want and need and your reasons for that, but only after sufficiently focusing on the other person's wants and needs.

- **C**ollect several alternative solutions that meet both of your needs.

- **T**ry the best alternative solution.

Returning to the example described earlier, using RESPECT, Steve might express the need for having friends to provide the social support and positive self-esteem that

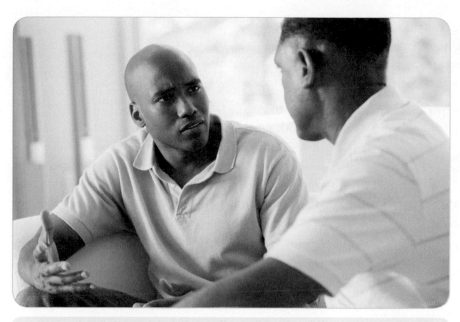

Conflict-resolution skills can help those in disagreement to resolve their differences to the satisfaction of both.

busy to discuss a course assignment with you outside of class. You pay for your professor's time outside of class and have a right to get that when you need it. You also have other basic human rights. For example, you have the right to be treated with respect, to decide what to do with your body and time, and to put yourself first sometimes.

When you act to protect a right, you can do that in several ways, and some ways are more effective than others. (1) You can yell at the professor or complain to the department chairperson. That behavior is called **aggressiveness**. You may get what you are entitled to, but you have violated the professor's right to be treated respectfully. (2) You could just accept the situation and attempt to complete the assignment to the best of your ability. That behavior is called **nonassertiveness**. You give up your rights so as not to bother someone else. (3) You could speak to the professor expressing your desire to meet and the reason why that is so important to you. That behavior is called **assertiveness**.

he needs. David might express his responsibility to do well in school, especially as his family is making sacrifices to pay the school bills. The conflict transfers from discussion of *wants* (I *want* to use the room for partying versus I *want* to use the room for studying) to an understanding of the *needs* involved (I *need* to maintain my friendships to feel good about myself versus I *need* to get good grades to do right by my family). Once needs are identified, a solution can be devised that satisfies both people. In this case, Steve can agree to have people over earlier, so that the room will be quiet after the library closes and David returns. In return, David can agree to give Steve advance notice of his needs for a quiet room in future.

Complete Health Check Up 3.5 to determine how well you can use these conflict-resolution strategies (see Health Check Up 3.5 on the companion website). After completing Health Check Up 3.5, place it in your Health Decision Portfolio.

Being Assertive

Most professors are available to students outside of class. They are concerned about their students' learning, and many even provide counsel regarding students' personal lives. Imagine, however, that one of your professors is too

RESPECT: a conflict resolution technique that **R**ecognizes a difference of opinion exists, **E**liminates thoughts about what you want, **S**cans and *listens* to what the other person is communicating in words and feelings, **P**araphrases the *words* and *feelings* of the other person, **E**xpresses what you want and your reasons, **C**ollects several alternative solutions, and **T**ries the best alternative solution.

Aggressiveness: a behavior whereby people get their entitlements but violate someone else's rights.

Nonassertiveness: a behavior whereby people give up their entitlements so as not to bother someone else.

Assertiveness: a behavior whereby people get their entitlements without violating anyone else's rights.

You affirm the right to which you are entitled and do so without violating anyone else's rights. To make an assertive statement, use a method developed many years ago called the **DESC form** (Bower and Bower, 1976):

■ **D**escribe the situation or the other person's behavior about which you are concerned.

■ **E**xpress your feelings regarding the situation or other person's behavior.

■ **S**pecify the change you would like to see regarding the situation or the other person's behavior.

■ **C**onsequences: Describe the consequences that will occur if the change is made versus if the change is *not* made.

Using the DESC form, you might say to your professor:

> When I am not allowed to meet with my professors outside of class to clarify assignments (Describe), I feel as though I am being cheated out of a good college experience and that I am being denied my rights as a student here (Express). Could you set up office hours so that you could be available outside of class (Specify)? If you did, I promise not to abuse the privilege—I will only contact you during office hours. If you can't offer office hours, I will raise my grievance with the department head (Consequences).

Communicate Effectively

When you are psychologically healthy, you communicate well. People understand what you tell them, and you express your messages appropriately. To achieve this level of communication, your words and your body language must be consistent.

Verbal Communication: Communicating in Words

FIG. 3.1 ▶ presents a model of communication consisting of a *sender* of a message, the *message* itself, the *medium* through which the message is sent, and the intended *receiver* of the message. Paying attention to these components can help you communicate more effectively.

The Sender

It should be clear who is sending the message. This seems obvious but is often not the case. For example, in this text it appears that the author is the sender of the message that you should make healthful decisions. Is this true? Or, is it health scientists and policy makers who are sending this healthful message using authors of books and college instructors as the media through which this message is conveyed? You should make it clear to those with whom you communicate whether you originated the message or are summarizing information from other sources and passing on that message. You will be trusted more if you are honest about this.

The Message

The message should be organized in a way that it is most likely to be understood. Several guidelines will help you do that:

■ Keep it short. If the message is clear, there is no reason to repeat it.

■ Only communicate what is necessary. Do not confuse the message with extraneous information that detracts from focusing on the message itself.

■ If the message contains several pieces of information, present the most important first, then the second most important, and so on.

■ Summarize the message after you present it.

■ Ask if the receiver understands the message or if clarification is necessary.

The Medium

Once it is clear who the sender is and the message is organized in the best possible way, it must be conveyed

---

DESC form: a method of making an assertive statement that involves **D**escribing the situation, **E**xpressing feelings, **S**pecifying the desired change, and identifying the **C**onsequences of making or not making the change.

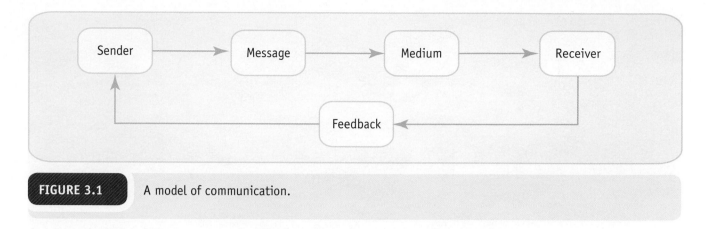

FIGURE 3.1   A model of communication.

through some medium. Media options include one-on-one discussion; group discussion; phone conversation; electronic communication such as email, text message, or social media post; or some written form, such as a letter or note. A face-to-face discussion, whether it be one on one or in a group, gives you the advantage of being able to observe the reaction of the receiver to your message. You can learn a lot from the physical reaction of the receiver to your communication. However, emails, instant messaging, and written forms of communication have the advantage of allowing the receiver to think longer before responding. In that way, a more thoughtful and appropriate response can be made. Somewhere between a face-to-face discussion and an electronic communication is a phone conversation. With phone calls you lose the ability to read body language but you may feel more comfortable discussing sensitive, personal matters without being observed and without forcing the receiver to be observed.

The Receiver

To communicate well, you need to understand the receiver. What will make this person angry? What are the receiver's motivations, interests, and needs? How valued are your opinions to the receiver? Whose opinions are valued by the receiver? When will the receiver be most receptive to your message? If you know the answers to these questions, you will be able to state your message to communicate effectively. You will avoid words or accusations that would anger the person with whom you wish to communicate. You will enlist the support of others whose opinions the receiver values. You will present your message through a medium with which the receiver interacts.

And, you will appeal to the motivations, interests, and needs of the receiver.

Feedback

Suppose you were asked to describe a diagram with enough detail that your classmates could draw it from your description. If they had their backs turned to you and were not allowed to ask questions, they would have difficulty drawing that diagram accurately. However, if you allowed them to ask questions to clarify your description, more of them would be able to draw the diagram accurately. This ability to ask questions and get feedback is the difference between one-way and two-way communication.

For effective communication, the receiver should be encouraged to ask questions of the sender to understand the message better. If you are the sender, recognize the importance of feedback; solicit questions even if none are initially asked by the receiver.

Nonverbal Communication: Communicating in Body Language

Body language comprises the nonverbal physical reactions and positioning of the body that relay information during communication. Consider some examples. (1) During your

> **Body language:** nonverbal physical reactions and positions of the body that relay information during communication.

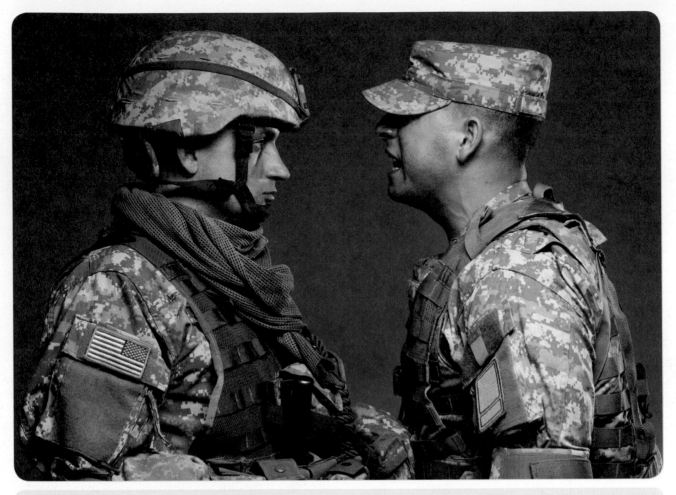

People often communicate more nonverbally than they do with words. It is clear, even without words, what this drill instructor is communicating.

next class, notice the body language of your classmates. Are they "into" what is going on? When they are, they lean toward (*into*) the instructor. If they are not interested in what is occurring, they lean back. (2) When you enter a professor's office and the desk is situated between you and the professor, this physical barrier sends a message that the professor is the authority figure and you are "on the other side of the desk." (3) When you cross your arms during a conversation, you are also separating yourself from that conversation, only you are doing so without a desk.

Often, body language communicates more effectively than words. Recall the example of communicating assertively to your professor. If you state those words exactly as suggested, using the DESC form, but your body language expresses nonassertiveness, the message is then

nonassertive. For example, if you look down and do not make eye contact, hesitate every couple of words, shift your weight, and nervously laugh, you are expressing nonassertiveness regardless of the words you use. In contrast, if you point your finger at the other person, glare, raise your voice, place your hands on your hips, or lean forward, you are expressing aggressiveness regardless of the words you use. To convey assertiveness, you need to combine a DESC form verbal response with nonverbal assertiveness. To do so, make eye contact with the other person, speak loudly enough to be heard, face the other person, be steady on your feet, and speak without hesitation.

To practice communicating effectively nonverbally, stand in front of a mirror and imagine you are speaking with someone. Pay attention to how your body expresses your

What I Need to Know

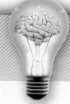

Humor and Psychological Health

Here are some questions to ponder: (1) Why are there interstate highways in Hawaii? (2) Why do we drive on parkways and park on driveways? (3) Why is it that when you transport something by car, it's called a shipment, but when you transport something by ship, it's called cargo? (4) If you are in a vehicle going the speed of light, what happens when you turn on the headlights?

Humor is an excellent way to alleviate psychological discomfort and promote psychological and physical health. For example, it helps with posttraumatic stress disorder, cancer, and grieving. Why should this be so? Laughter initially increases muscular and respiratory activity, oxygen exchange, heart rate, and production of endorphins, which are chemicals that can improve mood and reduce pain. Laughter is followed by a more relaxed state, in which breathing, heart rate, blood pressure, and muscle tension rebound to normal levels.

So, the next time something happens that might otherwise upset you, look for the humor in that situation.

This is often easier said than done but, with practice, you might mentally "step outside" a stressful situation to see that it is actually quite silly or trivial or notice how funny or ridiculous a person's mean comment is.

ADAPTED FROM: Phua, D. H., Tang, H. K., and Tham, K. Y. Coping responses of emergency physicians and nurses to the 2003 severe acute respiratory syndrome outbreak. *Academic Emergency Medicine* 12 (2005): 322–328; Davidson, J. R., Payne, V. M., Connor, K. M., Foa, E. B., Rothbaum, B. O., Hertzberg, M. A., and Weisler, R. H. Trauma, resilience and saliostasis: Effects of treatment in posttraumatic stress disorder. *International Clinical Psychopharmacology* 20 (2005): 43–48; Christie, W. and Moore, C. The impact of humor on patients with cancer. *Clinical Journal of Oncological Nursing* 9 (2005): 211–218; Ong, A. D., Bergeman, C. S., and Bisconti, T. L. The role of daily positive emotions during conjugal bereavement. *The Journals of Gerontology Series B, Psychological Sciences and Social Sciences* 59 (2004): 168–176.

message and whether it is consistent with the verbal message you are communicating. Make any adjustments that are necessary to communicate more effectively.

Complete Health Check Up 3.6 to test how well you can use these assertiveness skills (see Health Check Up 3.6 on the companion website). After completing Health Check Up 3.6, place it in your Health Decision Portfolio.

Understand Suicide and Recognize Suicidal Persons

It may surprise you to learn that in the United States, almost twice as many people die of **suicide**—the purposeful taking of one's own life—than die of homicide. In 2007,

18,4361 Americans died of homicide, whereas 34,598 died of suicide (U.S. Census Bureau, 2010). Four times as many men commit suicide as women, although women attempt suicide more often. Among those ages 25–34 years, suicide is the second leading cause of death with homicide being the third. Because suicide is so prevalent and its consequences so severe, you should learn how to recognize the warning signs that someone is thinking about taking his or her own life so that you are able to help whenever possible. Alternatively, if you have suicidal thoughts, you should know that help is available and how to get it. This section is devoted to these goals.

> **Suicide:** the purposeful taking of one's own life.

Myths *and* Facts
About Psychological Health

MYTH	FACT
If you are not mentally ill, you are psychologically healthy.	You may not experience a mental disorder such as clinical depression, panic disorder, or suicidal thoughts. However, to be psychologically healthy, you need also to be able to feel good about yourself, manage anxiety, control shyness, protect yourself from loneliness, resolve conflicts well, and communicate effectively.
What you think of yourself develops over a lot of years and is, therefore, resistant to change.	It is true that your self-esteem develops over a long period of time and through a large number of experiences. Still, self-esteem can be improved, especially if you focus on your strengths while learning from and improving on your weaknesses.
People who are exceptionally anxious need professional help.	When anxiety prevents people from engaging in activities that will increase the quality of their lives—such as flying to visit family—they may need to have a mental health professional work with them to overcome that anxiety. Yet, there are many effective self-help methods of managing anxiety that need not involve a professional. Among these are environmental planning, self-talk, thought stopping, and systematic desensitization.
Conflicts occur because different people want different things. To resolve conflict, one person has to give up what he or she wants.	Conflicts are about *needs*, not *wants*. To resolve conflicts, people should discuss not what they want, but what they need. Once these needs are identified, a solution can be selected that meets the needs of all people in conflict. No one should have to give up needs, although everyone should be willing to give up the way they thought these needs should be met; that is, their *wants*.

Why People Attempt Suicide

People attempt suicide for many reasons. Ninety percent of people who kill themselves have depression, another diagnosable mental disorder, or substance-abuse problems (Moscicki, 2001). Other risk factors include a prior suicide attempt, a family history of mental disorder or substance abuse, a family history of suicide, family violence such as physical or sexual abuse, and access to firearms (National Institute of Mental Health, 2010b). People contemplating suicide feel so miserable that they seek relief. A family history of suicide suggests a remedy to their misery, and access to instruments of suicide (e.g., firearms or pills) makes it easier for them to carry out their intention.

Signs of Suicide

There are often indications when people are thinking of ending their lives. They may state that their lives "stink," that they are failures, or that there is no hope in their futures. They may even joke about ending it all by suicide. An even more significant warning sign is if someone has already made plans for suicide. If a gun has been acquired or pills accumulated, this is a very serious indication that help is needed immediately.

There are other signs that may lead you to suspect that a college classmate or friend is thinking of suicide (Suicide Prevention Resource Center, 2008). These include:

- *A sudden worsening of school performance*, such as suddenly ignoring assignments and cutting classes.

- *A fixation with death or violence*, which may be expressed through poetry, doodling, and artwork, or a fascination with weapons.

- *Unhealthy peer relationships*, such as a lack of friends or sudden rejection of friends.

- *Violent mood swings or a sudden change in personality*, such as becoming sullen, withdrawn, or angry.

- *Indications of being in an abusive relationship*, such as unexplained bruises or other injuries.

- *Depression*, including expressions of sadness, hopelessness, or anger and rage; lowered self-esteem; lack of concentration; change in sleeping patterns; and fatigue.

Helping a Suicidal Friend or Relative

You can help someone thinking of suicide by being available to talk with him or her about his or her feelings, listening well, and being nonjudgmental. You should express your concern, but not belittle or deny the person's feelings. Rather than say, "Oh, life is not so bad," you might express acceptance and understanding—"It must be miserable to feel that way." Often, a friend or relative thinking about taking his or her own life will not initially be willing to discuss those feelings. You might have to encourage the person to talk, but he or she may eventually welcome the opportunity to express his or her feelings to someone else—someone who is really listening.

If you suspect someone is contemplating suicide, ask that person directly: "Have you been thinking of killing yourself?" "Have you thought about how you will take your own life?" Talking about suicide will not push someone into killing himself or herself. It is better to be safe than sorry. Imagine how you would feel if you suspected the person was thinking about killing himself or herself but you did nothing about it until it was too late and the person was dead?

If someone says they are thinking of taking his or her own life, you need to encourage the suicidal person to speak with a mental health professional. The best thing you can do is get that person help, even if he or she resists. Never promise to keep someone's suicidal thoughts a secret. If a suicidal person does not want you to share those feelings with anyone else and refuses to obtain professional help, you *must* raise your concerns with the person's family, a member of the clergy, or a mental health professional who will be able to get the person help. Most campuses have mental health counselors trained in suicide prevention. Antidepressant drugs and psychotherapy are common treatments. Additionally, the suicidal person may be committed to a hospital or other treatment facility to prevent him or her from committing self-harm.

If it is you who has suicidal thoughts, you need to get help as soon as possible. Speak with your family, a friend, or a professor, but also be sure you speak to a mental health professional. You can also contact the National Suicide Prevention Lifeline through a toll-free telephone number at (800) 273-TALK for referral to the nearest suicide prevention and mental health service provider.

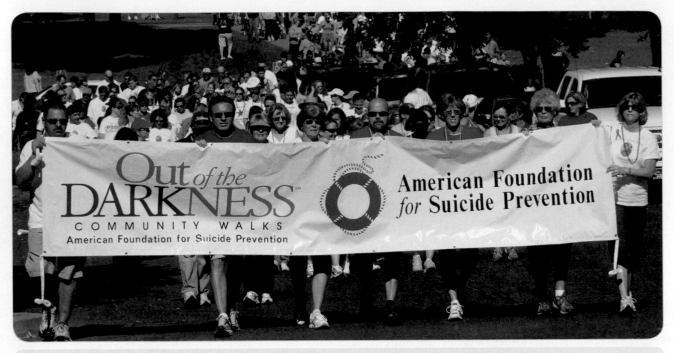

If suicidal thoughts occur, help should be sought immediately. Waiting can have drastic effects.

There are solutions to your problems, and there are people to help.

Complete Health Check Up 3.7 to determine how prepared you are to help someone who is at risk of suicide (see Health Check Up 3.7 on the companion website). After completing Health Check Up 3.7, place it in your Health Decision Portfolio.

Know Signs of Mental Illness and the Treatments Available

An estimated 57.7 million Americans age 18 years and older—26%—experience a diagnosable mental disorder in a given year (Kessler, Chiu, Demler, and Walters, 2005). And, nearly half—45%—of those with a mental disorder experience two or more disorders. Table 3.3 presents the prevalence, symptoms, and treatments for mental illness by order of prevalence.

Recognizing When Someone Needs Professional Help

You will know when professional help is needed when you can recognize the emotional and physical signs and symptoms of mental disorders (see Table 3.3). Emotional symptoms include persistently feeling sad, anxious, pessimistic, hopeless, guilty, and worthless. Physical symptoms include loss of appetite and weight loss or overeating and weight gain, insomnia, chronic fatigue, headaches, nausea, dizziness and fainting, and an inability to remember well. If you find yourself experiencing any of the symptoms listed in Table 3.3, you should contact your campus health center or arrange for private mental health counseling. If you notice these symptoms in friends or relatives, encourage them to seek professional help. Although mental disorders may be extremely debilitating, treatments for these disorders can be very effective. Delaying professional help only exacerbates the condition and makes a successful recovery more difficult.

Choosing a Therapist

If you recognize in yourself psychological symptoms that require professional help, you will need to choose a therapist. You may have symptoms of a disorder or you may just have persistent psychological health issues (such as low self-esteem or shyness) that can benefit from therapy. The following process is recommended when selecting a therapist (Lowery, 2001; Substance Abuse and Mental

TABLE 3.3	Mental Illness in the United States: Prevalence, Symptoms, and Treatment

Illness	Prevalence*	Symptoms	Treatment
Depression	20.9 million	Persistent sad, anxious, and "empty" mood; feelings of hopelessness, pessimism, guilt, worthlessness, and helplessness; lack of interest in activities that were once enjoyed; decreased energy and fatigue; loss of appetite and weight loss or overeating and weight gain; insomnia.	Antidepressant medications: SSRIs such as Prozac or Paxil, tricyclics, MAOIs. Psychotherapy. Electroconvulsive therapy (ECT) for individuals with severe or life-threatening depression.
Social phobia	15 million	Overwhelmingly anxious and excessively self-conscious in everyday social situations; intense, persistent, and chronic fear of being watched and judged by others; blushing, profuse perspiration, trembling, nausea, and difficulty talking.	Medications: clonazepam, beta-blockers (propranolol), SSRIs such as Prozac or Paxil. Psychotherapy.
Posttraumatic stress disorder	7.7 million	Develops after a terrible ordeal involving physical harm or the threat of physical harm; easily startled, emotionally numb, loss of interest in things that used to be enjoyable, trouble feeling affectionate, irritable, aggressive, flashbacks of the traumatic event.	Medications: SSRIs such as Prozac or Paxil, tricyclics. Cognitive behavior therapy.
Generalized anxiety disorder	6.8 million	Exaggerated worry and tension; worrying excessively about everyday problems; trouble falling asleep and concentrating; fatigue, headaches, muscle tension, muscle aches, trembling, twitching, irritability, nausea, lightheadedness.	Antidepressant medications: SSRIs such as Prozac or Paxil, tricyclics, MAOIs, clonazepam, Xanax, buspirone, beta-blockers (propranolol), MAOIs. Psychotherapy.
Panic disorder	6 million	Sudden attacks of terror accompanied by a pounding heart, perspiration, weakness, faintness, or dizziness; fear of impending doom; fear of losing control.	Medications: lorazepam (Ativan), beta-blockers (propranolol), tricyclics (Tofranil). Psychotherapy.
Bipolar disorder	5.7 million	Dramatic mood swings between mania and depression. Signs of mania: increased energy and restlessness, extreme irritability, euphoric mood, difficulty concentrating, little sleep needed. Signs of depression: feelings of sadness, anxiety, hopelessness, worthlessness, fatigue, sleeping too much, thoughts of death or suicide.	Medications: mood stabilizers such as lithium, anticonvulsants such as valproate. Cognitive behavior therapy.

(Continues)

TABLE 3.3 **Mental Illness in the United States: Prevalence, Symptoms, and Treatment (Continued)**

Illness	Prevalence*	Symptoms	Treatment
Borderline personality disorder	4 million	Intense anger, depression, and anxiety; aggression, self-injury, and drug and alcohol abuse; feeling lost and worthless; thoughts of suicide.	Medications: SSRIs such as Prozac or Paxil, mood stabilizers (lithium), antipsychotic drugs. Dialectical behavior therapy.
Schizophrenia	2.4 million	Hallucinations, delusions (false beliefs), loss or decrease in ability to speak, express emotion, or find pleasure. Cognitive symptoms: problems with attention, loss of memory, and loss of ability to plan.	Medications: older antipsychotics include Thorazine and Haldol. Newer antipsychotic drugs, such as Clozaril, produce fewer side effects. Cognitive behavior therapy.
Obsessive-compulsive disorder	2.2 million	Persistent upsetting thoughts (obsessions) and performance of rituals (compulsions) to control the anxiety these thoughts produce. Examples: washing hands, locking and relocking doors, and the need to check things or count things repeatedly.	Medications: SSRIs such as Prozac or Paxil. Psychotherapy.
Suicidal behavior	31,655	Speaking of thoughts of dying, planning how to die, depression, previous suicide attempt.	Confinement to prevent harm to the person. Antidepressant drugs. Psychotherapy.

*Adult cases in a given year.

DATA FROM: National Institute of Mental Health. *Anxiety Disorders*. Washington, DC: National Institute of Mental Health, 2006. Available at: http://www.nimh.nih.gov/pulicat/anxiety.cfm; Data from: National Institute of Mental Health. *Borderline Personality Disorder: Raising Questions, Finding Answers*. Washington, DC: National Institute of Mental Health, 2001. Available at: http://www.nimh.nih.gov/pulicat/bpd.cfm; Data from: National Institute of Mental Health. *Depression*. Washington, DC: National Institute of Mental Health, 2000. Available at: http://www.nimh.nih.gov/pulicat/depression.cfm; Data from: National Institute of Mental Health. *In Harm's Way: Suicide in America*. Washington, DC: National Institute of Mental Health, 2003. Available at: http://www.nimh.nih.gov/pulicat/harmsway.cfm; Data from: National Institute of Mental Health. *The Numbers Count: Mental Disorders in America*. Washington, DC: National Institute of Mental Health, 2006. Available at: http://www.nimh.nih.gov/pulicat/numbers.cfm.

Health Services Administration, 2003; Stoppler and Shiel, 2005; Cleveland Clinic, 2010):

- See a primary care physician to rule out a physical cause of the problems.

- Ask your health insurance company what mental health services are covered under your policy. Ask the insurance company for a list of providers.

- Ask the primary health care provider for a referral. Also ask friends and relatives who have used mental health providers for recommendations.

- Identify the age, sex, race, or religious background of therapists if those characteristics are considered important.

- Once two or three referrals are obtained, call the offices of the therapists to determine:
  - What are the office hours, and are appointments available? Where is the therapist located? What is the cost?
  - Will your health insurance be accepted?
  - What is the therapist's expertise, education, licensure, and number of years in practice?

- If satisfied with the answers, make an appointment.

- During the first visit, find out:
  - What kind of therapy/treatment program does the therapist recommend? What is the therapist's treatment approach and philosophy? Is group therapy an option?

- Has this approach been proved effective for dealing with similar problems?

- What are the benefits and side effects of this approach?

- How much therapy does the therapist recommend? Does this match the time you are willing to devote to therapy?

■ Be sure the therapist does not take the approach that what works for one person, works for another. Different psychotherapies and medications should be tailored to meet specific needs.

■ Although the role of a therapist is not to be a friend, rapport is a critical element of successful therapy. After the initial visit, decide whether that rapport will be likely.

■ If you are satisfied with the information you receive during your first visit, you can schedule your next appointment to begin the process of working together to understand and overcome your mental health issues. If your impression from the first visit is less than satisfactory, you can repeat the process with another therapist from your referral list.

■ Note that if the person needing a therapist is a friend or family member, he or she may be feeling too fragile or overwhelmed to find a therapist. With his or her permission, you can initiate many of the steps listed above (calling the insurance company and providers, setting up appointments, etc.).

The list of organizations that follows can provide information on finding psychological services in your area:

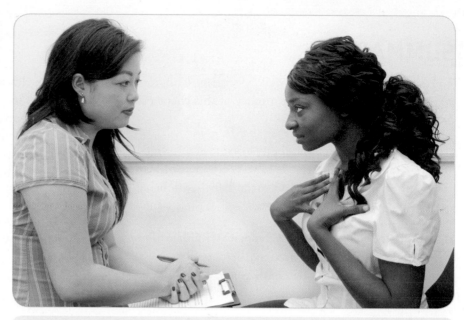

Not all therapists will be appropriate for all situations or for all people. Using the criteria in this chapter will help you choose the right therapist for the specific situation.

■ SAMHSA's (Substance Abuse and Mental Health Services Administration) National Mental Health Information Center
http://www.mentalhealth.samhsa.gov

■ American Association of Pastoral Counselors
http://www.aapc.org

■ American Psychiatric Association
http://www.psych.org

■ American Psychiatric Nurses Association
http://www.apna.org

■ American Psychological Association
http://www.helping.apa.org

■ National Association of Social Workers
http://www.naswdc.org

■ National Mental Health Association
http://www.nmha.org

Applying Behavior Theory

How can you use behavior change theory to become healthy and develop high-level wellness? Complete the Applying Behavior Change Theory for this chapter on the companion website. Once completed, place it in your Health Decision Portfolio.

SUMMARY

To facilitate your being able to make decisions to improve your psychological health, a summary of this chapter is provided.

- Psychological health is the ability to express, think, and behave appropriately relative to your emotions. There are emotional, physical, and social benefits to being psychologically healthy.

- Among the challenges to psychological health are low self-esteem, depression, anxiety, shyness, loneliness, and an inability to resolve conflicts and communicate well.

- Self-esteem—how high a regard or opinion you have of yourself—is an important component of psychological health. Self-esteem can be increased by focusing on your positive traits and learning from, but not dwelling on, your negative traits.

- Clinical depression is a mental health disorder characterized by chronic feelings of sadness, hopelessness, worthlessness, and helplessness. More than 10% of college students have at some time been diagnosed with clinical depression. Depression is a major cause of suicide and should be treated by a mental health professional with medication and psychotherapy.

- Anxiety includes three components: an unrealistic fear, physiological arousal, and either avoidance or withdrawal behavior. Self-help techniques include environmental planning, self-talk, thought stopping, and systematic desensitization. Anxiety can also be managed with medications and/or psychotherapy; in particular, cognitive behavior therapy.

- Among the self-help techniques for shyness are acknowledging the conflict between the need to belong and the fear of rejection, role playing of challenging situations in advance, developing constructive alternatives to negative thoughts, and recognizing that shyness and social anxiety are common and universal experiences for all people. When shyness becomes severe, it is referred to as social phobia.

- Chronic loneliness is an emotional state in which powerful feelings of emptiness and isolation and alienation from other people are experienced. Loneliness can result in physical illness, negatively affect memory and learning, and interfere with sleep patterns, thus affecting the ability to function in everyday life. Remedies for loneliness include joining campus groups and volunteering.

- Part of being psychologically healthy is the ability to interact with other people in a healthy way. That includes being able to resolve conflict, being assertive, and communicating effectively.

- One method of resolving conflict is the RESPECT technique: **R**ecognize that there is a difference of opinion, **E**liminate any thoughts from your mind about what you want, **S**can and *listen* to what the other person is communicating in words and feelings, **P**araphrase the *words* and *feelings* of the other person, **E**xpress what you want and your reasons for that, **C**ollect several alternative solutions that meet both sets of needs, and **T**ry the best alternative solution.

- Assertiveness is getting that to which you are entitled without violating anyone else's rights. To make a verbal assertive statement use the DESC form: **D**escribe the situation or the other person's behavior about which you are concerned, **E**xpress your feelings regarding the situation or other person's behavior, **S**pecify the change you would like to see, and state the **C**onsequences that will occur if the change is made and if the change is not made.

- One model of communication involves a sender, sending a message, through a medium, to a receiver. To communicate effectively, the identity of the *sender* of the message should be clear, the *message* should be short (communicate only what is necessary), the *medium* should be appropriate to the type of message being communicated, and a great deal should be known about the targeted *receiver*. In addition, the importance of nonverbal communication, or body language, should be recognized.

■ Among the most prevalent reasons for suicide are depression, other mental disorders, and substance abuse. People contemplating suicide need the help of a mental health professional as soon as possible. Assistance can be obtained from the National Suicide Prevention Lifeline through a toll-free telephone number at (800) 273-TALK.

■ Mental health disorders are prevalent, with 57.7 million Americans age 18 years and older diagnosed with one in a given year. When a mental disorder exists, professional help should be sought. Treatment may include medication and/or psychotherapy.

■ To choose the right therapist to treat a mental disorder, find out what your mental health coverage is under your health insurance policy; get two or three referrals specifying age, sex, race, or religious background if those characteristics are important to you; call to find out about appointment availability, location, and fees; and make sure the therapist has experience helping people whose problems are similar to yours.

REFERENCES

American Psychiatric Association. *Diagnostic and Statistical Manual of Mental Disorders, 4th ed.* Washington, DC: American Psychiatric Association, 1994.

APA Help Center. *Painful Shyness in Children and Adults.* Washington, DC: American Psychological Association, 2010. Available at: http://www.apa.org/helpcenter/shyness.aspx.

Balázs, J., Benazzi, F., Rihmer, Z., Rihmer, A., Akiskal, K. K., and Akiskal, H. S. The close link between suicide attempts and mixed (bipolar) depression: Implications for suicide prevention. *Journal of Affective Disorders* 91 (2006): 133–138.

Ballenger, J. C., Davidson, J. R., Lecrubier, Y., Nutt, D. J., Foa, E. B., Kessler, R. C., McFarlane, A. C., and Shalev, A. Y. Consensus statement on posttraumatic stress disorder from the International Consensus Group on Depression and Anxiety. *Journal of Clinical Psychiatry* 61 (2000): 60–66.

Bower, S. and Bower, G. A. *Asserting Yourself*, 2nd ed. New York: Perseus Book Publishers, 1976.

Chavira, D. A., Stein, M. B., and Malcarne, V. L. Scrutinizing the relationship between shyness and social phobia. *Journal of Anxiety Disorders* 16 (2002): 585–598.

Cleveland Clinic. *Mental Health: Choosing a Doctor and Therapist.* 2010. Available at: http://my.clevelandclinic.org/healthy_living/mental_health/hic_mental_health_choosing_a_doctor_and_therapist.aspx.

Grant, B. F., Hasin, D. S., Stinson, F. S., Dawson, D. A., Chou, S. P., Ruan, W. J., and Pickering, R. P. Prevalence, correlates, and disability of personality disorders in the United States: Results from the National Epidemiologic Survey on Alcohol and Related Conditions. *Journal of Clinical Psychiatry* 65 (2004): 948–958.

Hawkley, L. C., Masi, C. M., Berry, J. D., and Cacioppo, J. T. Loneliness is a unique predictor of age-related differences in systolic blood pressure. *Psychological Aging* 21 (2006): 152–164.

Henderson, L. and Zimbardo, P. Shyness, social anxiety, and social phobia. In Hofmann, S. G. and DiBartolo, P. M., eds. *From Social Anxiety to Social Phobia.* Boston: Allyn and Bacon, 2001, 46–64.

Hidalgo, R. B. and Davidson, J. R. Posttraumatic stress disorder: Epidemiology and health-related considerations. *Journal of Clinical Psychiatry* 61 (2000): 5–13.

Hoge, C. W., Castro, C. A., Messer, S. C., McGurk, D., Cotting, D. I., and Koffman, R. L. Combat duty in Iraq and Afghanistan, mental health problems, and barriers to care. *New England Journal of Medicine* 351 (2004): 13–22.

Horsch, L. M. Shyness and informal help-seeking behavior. *Psychological Reports* 98 (2006): 199–204.

Kessler, R. C. Posttraumatic stress disorder: The burden to the individual and to society. *Journal of Clinical Psychiatry* 61 (2000): 4–12.

Kessler, R. C., Chiu, W. T., Demler, O., and Walters, E. E. Prevalence, severity, and comorbidity of twelve-month DSM-IV disorders in the National Comorbidity Survey Replication (NCS-R). *Archives of General Psychiatry* 62 (2005): 617–627.

Loneliness. 2012. *Wikipedia.* Available at: http://en.wikipedia.org/wiki/Loneliness

Lowery, N. Choosing a mental health therapist. *International Primal Association Newsletter* (Fall 2001).

McLaughlin, C. R. Furry friends can aid your health. Discovery Health Channel. 2008. Available at: http://www.health.discovery.com/centers/aging/powerofpets/powerofpets_print.html.

Moscicki, E. K. Epidemiology of completed and attempted suicide: Toward a framework for prevention. *Clinical Neuroscience Research* 1 (2001): 310–323.

National Institute of Mental Health. *Anxiety Disorders.* Washington, DC: National Institute of Mental Health, 2009.

National Institute of Mental Health. *Older Adults: Depression and Suicide Facts (Fact Sheet).* 2010a. Available at: http://www.nimh.nih.gov/health/publications/older-adults-depression-and-suicide-facts-fact-sheet/index.shtml.

National Institute of Mental Health. *Suicide in the U.S.: Statistics and Prevention.* 2010b. Available at: http://www.nimh.nih.gov/health/publications/suicide-in-the-us-statistics-and-prevention/index.shtml.

National Institute of Mental Health. *The Numbers Count: Mental Disorders in America.* 2010c. Available at: http://www.nimh.nih.gov/health/publications/the-numbers-count-mental-disorders-in-america/index.shtml.

Nutt, D. J. The psychobiology of posttraumatic stress disorder. *Journal of Clinical Psychiatry* 61 (2000): 24–29.

PubMed Health. Major depression. 2010. Available at: http://www.ncbi.nlm.nih.gov/pubmedhealth /PMH0001941/.

Stoppler, M. and Shiel, W. C., Jr. *Questions to Ask When Choosing a Mental Health Care Provider and Doctor.* MedicineNet.com. 2005. Available at: http://www .medicinenet.com/script/main/art.asp?articlekey= 47440.

Substance Abuse and Mental Health Services Administration. *Choosing the Right Mental Health Therapist.* Washington, DC: SAMHSA's National Mental Health Information Center, 2003. Available at: http:// www.mentalhealth.samhsa.gov/publications/allpubs /KEN98-0046/default.asp#what.

Suicide Prevention Resource Center. *The Role of College Students in Preventing Suicide.* Newton, MA: Suicide Prevention Resource Center, 2008. Available at: http://www.sprc.org/featured_resources/customized/ college_student.asp.

U.S. Census Bureau. *Statistical Abstracts of the United States: 2011.* Washington, DC: U.S. Census Bureau, 2010.

INTERNET RESOURCES

National Institute of Mental Health
http://www.nimh.nih.gov

National Mental Health Association
http://www.nmha.org

National Alliance on Mental Illness
http://www.nami.org

Kristin Brooks Hope Center
Suicide Prevention Telephone Hotline Center
http://www.hopeline.com

The National Mental Health Consumer's Self-Help
Clearinghouse
http://www.mhselfhelp.org

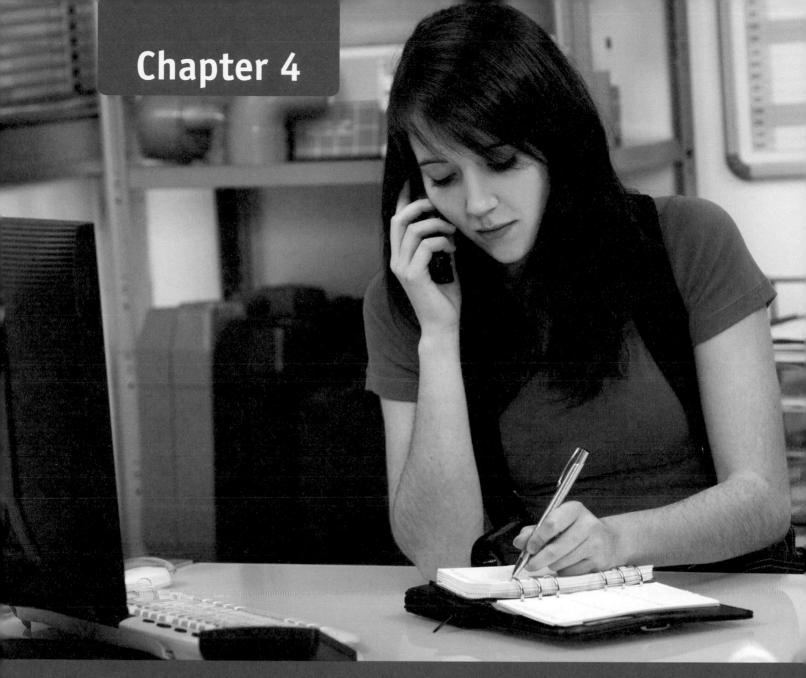

Chapter 4

Managing Stress, Rather Than Letting Stress Manage You

 Access Health Check Ups and Health Behavior Change activities on the Companion Website: **go.jblearning.com/Empowering.**

Learning Objectives

- Define stress and describe a model of stress.

- Discuss life interventions that can limit the amount of stress experienced.

- Cite effective stress-management strategies related to perception.

- Describe stress-management techniques that can be used to decrease emotional reactions to a stress.

For a million dollars (only kidding), can you guess what these famous people have in common? Abraham Lincoln (president), Winston Churchill (prime minister), Bill Russell (basketball star), Alanis Morisette (singer), Michael Jackson (singer), Howard Stern (radio host), and Oprah Winfrey (television host). The answer: They all suffered from stress and anxiety so much that it affected their behavior negatively. For example, Bill Russell of the Boston Celtics was voted one of the best professional basketball players of the century. Yet, before many games, he vomited from the stress of being expected to do well. The common characteristic shared by all these people was a lack of confidence. In spite of their talents in their respective fields, they had doubts about their abilities to perform well. They worried about being accepted by others and appearing competent.

If these highly successful people could be affected in this way, despite the acclaim they received on a daily basis, it should come as no surprise that the rest of us are also prone to stress reactions and their consequences. Think of how you feel when you experience the stress of being called on in class. Or, when you present your case to a professor for a higher grade on a paper. Or, when you ask someone out on a date. This chapter will help you understand these feelings and give you some tools to manage them.

What Is Stress?

In the early part of the 20th century, a Harvard Medical School physiologist named Walter Cannon first described the body's reaction to stress and coined the phrase *fight or flight response*. Later, Hans Selye further refined this response into three phases called the *general adaptation syndrome* (alarm reaction, stage of resistance, and stage of exhaustion). These researchers described much of what we know about the physiological response to stress. How might you define stress? Stress is like love—hard to define, but clearly recognizable when you feel it. Even experts define stress in different ways. For the purposes of this text, **stress** is physiological and psychological arousal in response to a life situation that is perceived as a threat (Greenberg, 2011). Individuals determine whether a stressor is interpreted as a (negative) threat or a (positive) challenge. In other words, your stress level is up to you.

Contrary to popular notion, stress is not always bad. Imagine you feel stressed out before having to make a presentation in front of the class. The anticipation causes you such concern that you make sure the presentation is well researched. Furthermore, you practice it several times to make sure it is interesting and informative. In this case, the stress associated with the presentation led to a positive outcome—a better presentation than you might have made otherwise. Stress that leads to a positive consequence is called **eustress**. Stress that leads to a negative consequence is called **distress**.

> **Stress:** the combination of a life situation perceived as a threat and the resulting physiological and psychological arousal.
>
> **Eustress:** stress that leads to positive, or welcome, consequences.
>
> **Distress:** stress that leads to negative, or unwelcome, consequences.

A **stressor** is something that occurs that has the *potential* to cause physiological or psychological arousal. Stressors may pose threats such as fear of doing poorly on a test or concern about appearing competent when speaking in front of a group of people. Stressors can occur in various parts of your life. You may experience stressors related to school (passing your courses, researching and writing term papers, meeting deadlines), finances (paying your tuition, buying textbooks), family (finding the time to spend with family members, managing family conflict), or your social life (finding someone to date, developing friendships).

Stressors do not automatically cause a stress reaction. Sometimes a stressor is present but is not interpreted as a threat. Instead, it is viewed as a challenge. Suppose you have a test in one of your courses. If you see the test as a challenge, as a way to demonstrate how competent you are

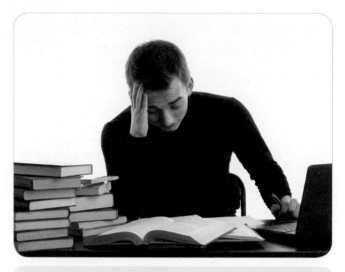

Your interpretation of potentially stressful events is even more important than the event itself. Because *you* decide how to interpret an event, you can decide whether or not you will experience a stress reaction.

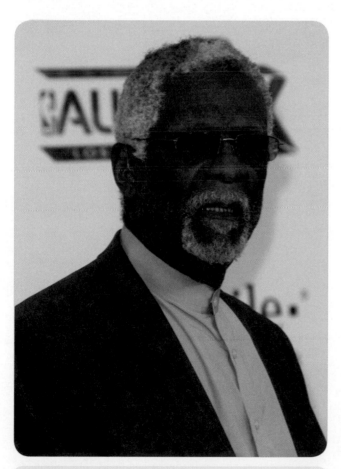

Even famous people (like Bill Russell) who often have to perform in front of others can experience stress as a result of trying to do well.

in that subject matter, you will not have a stress reaction. The point is that the interpretation of a potentially stressful event—perceiving it as a threat or a challenge—is even more important than the event itself.

If a stressor is perceived as a threat, a **stress reaction** occurs. Endocrine glands secrete hormones into the bloodstream, and as a result, heart rate and blood pressure increase, breathing becomes rapid and shallow, muscles tense, cholesterol increases in the blood, and fewer white blood cells are produced making the immunological system less effective and increasing susceptibility to illnesses and diseases.

A Model of Stress

The stress model in **FIG. 4.1 ▼** (Greenberg, 2011) shows how stress occurs in phases and how it can affect

Stressor: a life situation that has the potential to elicit physical or psychological arousal.

Stress reaction: changes in the body that occur when a stressor is perceived as a threat; for example, increased heart rate, blood pressure, and muscle tension.

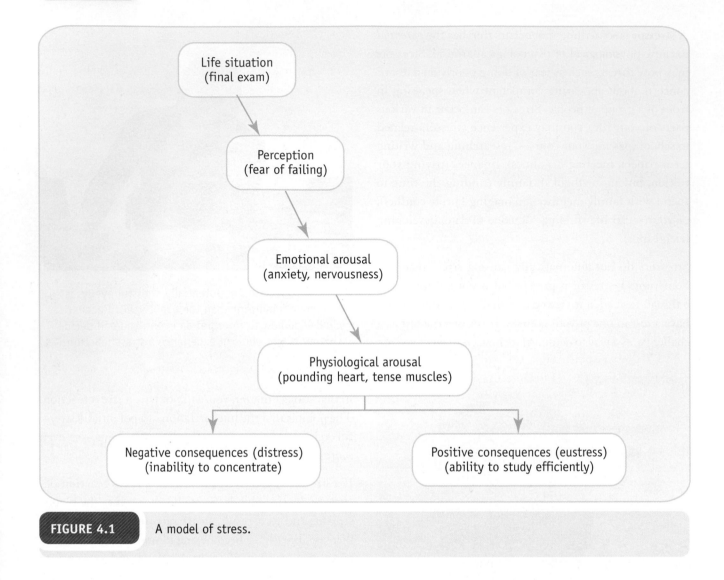

Life situation
(final exam)

Perception
(fear of failing)

Emotional arousal
(anxiety, nervousness)

Physiological arousal
(pounding heart, tense muscles)

Negative consequences (distress)
(inability to concentrate)

Positive consequences (eustress)
(ability to study efficiently)

FIGURE 4.1 A model of stress.

you. The starting point of the model is the **life situation level**. This point marks a significant event in your life to which you must adjust. You might lose a job, fail a test, argue with parents, or break up with a girlfriend or boyfriend.

At the **perception level**, you interpret that life situation as a threat. Perceiving the threat, you thus move to the **emotional arousal level**. At this level, you experience various emotions; for example, anger or nervousness. These emotions lead to the **physiological arousal level**: increases in heart rate, blood pressure, and muscle tension. When these emotional and physical changes occur, you are more likely to get ill, argue with other people, and not be able

Life situation level: the stage on the stress model at which a significant life event occurs to which one needs to adjust.

Perception level: the stage on the stress model at which a life situation is interpreted as a threat.

Emotional arousal level: the stage on the stress model at which feelings arise, such as anger, nervousness, or fear.

Physiological arousal level: the stage on the stress model at which the body reacts physically to a stressor, such as with increased heart rate, blood pressure, and muscle tension.

to focus on your schoolwork. Those are just some of the negative **consequences** of stress.

Notably, you experience these changes even when there are positive consequences of stress. However, the stress by-products, such as increased heart rate and muscle tension, are used to achieve the positive outcome. Therefore, the physical effects are dissipated; that is, they do not stick around long enough to damage the body and, as a result, do not pose a threat to your health.

Imagine you are all stressed out about a scheduled job interview. As a result of that stress, you practice responses to questions you anticipate being asked. You spend time making yourself look good by showering, deciding on the right clothes to wear, and grooming your hair. You organize a portfolio of your previous work experience and plan your travel route to the interview. These activities channel your stress toward creating a more effective you—that is, a better interviewee. This is a clear example of *eustress*.

Using the Stress Model to Manage Stress

Imagine the stress model maps a road that passes through the towns of Life Situation, Perception, Emotional Arousal, Physiological Arousal, and Consequences. As with any road, roadblocks could be set up along the way. For example, you could set up a roadblock between the towns of *Life Situation* and *Perception* to prevent a stressor from being interpreted as a threat. Because the model includes sequential phases, with each phase dependent upon the full development of the previous phase, any interruption of this sequence will short-circuit the process. That is stress management: setting up roadblocks on the stress model road map so negative consequences do not occur (see **FIG. 4.2 ▶**). Next, you will learn how to set up these roadblocks.

Life Situation Interventions

A change in a life situation starts the trip down the stress model road. Therefore, if nothing occurs to which you have to adjust, the trip never starts. The goal of stress management, however, is not to keep the trip from happening. (This would result in a very boring life!) Rather, the goal is to keep stress levels at an optimal level, one that welcomes challenges that make life interesting, but not so many challenges that they pile up and overwhelm you.

One way to do this is to eliminate unnecessary stressful life events in the first place. If you do that, you set up a roadblock before the Life Situation level, and some trips down the stress model road never begin. Recognize, however, that you cannot avoid all stressful events. You may become stressfully aroused when taking exams, but you still have to take exams. In contrast, there are some occasions when you may purposefully decide to take on a stressful event. Perhaps you decide to try out for a role in a play. Although you may experience stress arousal, you decide that the chance to be in the play is worth the fear you experience.

Complete Health Check Up 4.1 to identify the stressful life situations you routinely encounter (see Health Check Up 4.1 on the companion website). Then decide which you can eliminate and which you can deal with in a less stressful way. Once completed, place Health Check Up 4.1 in your Health Decision Portfolio.

Time Management

One factor that results in stress for a lot of college students is poor time management. What with school responsibilities (reading book chapters, studying for tests, etc.), family responsibilities (maintaining communication, visiting, etc.), and social responsibilities (hanging out with friends, going to games, etc.), there does not seem to be enough hours in the day. By using effective time-management strategies, however, there are plenty of hours to do it all.

Consequences: the stage on the stress model at which the overall results of stress are seen: there may be negative consequences (e.g., illnesses and diseases or impaired relationships) or positive consequences (e.g., improved grades or job performance).

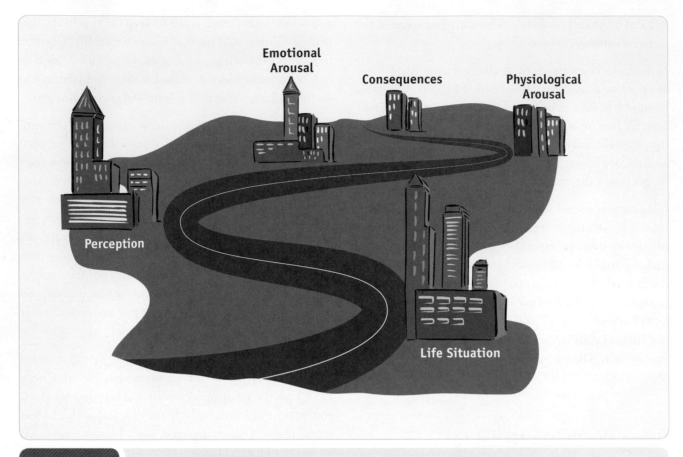

Emotional Arousal

Consequences

Physiological Arousal

Perception

Life Situation

FIGURE 4.2 Stress management is setting up roadblocks on the stress model road.

What it takes is just a little bit of organization and prioritization. Time-management skills are some of the most effective life situation interventions you can use.

Remember that time is your most precious possession. Time spent is time gone forever. In spite of what we often profess, we cannot save time. Time moves continuously and it is used—one way or another. If we waste time, there is no bank where we can withdraw time we previously saved to replace the time wasted. To come to terms with our mortality is to realize that our time is limited.

Assessing How You Spend Time

As a first step in managing time better, you might want to analyze how you spend your time now. To do this, divide your day into 15-minute segments. Then record what you

are doing every 15 minutes (Table 4.1). Afterward, review this time diary and total the time spent on each activity throughout the day (Table 4.2). For example, you might find you spent 3 hours playing a virtual reality game online, 1 hour exercising, 1 hour studying, and 2 hours shopping. Next, evaluate that use of time. On the basis of this evaluation, decide on an adjustment, and make it specific. For example, "I will play online for 1 hour and will study 2 hours." A good way actually to make this change is to draw up a contract with yourself that includes a reward for being successful.

Prioritizing

Once you have adjusted your use of time, you need to prioritize your activities. Not all of your activities will be equally important. Focus on those of major importance

TABLE 4.1	Daily Record of Activity

Activity Time (a.m.)	Activity Time (a.m.)	Activity Time (p.m.)	Activity Time (p.m.)
12:00 _____	6:00 _____	12:00 _____	6:00 _____
12:15 _____	6:15 _____	12:15 _____	6:15 _____
12:30 _____	6:30 _____	12:30 _____	6:30 _____

Note: This sample table does not present an entire 24 hours divided into 15-minute segments.

TABLE 4.2	Summary of Activities (Sample)

Activity	Total Time Spent on Activity
Talking on the phone	2 hours
Socializing	2 hours
Studying	1 hour
Playing online games	3 hours
Exercising	1 hour
Shopping	2 hours
Housework	2 hours
In class	5 hours
Sleeping	6 hours

to you, and work on the others secondarily. To help with this, develop *A, B, C lists* each day.

On the *A list* are those activities that must get done; they are so important that not to do them would be very undesirable. For example, if your term paper is due next week and today is the only day this week you can get to the library to do the research required for that paper, going to the library goes on your A list today.

On the *B list* are those activities you'd like to do today and that need to be done. However, if they do not get done today, it would not be too terrible. For example, if you have not been in touch with a close friend and have been meaning to email her, you might put that on your B list. Your intent is to email her today, but if you don't get around to it, you can always do it tomorrow or the next day.

On the *C list* are those activities you'd like to do if you get all the A and B list activities done. If the C list activities *never* get done, that would be just fine. For example, if a department store has a sale and you'd like to go browse, put that on your C list. If you do all of the A's and B's, then you can go browse; if not, it's no big loss.

In addition, you should make a list of things *not to do*. For example, if you tend to waste your time watching television, you might want to include that on your not-to-do list. In that way, you will have a reminder not to watch television today. Other time wasters should be placed on this list as well.

Saying No

I have a friend who says, "You mean I don't have to do everything I want to do?" What he means is that there are so many activities he would love to engage in that he overloads himself and winds up enjoying them less and feeling overburdened. Because of guilt, concern for what others might think, or a real desire to engage in an activity, we have a hard time saying no. The A, B, C lists will help you identify how much time remains for other activities and will make saying no easier.

Delegating

When possible, get others to do those things that need to be done but that do not need your personal attention. Conversely, avoid taking on chores that others try to delegate to you. A word of caution: This advice does not mean that you use other people to do work you should be doing, nor that you should not help out others when they ask. What it means is that you should be more *discriminating* about the delegation of activities. In other words: Do not hesitate to seek help when you are short on time and are overloaded, and help others only when they really need help and you have the time available.

Evaluating Tasks Once

As much as possible, deal with things only once. For example, many of us log in daily to our email accounts, read through our new emails, and then leave them there, piling up in our inboxes. Be prepared to respond quickly to emails that warrant a response. If it's really necessary to keep an email, file it in an appropriate place where you can easily find it.

Using the "Circular File"

Another way of handling accumulating emails and paper correspondence is to file them—in the garbage can. How many times do you receive junk mail that is obvious from its envelope—you know, the kind addressed to "Current Resident"? In spite of knowing what is enclosed in that envelope and that after we read its contents we will throw it out, we still take the time to open it and read the junk inside. We would be better off bypassing the opening-and-reading part and going directly to the throwing-out part.

Limiting Interruptions

Throughout the day, you are likely to be interrupted from what you have planned to do. Recognizing this fact, you can actually schedule-in times for interruptions. On the one hand, do not make your schedule so tight that interruptions would throw you into a tizzy. On the other hand, try to keep these interruptions to a minimum. There are several ways you can accomplish this. You can refuse to accept phone calls between certain hours. Just turn off your cell or turn off the volume on your landline and answering machine. Do the same for visitors. For example, post a note on your dorm door that says, "Studying. Do not disturb. Come back at 10:00." If you are serious about making better use of your time, you will need to adopt some of these means of limiting interruptions. Adhere to your schedule as much as you can.

Investing Time

The bottom line of time management is that you need to invest time *initially* in order to benefit from the good use of your time subsequently. You might be thinking, "I don't have the time to organize myself. That would put me farther in the hole." This is an interesting paradox. Those who believe they do not have time to plan the better use of their time probably need to take the time more than those who believe they do have the time. Confusing enough? Well, let me state it this way: If you are so pressed for time that you believe you do not even have sufficient time to get yourself organized, that in itself tells you that you are in need of applying time-management skills. The investment in time devoted to organizing yourself will pay handsome dividends by allowing you to achieve more of what is really important to you.

Notably, researchers inform us that in spite of making a time-management plan, people tend not to follow through on it (Konig and Kleinmann, 2005). Will you be one of those people or will you employ ways to use your time more efficiently?

Perception Interventions

Notably, although an event may not really pose a threat, people's perceptions alone—or how they view that event—can lead to stress arousal. If someone who is afraid of dogs encounters a small, friendly dog, stress arousal may occur. The reality, however, is that the dog is not a threat, therefore a stress response is inappropriate. It is the *perception* of a threat that creates the stress response. There are many ways to set up roadblocks at the perception level, including the development of an *attitude of gratitude*, understanding your *locus of control*, and improving your *self-talk*.

But first, consider the college student who wrote her parents the following letter:

Dear Mom and Dad:

I had an accident at school but am doing okay. My writing may be difficult to read because my right side is temporarily paralyzed, but the good news is that I am in love. His name is Eric and I met him when they

What I Need to Know

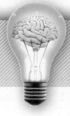

Issues of Diversity and Stress

Life situations have significant effects on levels of stress and, consequently, health. For example, it is known that hypertension rates are higher among African Americans than those among white Americans (National Center for Health Statistics, 2004). One proposed explanation for this disparity is racism. Called the John Henry syndrome, it is thought that stress from encountering racism results in increased blood pressure. When this happens often or is chronic, hypertension develops. Several researchers have found data to support this view (Spruill, 2010). There are many indications of the health disparities between minority and white Americans. The reasons for these disparities are varied, but one is stress. In a study of minority adults (Davis et al., 2005), fully 74% reported experiencing stress-provoking encounters of racial discrimination.

How can you use this information to make better health decisions? First of all, if you have been subjected to discrimination, you should be particularly watchful of stress reactions to racism and other biased behavior. Using the stress-management techniques presented in this chapter, you can prevent someone else's boorish behavior from taking over your physiology (heart rate, level of blood pressure, muscle tension, etc.). Second, if you are a white American, you have a responsibility to refrain from any action that can be interpreted as racist or discriminatory. Sometimes, behavior that is not intended as discriminatory is perceived that way. We all should be watchful of such behavior and to refrain from using it. The resulting health effects make this particularly important.

took me to the hospital. He is a hospital orderly. In fact, we care so much for one another that we have decided to get married. Now, we guessed you would disapprove because he is of a different religion, ethnicity, and culture than me, so we decided to elope. Don't worry though, I am convinced our marriage will work out because he learned from his two previous failed marriages and has a plan to get rich by investing in an alpaca farm in Australia.

Mom and Dad, don't worry. I did not get injured, I am not in a hospital, and I am not in love with nor marrying a two-time divorcee. However, I did fail chemistry, and wanted you to be able to put that in its proper perspective.

The purpose of this story is to illustrate an important truth—everything belongs in its proper perspective.

An Attitude of Gratitude

One roadblock you can use to manage stress is to develop an "attitude of gratitude." We can look one way and see

people with more money, better looks, and more friends. Or, we can look the other way and see people who face physical, emotional, or financial challenges that we do not. If we focus on those who have more and bemoan the fact that we do not have what they do, we will be dissatisfied with our lives and experience stress from that dissatisfaction. However, if we focus on being grateful for what we do have, we will be more satisfied with our lives and less stressed as a result.

Developing an **attitude of gratitude** is learning to be grateful for what you have. Certainly, strive to improve yourself. However, when doing so, be sure to appreciate the positive aspects of your life as they exist right now. Use Health Check Up 4.2 to make a list of as many of the positive aspects of your life as you can (see Health

> **Attitude of gratitude:** a focus on being grateful for what one has rather than bemoaning what one does not have.

Check Up 4.2 on the companion website). Place Health Check Up 4.2 in your Health Decision Portfolio when finished. Then, when you get stressed, take out this list and use it to focus on these good things. Cultivate an attitude of gratitude.

Internalizing Your Locus of Control

Another roadblock you can use concerns a concept called locus of control (Rotter, 1990). Before reading this section, however, complete Health Check Up 4.3 and place it in your Health Decision Portfolio (see Health Check Up 4.3 on the companion website). This section will make more sense if you complete the Health Check Up box first.

Julian Rotter (1990), the developer of the *locus of control* construct, defines it as the *perception* you have regarding the amount of control you exert over events in your life. People with an *external locus of control* believe that whatever happens to them is determined by luck, chance, fate, or by significant and powerful people (such as professors, doctors, or bosses). If you believe that others control your future, why would you ever go about trying to learn how to control it in the first place? Those with an *internal locus of control* believe they have a great deal of influence over their lives. If you have an internal locus of control, you will seek out information and learn skills you can use to take control over events in your life. For example, hospital patients who have an internal locus of control will learn about their illnesses, find out what the hospital staff can do to help them get better and what they can do for themselves, and figure out what behaviors they need to adopt once they leave the hospital. Those with an external locus of control will not seek out this information because they believe nothing they do will have an effect on their health.

Developing an internal locus of control, if you do not already have one, is important for stress management. With that perception, you will be more likely to learn how to develop an attitude of gratitude, how to use relaxation techniques, and how to diffuse stress by-products (e.g., muscle tension) once they develop so they do not make you ill. Health Check Up 4.3 will help you develop an internal locus of control.

Positive Self-Talk

Another way to set up a stress roadblock at the perception level is to use **self-talk**—saying things to yourself to help you feel less distressed (Meichenbaum, 1977). For example, if you experience stress when asking someone out on a date—as you worry about being rejected—you can say to yourself:

> The worst thing that can happen is the answer is NO. That's not so bad. I can always ask someone else out.

Practice self-talk statements by completing Health Check Up 4.4 (see Health Check Up 4.4 on the companion website), then place it in your Health Decision Portfolio.

Emotional Arousal Interventions

Setting up roadblocks at the emotional arousal level of the stress model involves engaging in relaxation techniques such as *meditation*, *imagery*, and *diaphragmatic breathing*. All relaxation techniques involve focusing on something that does not cause stress in order to avoid focusing on something that is stressful. As a result, these techniques elicit a **relaxation response**; that is, lowered heart rate and blood pressure, less muscle tension, a decrease in serum cholesterol, and an increase in white blood cells. Regular practice of these techniques also helps prevent unhealthy emotional and behavioral responses to stress. By using these techniques, a person will tend to react with less aggression and less panic to stressful situations.

Meditation

To meditate, you will need something on which to focus. **Meditation** requires focusing on something repetitive (such as a repeated word or your breathing) or something

---

Self-talk: saying things to oneself to be less distressed, such as focusing on the positive aspects of a potentially stressful situation.

Relaxation response: physiological changes that occur in the body as a state of relaxation is achieved; for example, decreased heart rate, blood pressure, and muscle tension.

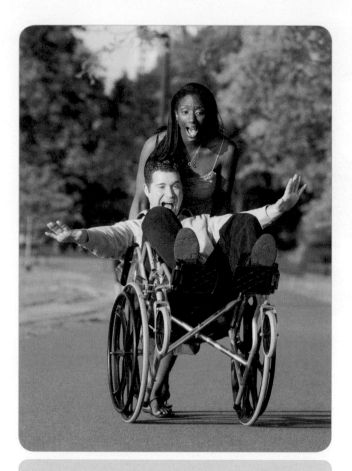

You can bemoan what you do not have or you can develop an attitude of gratitude and be thankful for what you do have. Although this person is physically challenged, he can be grateful that he has friends and an active social life.

unchanging (such as a spot on the wall). For our purpose, choose a relaxing word (also called a *mantra*) as your focus. Find a quiet place and follow these instructions:

■ Sit in a comfortable chair, with your buttocks against the back of the chair. This position will align your spine so you need very little muscle tension to maintain your posture. This posture will also help prevent you from falling asleep. (Sleep is a different physiological state than relaxation. If you sleep, you get the benefits of sleep but not the benefits of relaxation.)

■ Close your eyes. Let your head drop so your chin is on your chest, if that feels comfortable. If not, keep your head up, facing forward. Let your arms hang down or rest them in your lap.

■ Say the relaxing word to yourself every time you breathe out. Do this for 20 minutes. During that time, your mind will wander and you will stop repeating your mantra. Recognize this as normal, and return to focusing on the relaxing word with every exhaled breath.

■ Adopt a passive attitude. That is, do not try to relax. Just let the sensations that you feel happen. Be a passive observer, just repeating the mantra.

■ Once you are in a relaxed state, you do not want anything to shock you. Therefore, do not set an alarm clock to let you know when the time is up. When you think the 20 minutes is up, look at a watch. If it is up, stop meditating. If it isn't, go back to repeating the mantra.

■ Do not meditate immediately after eating. Part of the relaxation response is a dilation of the blood vessels in the arms and legs. As the blood vessels expand, more blood flows to your limbs. That is why your fingers and toes feel warmer after relaxation exercises. Immediately after eating, more blood pools in the abdomen to help with digestion, and less blood flows to the arms and legs.

■ Do not ingest stimulants—such as caffeine or nicotine—when meditating. By definition, they will stimulate you, not relax you.

As with all relaxation techniques, you should try meditation several times before determining if it is a method of relaxation you want to continue. If you only tried a relaxation technique once and it did not relax you, perhaps it was because you were particularly tense or anxious that day or maybe you just need to get the hang of it through repeated practice.

Meditation: a relaxation technique that requires focusing on something repetitive (such as breathing) or unchanging (such as a spot on the wall).

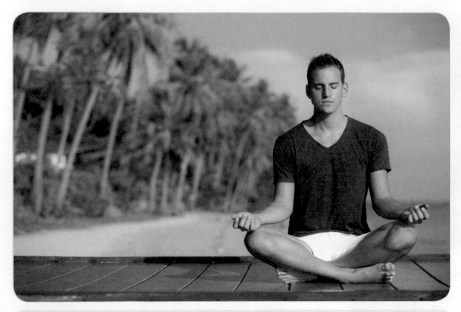

Meditation is a very effective method of managing stress, does not require special equipment, and does not cost anything.

After meditating several times, complete Health Check Up 4.5 to evaluate its potential as a form of relaxation for you (see Health Check Up 4.5 on the companion website). When completed, place it in your Health Decision Portfolio.

If you find that meditation does not relax you, don't worry. There are several other relaxation techniques you can try. One of these is imagery.

Imagery

Have you ever had such an enjoyable and relaxing day that you think back on it often? Imagining yourself back on that day—a technique called **imagery**—can be an effective stress-management strategy (Nelson et al., 2005); that is, if you recall the scene, the surroundings, the temperature, the activity, and as much other detail as possible. The more vivid your image of that day, the more effectively it will help you relax. You should see all the sights, hear all sounds, feel all feelings, and even *taste* the air. Use all of your senses to put yourself back there.

Ideally, you should use an image from a relaxing day you actually experienced for this exercise. If you do, it will be easier to recall the image vividly and to place yourself there. However, you can also use the example of the

relaxing image that appears in the accompanying box. To help you use imagery for stress management, complete Health Check Up 4.6 and place it in your Health Decision Portfolio (see Health Check Up 4.6 on the companion website). Then complete Health Check Up 4.7 to evaluate how effective imagery is as a relaxation technique for you (see Health Check Up 4.7 on the companion website). Place that, too, in your Health Decision Portfolio.

Diaphragmatic Breathing

Have you ever been nervous about asking someone out? You hover over the phone until, finally, you get up the courage to call. Then when you start to speak, you can hardly catch your breath. This shortness of breath is part of the stress response and happens because you expand your chest, rather than your diaphragm, to breathe. A more relaxing and healthier form of breathing, called **diaphragmatic breathing** (Krucoff and Krucoff, 2000), involves expanding your abdomen so you use your diaphragm, rather than your chest, to breathe. This allows you to take deeper breaths, more completely fill up your lungs, and decrease muscle tension in your chest.

To learn diaphragmatic breathing, lie on your back, with the palms of your hands placed on your lower stomach. As you breathe, expand your chest area while keeping your stomach flat. Recognize this as thoracic, or chest, breathing. Next, expand your abdomen so your stomach rises and falls with each breath while your chest remains relatively motionless (though it will expand some). You can

Imagery: a relaxation technique that requires thinking of a relaxing scene or event.

Diaphragmatic breathing: using the diaphragm rather than the chest muscles to breathe.

Myths and Facts

About Stressors

MYTH	FACT
Images in your mind do not affect your body.	The mind and the body are closely connected. What you think can have a profound effect on your body. To demonstrate this fact, determine your heart rate by taking your pulse at your wrist or at your temple (located just in front of the upper part of your ear). Now, spend 2 minutes thinking of someone you love or an experience you had that was very pleasing, and allow your imagination to place you with that person or back engaging in that experience. Recall details as vividly as your imagination will allow. After thinking of this person or experience for 2 minutes, take your pulse again. You should notice that your heart rate has increased, even though you did not engage in any physical activity. If you thought of someone you despised or a very unpleasant experience, your heart rate would similarly increase. The mind–body connection is a real one. Conversely, thinking negative thoughts results in distress. Use this information to reduce your stress. Try to focus on the positive.
To reduce your stress, you need to do anything it takes to stay ahead in school, including cheating when you need to.	Studies indicate that cheating and lying are indeed common behaviors among students. In a recent study (Kelley, Young, Denny, and Lewis, 2005), 48% of students reported cheating on exams. In another study (Josephson Institute of Ethics, 2002), the rate of cheating was even higher—75%. Many universities and colleges have strict honor codes that penalize cheating and other unethical behavior. The stress associated with being charged with cheating and the potential of suspension or expulsion from school is not worth the risk. Failing an exam is far better than having it noted on your permanent record that you cheated. Behaving unethically requires dishonest thoughts, actions to engage in the behavior, and attention paid to covering it up. The effort required to cheat, therefore, can be quite stressful. Aside from being a moral choice, refusing to cheat is a wise stress-management strategy.

An Imagery Exercise: A Relaxing Day at the Beach

Imagine you are in your car, driving to the beach with the windows down and the radio off. The wind is blowing through your hair, and the sun is warming your skin. As you approach the beach, you see people carrying beach chairs, blankets, picnic baskets, and coolers. You park your car and, as you are walking to the beach, you hear the surf rolling onto the shore and smell the ocean. You find a quiet spot of sand away from other people and spread your blanket. Because you are tired from the drive, you are relieved to allow your muscles to relax as you massage sun lotion into your arms and legs. Then you lie on the blanket, with your feet extending onto the warm sand.

As you relax, you can taste the salt in the air. Droplets of ocean seem to fall on you as you hear the surf pound and ever-so-gently roll back to sea. The bright white sunlight, contrasted with the relaxing tan color of the sand and the ocean's vivid blue, creates a feeling of serenity. You close your eyes and take in all the sensations.

The sun's warmth moves over your body. First your feet warm up from the intensity of the sun's rays on the sand. You can feel heat passing through them, relaxing your muscles. Next, the sun caresses your legs and they too become warm. The sun moves to your abdomen, bringing its relaxing warmth there. The sun moves to your chest now and your whole chest area becomes heated and relaxed. And, as though you've willed it, the sun next warms and relaxes your forehead. Your whole body now feels warm and relaxed as though you're sinking into the sand. Your body feels heavy and tingles from the sun's warmth.

You hear the seagulls flying over the ocean. They are free and light and peaceful. They are carrying your problems and worries with them as they fly out to sea. You think of nothing but your body's heaviness and warmth and the tingling sensation. You are totally relaxed. You have relaxed for hours like this, and now the sun is setting. As you feel the cool of evening start to creep in, you slowly open your eyes, feeling wonderfully content. You have no worries; you have no cares. You look at the seagulls, which have taken your problems and worries out to sea and you feel relieved. You stand and stretch, feeling the still warm—yet cooling—sand between your toes, and you feel terrific. You feel so good that you know the car ride home will be pleasant. You welcome the time to be alone in your car and at peace. You fold your blanket and leave your piece of beach, taking with you your sense of relaxation and contentment, knowing you can return anytime you like.

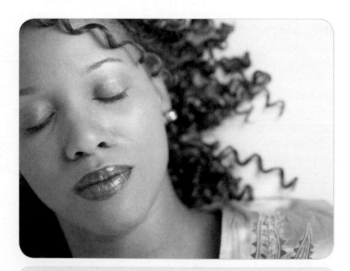

Imaging a relaxing setting can give you a relaxation response: lower heart rate, reduced muscle tension, lower blood pressure, and other beneficial physiological responses.

place a book on your stomach and watch it rise and fall as you breathe. Recognize this as diaphragmatic breathing. Practice it various times throughout the day (when seated doing schoolwork, for instance). Diaphragmatic breathing is basic to all forms of relaxation.

After trying diaphragmatic breathing for a week, complete Health Check Up 4.8 to evaluate its potential as a form of relaxation for you (see Health Check Up 4.8 on the companion website). When completed, place it in your Health Decision Portfolio.

Physiological Arousal Interventions

Imagine you are walking through a dark alley at night. Suddenly, a large, ferocious-looking dog approaches you. The dog's teeth are bared, saliva is streaming from its mouth, and it is barking loudly. The dog makes you fearful and anxious and causes you to look for a route of escape. In short, you perceive the dog as a threat. This perception of a threat causes changes in your body. Your muscles tense, your heart races, your blood pressure increases, you perspire, and the pupils in your eyes dilate. This is the stress response at the physiological arousal level of the stress model. It's called the **fight or flight** response; it prepares you either to fight the perceived threat or run away from it. In this situation, your body prepares to do something physical to protect you from the threat of being attacked by this dog.

The Fight or Flight Response

You can usually recognize when you've had a stress reaction. Your heart pounds in your chest (it speeds up), you start perspiring, your muscles become tense, your breathing becomes rapid and shallow, and you become more alert. As we stated earlier, this occurs to prepare you to respond to a threat physically—either fighting the threat or fleeing from it. There are also components of the stress response that occur of which you are unaware. For example, your blood pressure increases, you produce fewer T lymphocytes making your immunological system less effective, cholesterol levels in the blood increase, and your endocrine glands secrete hormones into the bloodstream. You do not feel these changes in your body, but they occur nonetheless. These physiological changes occur as a result of hormone secretions instructing various parts of the body to react in certain ways.

The significance of the fight or flight response depends on how it is used. If you need to respond to a threat physically—for example, if you did actually encounter a ferocious dog—then this response is beneficial. It allows you to fight the dog or run away from it. However, many of the threats we experience are only symbolic threats, for which a physical reaction is inappropriate. These threats pertain to how we think about ourselves and how others think of us—our self-esteem. For example, suppose you are stuck in traffic on the way to an important exam. You may grip the steering wheel tightly (increased muscle tension) and start to perspire. In this instance, fighting or fleeing are not appropriate reactions. Therefore, you are not using up the by-products of the stress you experienced. That is when the fight or flight response can be

harmful. The increased serum cholesterol, the increased blood pressure and heart rate, and the numerous other physiological changes accompanying a stress response remain with you.

If you are exposed often to the by-products of your stress reactions, you are more susceptible to illness and disease. The increased blood pressure can result in stroke. Over many years, increased cholesterol in your blood can lead to coronary heart disease. The decrease in T lymphocytes makes the immunological system less effective and subjects you to more infections and respiratory illnesses. Stress is not only psychologically disarming but also physically unhealthy (Table 4.3). This is why it is so important to manage stress well.

TABLE 4.3	**Stress-Related Diseases**

Physical Diseases
- Hypertension
- Stroke
- Coronary heart disease
- Headaches
- Cancer
- Allergies, asthma, and hay fever
- Common colds

Emotional Illnesses
- Anxiety
- Depression
- Panic attacks
- Posttraumatic stress disorder

Behavioral Manifestations
- Increased arguments
- Increased conflict and aggressiveness
- Inability to concentrate and be productive social withdrawal

There are many conditions caused by or exacerbated by stress. Some are physical diseases, some are emotional illnesses, and others are behavioral manifestations of stress.

Fight or flight: the preparedness of the body to fight or flee from a perceived threat.

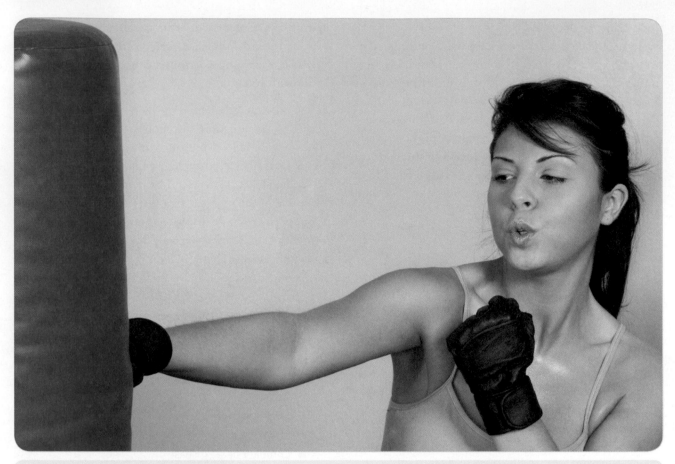

Exercise is an excellent way of using up stress by-products. The activity need not be a sport—pounding on a pillow or a mattress can do the job.

Physical Activity

One of the best strategies for preventing disease is to dissipate stress by-products by doing something physical, such as exercising (Greenberg, Dintiman, and Oakes, 2004). Even if you hate going to the gym or are bad at sports, there are other ways to be physical. Suppose you abhor exercise. Maybe you are athletically challenged. If this describes you, you can still use up the stress by-products in a physical activity. This activity need not require sport skill, such as for basketball, tennis, or swimming. Physical activities such as walking or jogging do not require much athletic skill, but they work just as well. Or you can punch a pillow or mattress until you are tired and use up the stress by-products in that way. Any vigorous physical activity will do.

Consequences

By now you know that stress is associated with poor physical health (stroke, heart disease, infection) and poor psychological health (anxiety, depression, low self-esteem). However, there are also other negative effects of stress that occur at the *consequences* level of the stress model. Have you ever been so stressed that you could not concentrate on your schoolwork or job? Or so stressed that you were easy to anger and maybe even responded aggressively by getting into an argument or actual fight? These are some of the behavioral consequences of stress.

Unfortunately, some people try to cope with stress in ways that just add negative consequences and exacerbate the situation. Some of your friends may exhibit some of these

Contributing to the Health of Your Community

None of us lives in a world alone. We are part of numerous communities: a university/college community, a town or city, a state, a country, and a global community. These communities provide us with comfort, services, education, medical care, and an array of other benefits. Consequently, we have an obligation to contribute to the health of these communities and to others who inhabit them with us. One way to contribute to the stress-management needs of a community is to share what you learn about managing stress with those with whom you live. For example, you could show others in your dormitory how to meditate. Or, you could help family members reduce their

stress levels by explaining the "attitude of gratitude" concept to them. Or, you could speak at a local school to teach self-talk skills to high school students. I have had students do all of this and more. They even helped cancer patients feel less stress about their disease.

You might be thinking what my students were thinking, "I'm no expert on stress. How can I teach stress management to others?" Yet once they got out there and tried it, they found that their grasp of stress-management skills was indeed pretty good. Now, please consider sharing what you know!

dysfunctional coping strategies. They may drink alcohol or take other mood-altering substances to escape the reality of their stressful condition or they may ignore actions they can take to remedy the situation and instead take a head-in-the-sand approach.

Avoid these dysfunctional coping strategies in your own life, and try to talk your friends out of using them, too.

Applying the stress-management techniques presented in this chapter is a much better way to prevent these negative consequences.

Recognize, however, that there are also positive consequences of the stress response. For example, if you are stressed about having to speak to a professor to complain about a grade you believe to be unfair, that stress might lead you to practice how you will present your argument. As a result, you will be more effective in that interaction and, therefore, have a better chance of the grade being changed. The stress, then, is beneficial. It leads to positive consequences. If you use stress to prepare better for an oral presentation or to meet a challenge head-on and find out more about your talents and potential, then the stress has positive outcomes. This *eustress* is to be welcomed, not avoided.

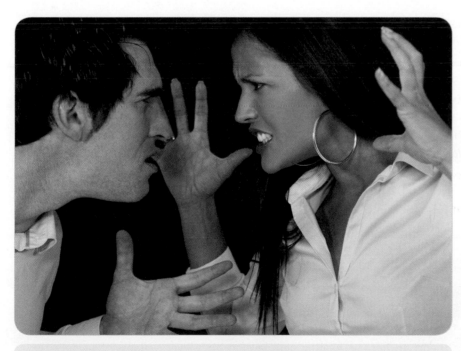

Negative effects of stress include arguing with friends and relatives more frequently. The consequence may be loss of friends or distancing yourself from loved ones.

Your Health Commitment

Learning how to manage stress is one thing; taking charge of your own stress level and choosing to be healthier is quite another. Having

What I Need to Know

Using Behavior Change Theory to Manage Stress

You can use the health belief model to organize your behavior change strategy.

- List the illnesses, diseases, and other negative consequences of stress to which you are *susceptible* if you do not manage stress well.

- Describe why these illnesses, diseases, and other consequences are significant. For example, how *severe/serious* is it to develop heart disease?

- Cite the *perceived benefits* of the various coping techniques you could use. For example, if you exercised regularly, what benefits would you expect?

- Identify *barriers* to engaging in these coping techniques. For example, one barrier might be finding the time to fit exercise into your busy schedule.

- For the barriers identified, brainstorm strategies you could use to overcome them. For example, write your intention to swim three times a week in your weekly schedule. Having it written down will help you adhere to that behavior goal.

- Develop *cues to action* that will remind you to engage in a stress-coping technique. For example, you might set up an automatic text message reminder.

How might you use other behavior change theories to better cope with stress? Complete the Applying Behavior Change Theory activity using a different theory than the health belief model (see the companion website). Once completed, place it in your Health Decision Portfolio.

read how to organize roadblocks to stress, are you willing to commit to identifying behavior changes to cope with stress more effectively and implementing those changes? A behavioral change contract, *My Health Commitment*, is found on the companion website. Use the contract to determine and state your stress-related goals, and commit to a timetable for reaching them. Complete the contract and place it in your Health Decision Portfolio. You can then review the contract on the date you specify to determine whether you have been successful at changing the stress-related behavior. If you are successful, reward yourself as specified in the contract. If not, make whatever adjustments are necessary, and form a new contract. You can take charge of your stress-related behavior and, as a result, be healthier and more fulfilled. Your health is in your hands.

Applying Behavior Theory

How can you use behavior change theory to become healthy and develop high-level wellness? Complete the Applying Behavior Change Theory for this chapter on the companion website. Once completed, place it in your Health Decision Portfolio.

SUMMARY

Knowledge for knowledge's sake is not the mission of this text. The reason health knowledge is presented here is because it is necessary for you to make meaningful health-related decisions. To make these decisions without health knowledge is like driving somewhere without directions—you might never get where you want to be. Or, if you get there, it will take you longer, you may drive through unnecessary hazards, and you could create wear and tear on your vehicle (in this case, your body and mind). With this in mind, a summary of the information presented in this chapter appears below to help you better organize stress-related knowledge and thereby use it more effectively in making health decisions.

- Stress is a combination of a *stressor* (a stimulus that, if perceived as a threat, has the *potential* to cause physiological and psychological arousal) and a *stress reaction* (physiological arousal such as increased heart rate, muscle tension, and rapid and shallow breathing). However, stressors do not necessarily cause a stress reaction. There are techniques you can use to prevent a stress response from occurring.

- A model of stress starts with a *life situation* that has the potential of being *perceived* as a threat and can, therefore, lead to *emotional arousal* (e.g., anxiety, anger, nervousness). The emotional arousal incites *physiological arousal* (e.g., increased muscle tension and heart rate) that, if unabated and if chronic, can result in *consequences*.

- Consequences on the stress model may be *negative* (such as various illnesses like stroke and hypertension) or *positive* (such as presenting an outstanding presentation in front of the class or earning a high grade on an examination). Stress leading to negative consequences is called *distress*, and stress leading to positive consequences is called *eustress*.

- The stress model can be used to prevent negative consequences from occurring. Interventions can be used at each of the levels of the stress model, thereby preventing the situation from proceeding to the next level on the model.

- Examples of interventions on the stress model include those at the life situation level (eliminating stressful events in the first place or altering them so they are less stressful) and at the perception level (developing an attitude of gratitude, adopting an internal locus of control, and using self-talk). Interventions can also be established at the emotional arousal level (meditation, imagery, diaphragmatic breathing) and at the physiological level (engaging in physical activity and thereby using up the stress by-products).

REFERENCES

Davis, S. K., Liu, Y., Quarells, R. C., Din-Dzietharn, R., and the Metro Atlanta Heart Disease Study Group. Stress-related racial discrimination and hypertension likelihood in a population-based sample of African Americans: The Metro Atlanta Heart Disease Study. *Ethnicity and Disease* 15 (2005): 585–593.

Greenberg, J. S. *Comprehensive Stress Management*, 12th ed. New York: McGraw-Hill, 2011.

Greenberg, J. S., Dintiman, G. B., and Oakes, B. M. *Physical Fitness and Wellness: Changing the Way You Look, Feel, and Perform*, 3rd ed. Champaign, IL: Human Kinetics, 2004.

Josephson Institute of Ethics. *2002 Report Card: The Ethics of American Youth*. 2002. Available at: http://www.josephsoninstitute.org/Survey2002-pressrelease.htm.

Kelley, R. M., Young, M., Denny, G., and Lewis, C. Liars, cheaters, and thieves: Correlates of undesirable character behaviors in adolescents. *American Journal of Health Education* 36 (2005): 194–201.

Konig, C. J. and Kleinmann, M. Deadline rush: A time management phenomenon and its mathematical description. *Journal of Psychology* 139 (2005): 33–45.

Meichenbaum, D. H. *Cognitive-Behavior Modification*. New York: Plenum Press, 1977.

National Center for Health Statistics. *Health, United States, 2004*. Hyattsville, MD: National Center for Health Statistics, 2004.

Nelson, C., Franks, S., Brose, A., Raven, P., Williamson, J., Shi, X., McGill, J., and Harrell, E. The influence of hostility and family history of cardiovascular disease on autonomic activation in response to controllable versus noncontrollable stress, anger imagery induction, and relaxation imagery. *Journal of Behavioral Medicine* 28 (2005): 213–221.

Rotter, J. B. Internal versus external control of reinforcement: A case history of a variable. *American Psychologist* 45 (1990): 489–493.

Spruill, T. M. Chronic psychosocial stress and hypertension. *Current Hypertension Reports* 12 (2010): 10–16.

INTERNET RESOURCES

The American Institute of Stress
   http://www.stress.org
Stress Education Center
   http://www.dstress.com/
National Center for Post Traumatic Stress Disorder
   http://www.ptsd.va.gov/

MEDLINE Plus—Stress
   http://www.nlm.nih.gov/medlineplus/stress
   .html
World Wide Meditation Center
   http://www.meditationcenter.com

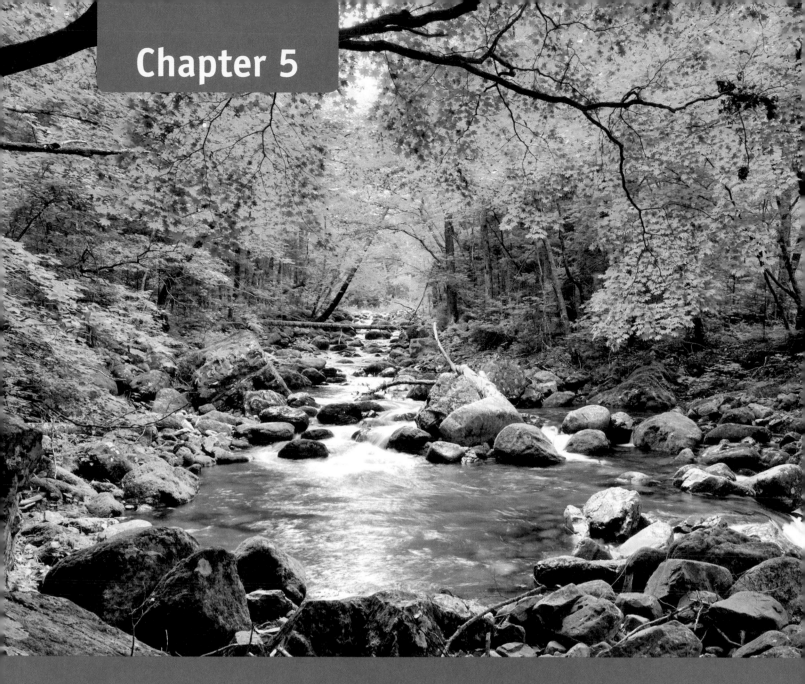

Chapter 5

Expressing Your Spirituality for Better Health

 Access Health Check Ups and Health Behavior Change activities on the Companion Website:
go.jblearning.com/Empowering.

Learning Objectives

- Describe the difference between spirituality and religion.

- Explain the relationship between spirituality and health.

- Discuss the relationship between forgiveness, spirituality, and health.

- Discuss volunteerism as an expression of spirituality.

- Describe strategies that tap into spirituality to improve overall health.

- Describe the grieving process.

- Discuss how to get help for someone who is dying.

- List preparations people can take so that their own death is less traumatic for their loved ones.

I f you want to know how someone can combine spirituality with health, you need go no further than Rabbi Hirshel Jaffe. When Rabbi Jaffe was diagnosed with cancer, he decided to use marathon running as a means of fighting back. When he recovered, he thanked God—and his doctors—by expressing his spirituality in his unique way. He devoted himself to helping others overcome their own adversity.

Rabbi Jaffe began counseling cancer patients, became a co-editor of a book distributed to hospital patients called *Gates of Healing*, wrote a highly acclaimed book called *Why Me? Why Anyone?*, and developed a video entitled *Hanging on to Hope*. In honor of these efforts, he received the American Cancer Society's Award of Courage.

Those who knew him best called him the *Running Rabbi*, both for his running marathons and his tireless efforts on behalf of others. Rabbi Jaffe demonstrates how the expression of one's spirituality can improve physical, psychological, emotional, and social health.

Know the Difference Between Religion and Spirituality

Religion is a formal, organized activity that involves beliefs, practices, and rituals related to a supernatural being or God or, in some Eastern religious traditions, the ultimate truth or reality. Religions usually describe what happens after death and codify rules to guide moral behavior. Religion usually involves groups of people congregating to express their similar religious beliefs. Table 5.1 lists the religious composition of the United States.

TABLE 5.1 **Religious Composition of the United States**

Religion	Number of People	Percentage (%) of U.S. Population
Catholic	50,873,000	24
Baptist	33,830,000	17
Methodist	14,150,000	6
Lutheran	9,580,000	5
Presbyterian	5,596,000	3
Jewish	2,831,000	2
Mormon	2,787,000	2
Buddhist	1,082,000	0.7
Muslim/Islamic	1,104,000	0.6
Hindu	766,000	0.4
Atheist	902,000	0.4
No religion	27,486,000	16

REPRODUCED FROM: The Pew Forum on Religion and Public Life: U.S. Religious Landscape Survey. http://religions.pewforum.org/reports.

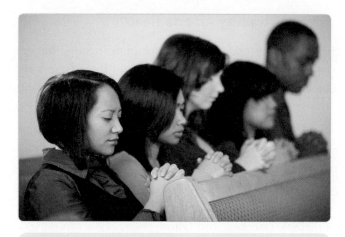

Religion usually involves groups of people congregating to express their similar religious beliefs.

Spirituality, in contrast, is more personal than religion in that it is something people define for themselves rather than being prescribed to them by others. Spirituality is largely devoid of the rules, conventions, and responsibilities typical of religions. People decide for themselves what is moral and when acting in accordance with that definition consider themselves spiritual. You may be religious or you may consider yourself spiritual but not religious. In being either religious or spiritual, you are likely to consider the meaning and purpose of life, connections with others both from the past and those who will follow, and to the natural world. Thereby, you may achieve a greater feeling of peacefulness and comfort with life events and life choices.

Spirituality in the Modern World

Ninety percent of the world's population is involved in some form of religious or spiritual practice (Barrett and Johnson, 2007). Only eight of 238 countries have populations where more than 25% say they are not religious, and those are countries in which the government has placed limitations on religious freedoms (Koenig, 2009). Atheism is actually rare, making up more than 5% of the population in only 12 of 238 countries. In America, 45% used prayer for health reasons within the past year—43% prayed for their own health, and 25% had others pray for them (National Center for Complementary and Alternative Medicine, 2005). Among these Americans, older

people and African Americans are more likely than others to use prayer (Bell et al., 2005; Goldstein et al., 2005).

How spiritual are you? Complete Health Check Up 5.1 to find out (see Health Check Up 5.1 on the companion website). Once completed, place Health Check Up 5.1 in your Health Decision Portfolio.

Spirituality and Health

Your consideration of religion and spirituality is more than merely an academic exercise. You can actually affect your health by being spiritual. For example, spirituality helps people cope with tragic events. After the September 11, 2001, attacks on the World Trade Center and the Pentagon, 90% of Americans coped with the stress by turning to religion (Schuster et al., 2001), 60% attended a religious or memorial service, and Bible sales rose 27% in the weeks after these attacks (Biema, 2001). Numerous other studies have also found that patients with physical health conditions and those with mental illnesses tend to cope by turning to religion.

Spirituality is also related to depression, which is a condition not uncommon among college students. Among depressed patients, depressive symptoms were most severe for those who were less religious and less severe for those who were more religious (Koenig, 2007). Furthermore, the most religious patients recovered from depression 50% faster than other patients.

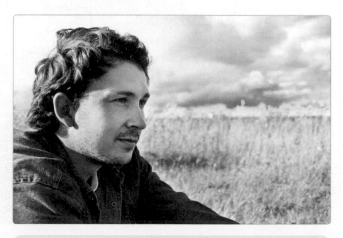

Spirituality can be expressed by focusing on the wonders of nature and the peace it can provide.

Other medical conditions are also related to spirituality and religion. When more than 2,000 cancer survivors were asked, 69% stated they had used prayer for their own health. This practice was most common among minority populations, with 81% of African Americans and 73% of Hispanics using prayer (Ross, Hall, Fairly, Taylor, and Howard, 2008). Spirituality has also been shown to help buffer the negative effects of stress (Delgado, 2007) and is even related to mortality. For example, a study conducted by the Centers for Disease Control and Prevention found people who did not attend religious services were 1.87 times more likely to have died over an 8-year period of time than were those who attended services more than weekly (Payne, 2008).

How Spirituality Affects Health

There are several factors that explain the relationship between spirituality and health. Some of these factors are biological, some sociological, and others psychological (Baetz and Toews, 2009).

Biological Factors

Religious expression lowers secretions of cortisol (a stress hormone) and blood pressure during stressful events (Tartaro, Luecken, and Gunn, 2005). This can prevent the harmful physiological effects of stress. Religious and spiritual activities are also associated with improved

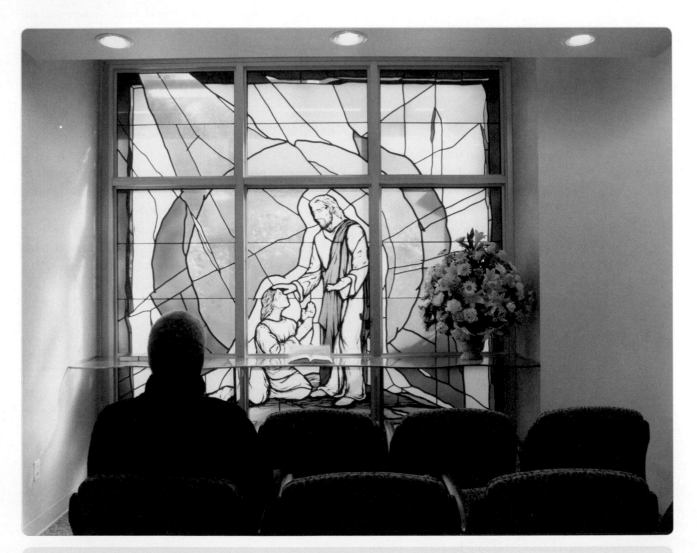

Religious expression, such as prayer and other spiritual activities, can help medical patients cope with the stress associated with their illnesses.

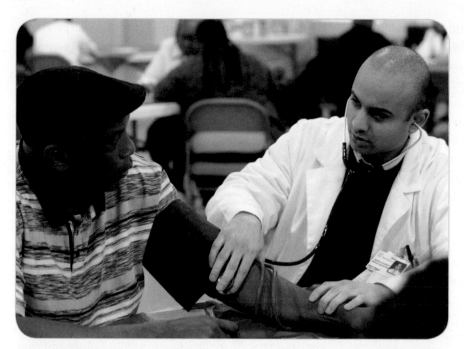

Religious and spiritual organizations offer many health-related activities to improve their members' health. These activities are a form of social support.

that when someone helps others, the volunteer's health status improves.

Psychological Factors

Religion and spirituality provide a sense of meaning in life. By decreasing self-focus, by redirecting attention to helping others or to contemplative prayer or meditation, they also invoke a calming effect. Religion and spirituality can also promote forgiveness, gratitude, and compassion and can provide hope that the future will be better than the present.

Theories to Explain the Relationship Between Spirituality and Health

Several theories have been proposed to explain how spirituality affects health. Among these are **control theory**, **social support theory**, and **placebo theory**.

Control Theory

Studies have consistently found that when someone perceives control over a stressful situation, that person's health

effectiveness of the immune system, thereby helping people ward off diseases (Koenig et al., 1997). In addition, religious expression and spirituality increase blood flow to the frontal lobes of the brain— structures that function in the development of empathy and compassion (Seybold, 2007).

Social Factors

Religious and spiritual practices and activities can encourage positive health behaviors that result in improved health. An example is the proscription (banning) of smoking and alcohol consumption by Seventh-day Adventists, Mormons, and other religious groups. In addition, many religious congregations and spiritual groups offer preventive healthcare such as blood pressure screening, organize health fairs that disseminate useful information, or encourage physical activity (such as hosting a youth dance or bowling night). Perhaps most important, however, is the social support provided by religious and spiritual organizations. Social support is highly correlated to health status. Lastly, these organizations offer opportunities for volunteer service—research indicates

Control theory: an explanation for the way in which spirituality affects health: control can be *primary control* (activities designed to change the situation) or *secondary control* (activities designed to take charge of oneself).

Social support theory: support provided by others; composed of emotional support, esteem support, tangible support, informational support, and advice support.

Placebo theory: when people believe something (e.g., being affiliated with a religious or spiritual organization) will help them, they often report that it actually does help them.

is less negatively affected than the health of someone who does not perceive such control. Control can be either primary or secondary. *Primary control* involves activities directed toward changing the situation. *Secondary control* involves activities directed toward changing oneself—for example, one's emotions—even when the situation cannot be changed. Praying for your health to improve is an example of primary control, whereas engaging in mediation to feel less disturbed by the situation is an example of secondary control.

There are several approaches you might take to control your health, which are described in the list that follows (Pargament et al., 1990). Once you are aware of these approaches, you can choose the one best suited for your situation.

Self-directing: You believe you are in control of your health. What you do is most important and, therefore, it is up to you to behave in a way that is health enhancing.

Collaborative: You believe that you work with God or forces of nature to control your health. You have some responsibility, and God or forces of nature have a role to play as well.

Deferring: You believe your health is in the hands of God or forces of nature and there is nothing you can do to change that. You do nothing, letting these forces take charge.

Pleading: You believe you need to beg God or forces of nature to intervene for you to be healthy.

Self-directing and *collaborative* approaches are most associated with a healthy status; in particular, when you really do have control. For example, whether you exercise regularly or not is in your control. In this instance, you would be better off adopting a self-directing or at least a collaborative approach—either approach will encourage you to engage in the healthy behavior. These are, therefore, primary control focuses.

In contrast, there are health-related situations in which you have little or no control; for example, the outcome of surgery. In this case, you would be best served by adopting a *deferring* or *pleading* approach. This secondary control approach would help you manage your emotions regarding the surgery. In that way, unhealthy consequences associated with negative emotions can be avoided.

Social Support Theory

Some experts believe that religious and spiritual organizations affect health because association of like-minded people provides social support.

Social support is usually thought of as actions to help people feel better so they can get through a major event. There are several different types of social support: emotional support, esteem support, tangible support, informational support, and advice support.

Emotional Support

Emotional support includes empathy, concern, caring, love, and trust; it generally comes from family and close friends. Religious and spiritual organizations provide emotional support when they organize groups whose members share their feelings about particular events or choices in their lives. Emotional support is the most commonly recognized form of social support.

Esteem Support

The purpose of **esteem support** is to make people feel better about themselves. This can take the form of expressions of confidence or encouragement, affirmation of an individual's strengths, or just the knowledge that others believe an the individual. The goal is to get people eventually to believe in themselves. An example of esteem support is when religious clergy and spiritual organization leaders counsel members by encouraging them to have confidence in themselves.

> **Emotional support:** expressions of empathy, concern, caring, love, and trust that generally come from family and close friends.
>
> **Esteem support:** expressions of confidence or encouragement, affirmation of an individual's strengths, or just the knowledge that others believe in an individual in order for the individual to feel better about himself or herself.

Tangible Support

Sometimes emotional or esteem support is not enough. **Tangible support** includes offerings of financial assistance, services, or material goods. For example, religious and spiritual organizations that lend or give money to members experiencing financial crisis (such as being behind in the rent), help with child care, or provide meals for homeless or housebound members are providing tangible support.

Informational Support

Sometimes social support takes the form of information; for example, the names and contact information of social service agencies that can be accessed in times of need. Religious and spiritual organizations often offer **informational support** by providing pamphlets from social service agencies or by maintaining a list of referrals.

Advice Support

Sometimes a person may be confused about what course of action to take and needs support in the form of advice. For example, a friend who has problems with his or her family may need advice about how to respond in a way most likely to resolve the issue. Religious clergy and spiritual organization leaders offer **advice support** by counseling members and recommending the best actions for them to take given their circumstances.

We all need social support at one time or another, and we all can provide social support to others for whom we care. Complete Health Check Up 5.2 to identify when you needed social support and when you provided it to others (see Health Check Up 5.2 on the companion website). Once completed, place Health Check Up 5.2 in your Health Decision Portfolio.

Placebo Theory

There are some who argue that neither religious nor spiritual organizations have any effect on health. Instead, they believe that the positive health effects associated with being a member of these organizations is akin to the placebo effect found by health researchers. That is, when people believe something will help them, they often report that it actually does help them. Some supporters of placebo theory, however, say it is immaterial if the health effects are similar to a placebo. What is important, they argue, is that the effects occur, regardless of the cause. They advise that whether the effects are direct or the result of a placebo effect, people ought to become affiliated with religious and spiritual organizations because it enhances their health.

Forgiveness, Spirituality, and Health

Part of being spiritual is being able to forgive others and yourself. If you believe you are connected to others, you understand that everyone makes mistakes and needs forgiveness to feel whole. Forgiveness is not to be misunderstood as excusing, justifying, condoning, or pardoning a transgression (Worthington, Witvliet, Pietrini, and Miller, 2007). Instead, **forgiveness** is a sincere intention not to seek revenge on or avoid the transgressor and to replace negative emotions, such as resentment, hate, and anger, with positive emotions such as compassion, empathy, and sympathy (Worthington, Witvliet, Lerner, and Scherer, 2005). One way to become more forgiving is to recognize in ourselves that we, too, have done things for which we wish to be forgiven. Feeling gratitude for having been forgiven ourselves or wishing we were forgiven when we were not should help us to forgive others. No one said it was easy—but forgiveness is worth striving toward, if for no other reason than it is good for your health.

Tangible support: providing for tangible needs such as money, time, clothing, food, and the like.

Informational support: providing information that will help a person make good decisions and improve that person's life.

Advice support: providing advice that will help a person make good decisions and improve that person's life.

Forgiveness: a sincere intention not to seek revenge on or avoid the transgressor and to replace negative emotions such as resentment, hate, and anger with positive emotions such as compassion, empathy, and sympathy.

What I Need to Know

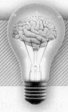

Spirituality and Unethical Behavior

Consider these three scenarios. (1) Lisa is so busy she has no time to work on the term paper that is due next week. So she decides to pay a friend to write the paper for her. (2) Juan is taking a health education course in which students are assigned to groups to develop an outline and conduct a health skills workshop for people in the wider community. However, Juan is studying for the MCATs for entrance to medical school and does not think he has time to spend on the health project. He decides to study for the exam rather than attend planning meetings scheduled by his group or participating in the development of the group's workshop outline. At the end of the semester, Juan asks the group to put his name on their project paper even though he hardly contributed to it. The professor will never know, he argues. (3) Jenna and Audrey are good friends. Both recognize that Audrey learns more easily and is a more conscientious student. So when it comes to taking the midterm exam in the course for which they are both enrolled, Jenna, relying on their friendship, expects Audrey will let her copy off of her answer sheet.

The situations described above all describe ethical violations by college students. Each scenario involves a student taking credit for work that was not his or her own. Cheating by students is a common problem: 75% of high school and college students admit to some form of cheating (Lies, damn lies, and statistics, 2004). Ethical behavior isn't just a problem on campuses. It has been highlighted by corporate scandals, such as the financial crisis associated with Legg Mason, AIG, Bank of America, and Citigroup.

However, the rest of us too often do not realize that some of our common behaviors are also unethical. Forty-four percent of Americans have lied about their work history when applying for a job, 25% have downloaded music illegally, and 30% own pirated software. Furthermore, 79% of workers say they would steal from their employers, 17% lie on their tax returns, and 3% of scientists admit to unethical scientific conduct such as fabrication of data.

Acting unethically is at odds with being spiritually healthy. There is the guilt associated with the behavior itself. In addition, there are the potential consequences if the unethical behavior is uncovered. Many universities and colleges have honor codes, and violations can result in suspension, expulsion, and/or notations on a violator's permanent record. The loss of trust, respect, and social support from family, friends, and classmates who know about the unethical behavior can take a heavy toll on one's spiritual health. One's emotional and psychological health also suffer.

Being angry and unforgiving is unhealthy. Studies have found that being unforgiving evokes brain activity consistent with stress, anger, and aggression (Pietrini, Guazzelli, Basso, Jaffe, and Grafman, 2000) and an increase in blood pressure (Witvliet, Ludwig, and Vander Lann, 2001). It also negatively affects psychological health (Berry et al., 2005) and makes your immunological system less effective (Temshok and Wald, 2005). In contrast, adopting a forgiving attitude results in lower levels of anxiety, depression, and stress (Lawler et al., 2003; Friedberg, Suchday, and Srinivas, 2009), fewer illnesses (Lawler et al., 2005), less back pain (Carson et al., 2005),

and spiritual well-being (Worthington, 2005). Now, who do you need to forgive?

In addition to wishing others to forgive us, we need to be willing to forgive ourselves. **Self-forgiveness** is "the willingness to abandon self-resentment in the face of one's own acknowledged objective wrong, while fostering compassion, generosity, and love toward oneself" (Enright and Human Development Study Group, 1996); or, in other words, "releasing resentment toward oneself for a perceived transgression and wrongdoing" (Tangney, Boone, and Dearing, 2005). Self-forgiveness is aided by the knowledge that *all* of us say and do things we regret. Such missteps are part of the human condition. Self-forgiveness does not mean we forget the past. Rather, it means that we remember it, learn from it, but then let it go. The ability to forgive oneself improves health; it has been shown to raise self-esteem, decrease anxiety and depression, and reduce stress (Mauger et al., 1992; Lawler et al., 2005).

Lastly, sometimes we blame events in our lives on God or a Supreme Being. We may experience a life tragedy (such as the death of a loved one or a chronic painful illness) and ascribe that to God or a Supreme Being. Consequently, we assume an unforgiving attitude toward that deity. This, too, can be unhealthy. When college students were studied, their difficulty in forgiving God was associated with anxiety and depression (Exline, Yali, and Lobel, 1999). However, researchers also found the reverse to be true: When people forgive God, they improve their health status (Enright and Human Development Study Group, 1996; Sells and Hargrove, 1998).

How forgiving are you? Complete Health Check Up 5.3 to find out (see Health Check Up 5.3 on the companion website). Once completed, place Health Check Up 5.3 in your Health Decision Portfolio.

Volunteerism as an Expression of Spirituality

Volunteering to help others would seem like a selfless spiritual activity. And yet, you can't but help benefit yourself when you volunteer to help others. Your self-esteem improves, you use skills you may not have known you had, and you develop an appreciation for what you have rather than bemoan what you do not have.

Volunteerism in the Corporate World

Even business leaders recognize the value of volunteerism. Businesses are some of the biggest contributors of money and volunteers to charitable causes. Sometimes, a business leader first develops empathy for a cause when a family member develops a condition, such as HIV or breast cancer. Beyond their personal motivations, business leaders may promote charitable giving because they want to be

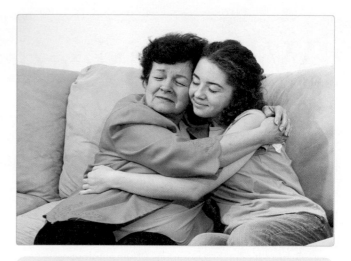

Learning to forgive others will help you to be healthier.

perceived as socially responsible. It is also good for public relations, and it is good tax policy. Regardless of the reasons, corporate contributions are welcomed by those in need of them.

Service Learning and Spirituality

Students in my stress-management course were required to teach stress-management skills to groups of people off-campus. They worked with nursing home residents to help them cope with moving into a group facility after living in their own homes or apartments for most of their lives. They helped cancer patients cope with their changed lives after their diagnoses. And, they helped prisoners manage their incarceration in the most productive way possible. This activity allowed them to use the knowledge and skills they learned in class to improve the lives of other people. This is called **service learning**, and it can

Self-forgiveness: the willingness to abandon self-resentment in the face of one's own acknowledged objective wrong while fostering compassion, generosity, and love toward oneself.

Service learning: using the knowledge and skills learned in class to improve the lives of other people, thereby learning more oneself and feeling a sense of spirituality.

What I Need to Know

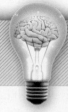

Corporate Charitable Activity

Following is a list of some of the corporations that contribute their time, money, and expertise to charitable causes. Many other examples could have been included.

Booz Allen Hamilton: In a 3-year period, 180 employees at this technology consulting firm volunteered their time to participate in a Girl Scouts leadership program. Other employees devoted their time to Neediest Kids, tutored and mentored unemployed workers and those stuck in dead-end jobs, and raised more than $50,000 for the Special Olympics.

Raffa: In one year, 195 employees from this accounting firm each dedicated an average of 52 hours to philanthropic activities, or more than 10,000 hours in all.

Men's Wearhouse: This retail chain collected business clothing to help former prisoners transition back into the workforce. More than 1,000 suits, 400 sports coats, 66 pairs of shoes, 31 overcoats, and 596 belts were donated.

Citigroup: This bank donated $25,000 to fund classes in English and for financial aid at a housing project and $100,000 for a high school program designed to increase the number of students going on to college.

Outback Steakhouse: One Outback restaurant provided cocktails, steaks, chicken, and cheesecake (and dedicated half its staff to cook, serve, and clean up) for a fundraiser that raised more than $55,000 for a local high school.

Roy Rogers Restaurants: In greater Washington, DC, when a franchise owner's mother needed hospice care, local Roy Rogers Restaurants placed collection boxes next to their cash registers, collecting more than $55,000 for the hospice. They also planned other fundraising activities for the hospice, such as golf tournaments, sailing regattas, and evening galas.

What charitable contributions have local businesses made where you live?

---

be quite a spiritual experience. Service learning combines class work with service, thereby helping those that need the service provided and, at the same time, enhancing learning on the part of students. After all, one does not want to teach others without being sure one knows what one is teaching.

You, too, can organize service-learning activities even if they are not a regular part of your courses. Health Check Up 5.4 helps you plan to do just that (see Health Check Up 5.4 on the companion website). Once completed, place Health Check Up 5.4 in your Health Decision Portfolio. If you do engage in a service-learning activity or organize your classmates to do so, you can expect to feel a strong sense of spiritualism as a result.

How You Can Use Spirituality to Be Healthier

Just learning about the relationship of spirituality to health may be interesting, but it is not enough. That knowledge has to be applied to have the desired effect; that is, you must use what you know about spirituality to improve your health. Some strategies are presented in the sections that follow.

Use Control Theory to Your Advantage

Realistically evaluate the control you have over events that affect your health. If you have a good deal of control, use primary control methods (e.g., self-directing or collaborative) to exercise that control. If you have little or no

What I Need to Know

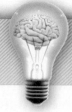

Faith-Based Health Programs

The health ministry concept originated in the 1800s in churches of predominantly African-American membership. Back then, the primary role of *church nurses* was to comfort family members of the deceased at funerals by distributing tissues and water for the grieving family. They also fanned parishioners who were overcome by their spiritual experiences during the church service (Townsend, 2004).

In modern times, the health ministry concept has become much more widespread—churches of many denominations, as well as synagogues and mosques, have embraced it. Many religious organizations provide home health visits, offer blood pressure screen-ings at worship services, organize support groups for congregants with chronic illnesses, conduct health education programs, organize health fairs, and conduct running and jogging events. Some congregations have even added full-service fitness facilities to their buildings. By way of example, a church in a Dallas suburb provides basketball cages, a rock climbing wall, and a walking trail around a lake (Brinton, 2008). The rationale for these programs is that God has given each person the gift of a body, and it is the responsibility of everyone to care for that gift. Furthermore, it is argued, spiritual vitality is not much good without physical health.

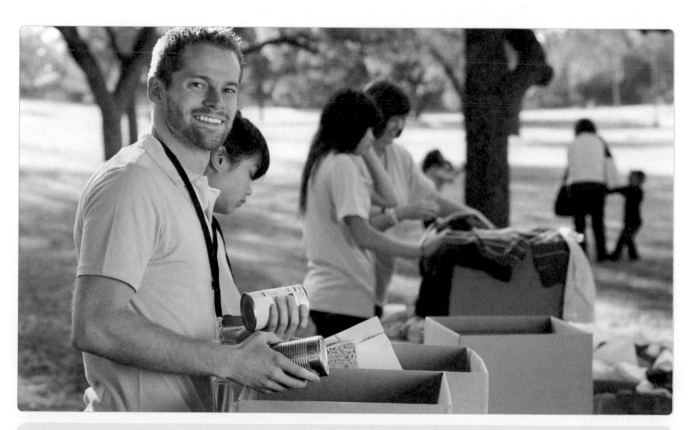

Helping your community is a spiritual activity that will provide you with a sense of accomplishment and improved health.

control, use secondary control methods (e.g., deferring or pleading) to manage emotions so as to limit negative health effects.

Join a Religious or Spiritual Organization

Whether it is because of social support or the placebo effect, studies have determined that affiliation with a religious and spiritual organization is likely to have a positive effect on your health. You can obtain a list of organizations you are potentially interested in joining from your campus community service office or from someone affiliated with the campus ministry. Make sure you consider any costs involved (such as membership fees), travel distance required, focus of the organization, and the kind of people who are members.

Take Advantage of the Support Offered by Religious and Spiritual Organizations

Joining a religious or spiritual organization will not miraculously result in your being healthy. You will need to take advantage of what the organization offers by participating in several of its events. For example, attend religious services, volunteer to serve on a committee, join a group session related to your needs and interests, or schedule a meeting with leaders of the organization to identify the type of support you need.

Adopt a Forgiving Attitude

Completing Health Check Up 5.3 will disclose how forgiving you tend to be. Perhaps you learned that you need to be more forgiving. Even if that is not the case, however, there probably are people whom you have yet to forgive. Use this knowledge of forgiveness to become healthier. Make a list of who you need to forgive. Next, write down specifically *how* and by *when* you will forgive these people. (Remember self-forgiveness, too.) Once you implement this plan, you will feel more spiritual and both emotionally and physically healthier.

Help Others

When you help other people whose situation is more dire than yours, you are better able to view your situation in

its proper perspective. That is good for your spiritual and emotional health and, consequently, your physical health. You can identify volunteer opportunities by consulting with your campus community/volunteer office, speaking with someone at your local health department or school system, or inquiring through your church, synagogue, or mosque.

Death and Dying

The deaths of loved ones are some of the most intense spiritual experiences we will ever encounter. After the death of a close friend or relative, there is a grieving process you can anticipate experiencing. Did you know that other losses—graduating from school and no longer seeing familiar surroundings or school buddies, the death of a pet, or the breakup of a relationship—can also elicit a grieving response? Of course, these losses are not experienced to the extent that the death of a loved one is experienced. However, you still grieve. Table 5.2 depicts the grieving process.

This section is designed to help you make decisions when faced with the death of a loved one. That includes making arrangements in the best interest of the dying person and doing what is best for you to recover from such a traumatic experience. Determine your attitude toward death by completing Health Check Up 5.5 (see Health Check Up 5.5 on the companion website). Once completed, place Health Check Up 5.5 in your Health Decision Portfolio. Your attitude toward death has a lot to do with how you choose to live your life.

Help for Those in Mourning

Help is available for people going through the grieving process. Many hospitals offer support groups for people in mourning. Churches, synagogues, and mosques may offer similar support groups. Relatives and friends can be called upon to offer different types of social support. Also, do not forget the help available from campus health centers.

Hospice Care

What should you do when someone you love is dying? Perhaps all you can do is arrange for that person to be

TABLE 5.2 **Stages of Grief**

When experiencing a death or another significant loss, we go through the following grieving process.

Stage 1: Shock. May last for hours, even up to weeks.

- An initial period of shock, or numbed disbelief.
- Unable to function or perform even simple tasks or make decisions.
- Physical symptoms such as agitation, weakness, crying, and aimless activity.

Stage 2: Suffering. May last for months or even a year.

- Physical symptoms may include a loss of appetite and weight, chest pain, insomnia, and extreme fatigue.
- Emotional symptoms such as sadness, anger, guilt, anxiety, restlessness, and agitation.
- Rapid mood swings, intense emotions, and sense of loss of control.
- Feelings of loneliness and depression.

Stage 3: Recovery. May occur after several months or a year.

- Ability to function and reconnect to the interesting and happy parts of life.
- Improvement in emotions.
- Diminished depression and despair.
- A new appreciation for the preciousness of life and a newfound ability to live life in the moment.

REPRODUCED FROM: *The New Grief Stages: Finding Your Way Through the Task of Mourning*. Recover-from-grief.com, 2009. Available at: http://www.recover-from-grief.com/new-grief-stages.html.

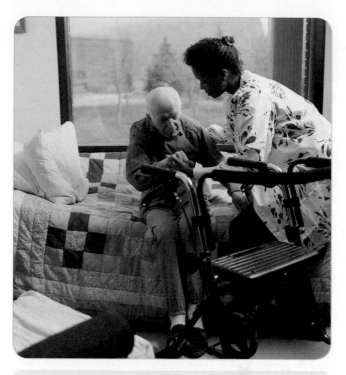

Hospice care can assist the patient to feel more comfortable, as well as help the family deal with the impending death of their loved one.

Americans who died received hospice care. This allowed 69% of these patients to die at home, in a nursing home, or in some other residential facility rather than in a hospital (National Hospice and Palliative Care Organization, 2009). This is significant, as the great majority of Americans state they would prefer to die at home. If you can help by arranging for a dying person to be pain-free and to die at home, you have been a blessing in the life of that person. A hospice can help you achieve that goal.

Making Preparations

Preparing for one's death, whether imminent or of a date unknown, is of help to family and friends left behind. Rather than loved ones being required to make funeral

as comfortable as possible. Sometimes no treatment is available to prevent death; for example, when someone is dying of an incurable form of cancer. In these instances, there are organizations that can help the dying person be more comfortable, which may entail administering pain-relieving medications or providing help in planning for the family's needs. Such an organization is called a **hospice**. Hospice care can be provided in a separate facility or in the home. In 2008, approximately 39% of all

Hospice: an organization that cares for dying patients by comforting them, administering pain medications, and that provides counseling and comfort for families of the patients.

arrangements while grieving or having to search through papers for a will or other important documents, all of this can and should be arranged beforehand. The preparations you and others in your family can make are given in the list that follows. Make sure that others know where these important papers are kept.

1. Have a will that identifies what should be done with your belongings and estate.

2. Write funeral and burial instructions such as who should officiate, where you want to be buried or whether you want to be cremated, and who you want as pallbearers.

3. Develop a list of names, addresses, and telephone numbers of people who should be contacted, such as friends, relatives, clergy, attorney, insurance agent, or stockbroker.

4. Organize a record of bank accounts and their numbers, as well as credit card numbers and billing addresses.

5. Identify any safe deposit boxes and who has access to them.

6. Among other records that could be provided are certificates of deposit, outstanding loans, past income tax returns, and insurance policy information.

Deciding about Organ Donation

You may decide that you want to help others, even in death, by donating your organs. Some people view this as the opportunity to ensure that their lives have had a beneficial purpose, regardless of what else they might do. Others feel awkward about having their organs removed from their bodies and placed in someone else's body. If you decide to be an organ donor, you will need to sign a donor registration form provided by the state in which you live. **FIG. 5.1 ▶** shows a sample donor registration form.

Applying Behavior Theory

How might you use behavior change theory to better express your spirituality? Complete the Applying Behavior Change Theory for this chapter on the companion website. Once completed, place it in your Health Decision Portfolio.

ORGAN AND TISSUE DONOR REGISTRATION FORM

State Driver License # _____

Social Security # _____

Date of Birth (ex. 01/15/2012) _____

Sex: _____ M _____ F

Name _____

Address _____

City _____ State _____ Zip _____

Signature of Donor _____

Date signed _____

In the hope that I may help others, I hereby make this organ and tissue gift, if medically acceptable, to take effect upon my death. The words and marks (or notations) below indicate my desires.
Default choice is (a).
I give:
(a)_____ any needed organ or tissue
(b)_____ only the following organs or tissue for the purpose of transplantation, therapy, medical research or education: _____
(c) _____ my body for anatomical study if needed.

Limitations or special wishes, if any, list below:
_____

NEAREST RELATIVE INFORMATION

Name _____

Address _____

City _____ State _____ Zip _____

Telephone # _____

WITNESS INFORMATION

Witness _____

Date signed _____

Witness (Parent or Guardian if under 18)

_____

Date signed _____

FIGURE 5.1   Sample donor registration form.
REPRODUCED FROM: the Agency for Health Care Administration and Department of Highway Safety and Motor Vehicles, Tallahassee, FL.

SUMMARY

The goal of this chapter is to provide you with the tools you need to be spiritually healthy. To help you do that, a summary of important information included in this chapter is provided.

- Religion describes what happens after death, codifies rules to guide moral behavior, and usually involves groups of people congregating to express their religious beliefs.

- Spirituality is largely devoid of rules, regulations, and responsibilities typical of religions. Important considerations include the meaning and purpose of life, connections to others both from the past and those who will follow, and to the natural world.

- Ninety percent of the world's population is involved in some form of religious or spiritual practice. Atheism is actually rare with atheists making up more than 5% of the population in only 12 of 238 countries.

- You can actually affect your health by being spiritual. Spirituality helps people cope with tragic events, alleviates depression, eases the stress of cancer survivors, and is related to fewer deaths.

- Spirituality affects health through biological factors (such as lowering blood pressure), social factors (such as preventive health services offered by religious and spiritual organizations), and psychological factors (such as promoting forgiveness, gratitude, and compassion).

- Control theory, support theory, and placebo theory are all explanations for how spirituality affects health.

- Social support can take different forms: emotional support, esteem support, tangible support, informational support, and advice support.

- You can use spirituality to improve your health by joining a religious or spiritual organization, taking advantage of what the organization offers by participating in several of its events, adopting a forgiving attitude, using control theory to your advantage, and helping others.

- Forgiveness results in improved health. Forgiveness is a sincere intention not to seek revenge or avoid the transgressor and to replace negative emotions such as resentment, hate, and anger with positive emotions such as compassion, empathy, and sympathy.

- Self-forgiveness is the willingness to abandon resentment toward oneself for a perceived transgression or wrongdoing.

- Volunteerism is a spiritual activity that improves the health of both the people receiving service and the volunteer. Many corporations are involved in volunteerism with benefits to those served as well as for the corporation.

- Service learning is a spiritual activity that involves students applying the knowledge and skills they learned in class to improve the lives of other people. Whereas the recipients of the service-learning activity benefit, so do students by enhanced learning and the development of a sense of spirituality.

- A hospice is an organization that helps dying people be more comfortable by administering pain-relieving medications or that provides help in planning for the family's needs. Hospice care can be provided in a separate facility or in the patient's home.

- It is important to prepare for one's death, even if the time of death may be far in the future. Among the preparations are making a will, identifying where important papers are kept, and writing funeral and burial instructions.

REFERENCES

Baetz, M. and Toews, J. Clinical implications of research on religion, spirituality, and mental health. *Canadian Journal of Psychiatry* 54 (2009): 292–301.

Barrett, D. B. and Johnson, T. M. World Christian Database: Atheist/nonreligious by country: World Christian trends. William Carey Library, 2007. Available at: http://www.worldchristiandatabase.org/wcd.

Bell, R. A., Suerkin, C., Quandt, S. A., Grzywacz, J. G., and Arcury, T. A. Pray for health among U. S. adults: The 2002 National Health Interview Survey. *Complementary Health Practice Review* 10 (2005): 175–188.

Berry, J. W., Worthington, E. L., O'Connor, L. E., Parrot, L., and Wade, N. G. Forgiveness, Vengeful Rumination, and Affective Traits. *Journal of Personality* 73 (2005): 1–43.

Biema, D. Faith after the fall. *Time*, October 8, 2001: 76.

Brinton, H. G. Redeeming both body and soul. *Washington Post*, June 10, 2008: HE01.

Carson, J. W., Keefe, F. J., Goli, V., Fras, A. M., Lynch, T. R., Thorp, S. R., and Buechler, J. L. Forgiveness and chronic low back pain: A preliminary study examining the relationship between forgiveness to pain, anger, and psychological distress. *Journal of Pain* 6 (2005): 84–91.

Delgado, C. Sense of coherence, spirituality, stress and quality of life in chronic illness. *Journal of Nursing Scholarship* 39 (2007): 229–234.

Enright, R. D. and the Human Development Study Group. Counseling within the forgiveness triad: On forgiving, receiving forgiveness, and self-forgiveness. *Counseling and Values* 40 (1996): 107–126.

Exline, J., Yali, A. M., and Lobel, M. When God disappoints: Difficulty forgiving God and its role in negative emotions. *Journal of Health Psychology* 4 (1999): 365–379.

Friedberg, J. P., Suchday, S., and Srinivas, V. S. Relationship between forgiveness and psychological and physiological indices in cardiac patients. *International Journal of Behavioral Medicine* 16 (2009): 205–211.

Goldstein, M. S., Brown, E. R., Ballard-Barbash, R., Morgenstern, H., Bastani, R., Lee, J., Gatto, N., and Ambs, A. The use of complementary and alternative medicine among California adults with and without cancer. *Evidence Based Complementary and Alternative Medicine* 2 (2005): 557–565.

Koenig, H. G. Religion and depression in older medical inpatients. *American Journal of Geriatrics and Psychiatry* 15 (2007): 282–291.

Koenig, H. G. Research on religion, spirituality, and mental health: A review. *Canadian Journal of Psychiatry* 54 (2009): 283–291.

Koenig, H. G., Cohen, H. J., George, L. K., Hays, J. C., Larson, D. B., and Blazer, D. G. Attendance at religious services, interleukin-6, and other biological parameters of immune function in older adults. *International Journal of Psychiatry and Medicine* 27 (1997): 233–250.

Lawler, K. A., Younger, J. W., Piferi, R. L., Billington, E., Jobe, R., Edmondson, K., and Jones, W. H. A change of heart: Cardiovascular correlates of forgiveness in response to interpersonal conflict. *Journal of Behavioral Medicine* 26 (2003): 373–393.

Lawler, K. A., Younger, J. W., Piferi, R. L., Jobe, R., Edmondson, K., and Jones, W. H. The unique effects of forgiveness on health: An exploration of pathways. *Journal of Behavioral Medicine* 28 (2005): 157–167.

Lies, damn lies, and statistics. *Wired*, March 24, 2004: 60–61.

Mauger, P. A., Perry, J. E., Freeman, T., Grove, D. C., McBride, A. G., and McKinney, K. E. The measurement of forgiveness: Preliminary research. *Journal of Psychology and Christianity* 11 (1992): 170–180.

National Center for Complementary and Alternative Medicine. Prayer and spirituality in health: Ancient practices, modern science. *CAM at the NIH: Focus on Complementary and Alternative Medicine*, Winter 2005.

National Hospice and Palliative Care Organization. *NHPCO Facts and Figures—2009 Findings*. Alexandria, VA: National Hospice and Palliative Care Organization, 2009.

Pargament, K. I., Ensing, D. S., Falgout, K., Olsen, H., Reilly, B., Van Haitsma, K., and Warren, R. God helps me: Religious coping efforts as predictors of the outcomes of significant negative life events. *American Journal of Community Psychology* 18 (1990): 793–825.

Payne, J. W. A matter of belief or evidence. *Washington Post*, June 10, 2008, HE01.

Pietrini, P., Guazzelli, M., Basso, G., Jaffe, K., and Grafman, J. Neural correlates of imaginal aggressive behavior assessed by positron emission tomography in healthy subjects. *American Journal of Psychiatry* 157 (2000): 1772–1781.

Ross, L. E., Hall, I. J., Fairly, T. L., Taylor, Y. J., and Howard, D. L. Prayer and self-reported health among cancer survivors in the United States, National Health Interview Survey, 2002. *Journal of Complementary and Alternative Medicine* 14 (2008): 931–938.

Schuster, M. A., Stein, B. D., Jaycox, L. H., Collins, R. L., Marshall, G. N., Elliott, M. N., Zhou, A. J., Kanouse, D. E., Morrison, J. L., and Berry, S. H. A national survey of stress reactions after the September 11, 2001 terrorist attacks. *New England Journal of Medicine* 345 (2001): 1507–1512.

Sells, J. N. and Hargrove, T. D. Forgiveness: A review of the theoretical and empirical literature. *Journal of Family Therapy* 20 (1998): 21–36.

Seybold, K. S. Physiological mechanisms involved in religiosity/spirituality and health. *Journal of Behavioral Medicine* 30 (2007): 303–309.

Tangney, J. P., Boone, J. L., and Dearing, R. Forgiving the self: Conceptual issues and empirical findings. In Worthington, E. L., ed. *Handbook of Forgiveness*. New York: Brunner-Routledge, 2005, 143–157.

Tartaro, J., Luecken, I. J., and Gunn, H. E. Exploring heart and soul: Effects of religiousity/spirituality and gender on blood pressure and cortical stress responses. *Journal of Health Psychology* 10 (2005): 753–766.

Temshok, I. and Wald, R. I. Forgiveness and health in persons living with HIV/AIDS. In Worthington, E. L., ed. *Handbook of Forgiveness*. New York: Brunner-Routledge, 2005, 335–348.

Townsend, H. Fanning and praying parish nursing is deeply rooted in tradition. *Nursing Spectrum*, May 3, 2004.

Witvliet, C. V. O., Ludwig, T. E., and Vander Lann, K. Granting forgiveness or harboring grudges: Implications for emotion, physiology, and health. *Psychological Science* 12 (2001): 117–123.

Worthington, E. L. (Editor). *Handbook of Forgiveness*. New York: Brunner-Routledge, 2005.

Worthington, E. L., Jr., Witvliet, C. V., Lerner, A., and Scherer, M. Forgiveness in health research and medical practice. *Explore* 1 (2005):169–176.

Worthington, E. L., Jr., Witvliet, C. V., Pietrini, P., and Miller, A. J. Forgiveness, health, and well-being: A review of evidence for emotional versus decisional forgiveness, dispositional forgivingness, and reduced unforgiveness. *Journal of Behavioral Medicine* 30 (2007): 291–302.

INTERNET RESOURCES

Handling Forgiving and Forgetting. Livestrong.com
http://www.livestrong.com/
article/14679-handling-forgiving-and-forgetting/

Spirituality and Health
http://www.spirituality-health.com/spirit/

Faith
http://www.faith.com

About Religion and Spirituality
http://www.about.com/religion

Spirituality and Practice
http://www.spiritualityandpractice.com/practices/

Chapter 6

Building a Lifetime of Physical Fitness

 Access Health Check Ups and Health Behavior Change activities on the Companion Website: **go.jblearning.com/Empowering**.

Learning Objectives

- Describe the components of physical fitness.
- Explain the benefits of being physically fit.
- Explain how to develop a physical fitness program.
- Discuss how to maintain a physical fitness program once it is started.
- Describe how to prevent and treat exercise injuries.

On college campuses, there is a wide array of body types. Among them are some well-toned bodies: six-pack abs, arms that show tight muscles without jiggle, and rear ends that can accommodate tight shorts. Can't we all attain that look? Under the category "Life is Unfair," the answer is NO. Some of us possess genetic limitations or physical challenges that prevent us from developing this look. Others of us are not willing to devote the time required to body building or body sculpting—doing this might leave us too little time to spend with our families, on our studies, or in spiritual activities. What we all *can* obtain, however, is a healthy level of physical fitness that develops our bodies in ways that make us capable of going through our days comfortably and with energy to spare. We can also develop our bodies for better long-term health, preventing or delaying the onset of such illnesses as coronary heart disease, stroke, hypertension, and diabetes. This chapter is devoted to giving you the knowledge and skills to develop a healthy level of physical fitness and to maintain that level throughout your life.

Understand the Components of Physical Fitness

Physical fitness is the ability to meet daily physical demands and unexpected physical challenges without being overly fatigued. It also includes having the energy to participate in leisure and recreational activities after meeting these life demands. In other words, physical fitness is the ability of your body to function effectively and efficiently.

There are different components of physical fitness, including cardiorespiratory fitness, muscular strength and endurance, flexibility, and body composition (Greenberg, Dintiman, and Oakes, 2004).

Cardiorespiratory Fitness

To be physically active, you need to transport oxygen to cells throughout your body. The heart, lungs, and blood vessels perform this function. When you breathe, oxygen enters your lungs and is absorbed into your bloodstream. That oxygenated blood then travels to your heart, where it is pumped out to supply the cells of your body. The more efficiently and effectively your heart and lungs work when transporting oxygen, the greater is your **cardiorespiratory fitness** (*cardio* for heart and *respiratory* for lungs and breathing). Complete Health Check Up 6.1 to assess your cardiorespiratory fitness (see Health Check Up 6.1 on the companion website). Once completed, place Health Check Up 6.1 in your Health Decision Portfolio.

Physical fitness: having the energy to meet daily demands and unexpected challenges effectively and efficiently. It is composed of four components: cardiorespiratory fitness, muscular strength and endurance, flexibility, and body composition.

Cardiorespiratory fitness: the efficiency and effectiveness of the heart and lungs to transport oxygen to cells throughout the body.

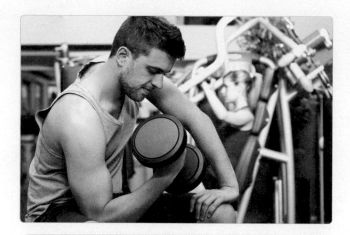

Weight training involves exercises that develop and maintain both muscular strength and muscular endurance.

Muscular Strength and Endurance

The force with which a muscle can contract is called **muscular strength**. The ability of a muscle to contract *repeatedly* or for a *sustained* period of time is called **muscular endurance**. Both are significant components of physical fitness. Sometimes you need to move a heavy object, such as a heavy couch—this requires muscular strength. At other times you need to maintain muscular force, such as when moving numerous pieces of lightweight furniture—this requires muscular endurance. Complete Health Check Ups 6.2 and 6.3 to assess your muscular strength and endurance (see Health Check Ups 6.2 and 6.3 on the companion website). Once completed, place Health Check Ups 6.2 and 6.3 in your Health Decision Portfolio.

Flexibility

Flexibility refers to the range of motion around a joint; for example, how much bend you have in your knees, how far you can lower your head from your neck, or how far you can reach from your shoulders. If you have limited range of motion, you are more susceptible to fitness injuries such as muscle strains and ligament tears. Flexibility improves posture, increases physical and mental relaxation, releases muscle tension and soreness, and reduces risk of injury (American Council on Exercise, 2010b). Complete Health Check Up 6.4 to assess your flexibility (see Health Check

Up 6.4 on the companion website). Once completed, place Health Check Up 6.4 in your Health Decision Portfolio.

Body Composition

Body composition refers to the amount of body fat compared to other body components (called *lean body mass*). We are all familiar with height–weight charts that advise us how much we should weigh for our height. For example, if Terry and Pat are both 5 feet 8 inches tall, the chart would recommend they weigh the same. Yet, suppose Terry is very muscular with a low percentage of body fat, and Pat has poor muscle tone with a higher percentage of body fat. Because muscle weighs more than fat, Terry may weigh more than Pat even though Terry is more fit. Body composition looks at the fitness of the body in terms of body fat, not just weight.

Know the Advantages of Being Physically Fit

A friend of mine likes to joke that he gets his exercise by serving as a pallbearer at the funerals of all his physically fit friends. Aside from simply being contentious, he raises an interesting and valid point. Exercise is no guarantee of a long life. Heredity plays an important role in how long you live. Still, exercise can help you live to the higher end of your inherited longevity range and to have an increased quality of life during those years. The benefits of physical fitness are physical, psychological, and social.

Muscular strength: the maximum force a muscle can contract.

Muscular endurance: the ability of the muscle to contract repeatedly or for a sustained period of time.

Flexibility: the range of motion around a joint.

Body composition: the amount of body fat compared to other body components (called *lean body mass*).

What I Need to Know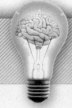

Overcoming Physical Challenges to Fitness

Bob Weiland lost his legs serving in the Marine Corps. He did not let that stop him, however. Propelling himself with just his hands—no wheelchair—he completed the Marine Corps marathon. It took him 79 hours 57 minutes to traverse the 26-plus miles, but he did it.

We all have physical challenges, although admittedly some of us have greater challenges than others. You may be overweight, lacking in athletic skill, allergic to substances in the air, or have some other limitation affecting your ability to achieve and maintain physical fitness. Still, you can develop strategies—taking your specific limitations and challenges into consideration—to become fit. Certainly, if Bob Weiland can do it, you can.

Recognizing the fitness potential of every person, several organizations have formed to encourage people facing severe challenges to engage in physical activity. For example, many schools and communities support wheelchair sports competitions. And, every 4 years, in conjunction with the Olympic Games, the Paralympics takes place, featuring physically challenged athletes competing in events such as wheelchair basketball, track (throwing, running), a marathon, wheelchair fencing, weight lifting, and goalball (football for blind athletes in which the ball contains small bells so athletes can determine where it is). The highly trained and skilled athletes of the Paralympics have learned that they do not necessarily need arms or legs, or even sight, to reach a high level of fitness. There is a lesson in that for all of us.

What are your limitations and challenges to becoming physically fit? And, how will you become fit in spite of these limitations and challenges?

Physical Benefits

Moderate daily physical activity can substantially reduce your risk of developing or dying from cardiovascular disease, type 2 diabetes, and certain cancers, such as colon cancer. Furthermore, daily physical activity helps to lower blood pressure and serum cholesterol, helps prevent or retard osteoporosis, and helps reduce obesity and symptoms of arthritis. Here are some specific examples: (1) Strength training (using mild to moderate resistance) reduces blood pressure, lowers low-density lipoproteins, or LDLs ("bad" cholesterol), raises high-density lipoproteins ("good" cholesterol), and improves the body's processing of sugar, reducing the risk of diabetes (American Council on Exercise, 2010d). (2) Physically active people are half as likely to develop coronary heart disease as are inactive people (President's Council on Physical Fitness and Sports, 2010). This is significant because heart disease is the leading cause of death among men and women in the United States. (3) Regular exercise can help a person maintain a healthy weight. Table 6.1 lists the number of calories expended for various physical activities.

Psychological Benefits

Regular exercise helps reduce feelings of anxiety and depression and can be effective in control of stress. It can make you feel better about yourself—increase your self-esteem—and help you relax. In general, exercise encourages feelings of well-being and good health (American Council on Exercise, 2010a). One of the reasons for these benefits is the release of brain neurotransmitters during exercise (*endorphins* and others). These chemicals attach to receptors in the brain that affect mood and emotion.

Social Benefits

People often exercise with others. Whether it is play on a team (e.g., pickup basketball) or with one other person (e.g., a tennis match), exercise can have a social health

TABLE 6.1	Calories Expended per Hour for Various Physical Activities

	Weight in Pounds											
	90	**110**	**130**	**150**	**170**	**190**	**210**	**230**	**250**	**270**	**290**	**310**
Activity						**kcal**						
Baseball												
Player	162	204	246	282	318	351	396	438	480	522	564	606
Pitcher	210	258	306	354	402	444	492	540	588	636	684	732
Badminton (singles)	246	294	342	396	450	498	554	612	672	732	796	860
Basketball (full court)	450	474	486	564	636	714	765	798	822	840	864	888
Half court	174	198	234	270	306	342	389	432	474	501	546	588
Bowling	162	188	210	246	276	312	342	378	420	462	504	546
Boxing	546	666	786	906	1,026	1,146	1,272	1,372	1,512	1,632	1,752	1,872
Calisthenics	162	216	268	306	348	374	423	462	510	546	582	618
Carpentry (general)	126	156	186	210	240	270	294	318	342	366	390	414
Circuit training	414	558	654	756	852	954	1,056	1,128	1,200	1,272	1,344	1,404
Cycling												
Leisure 5.5 mph	168	192	228	264	300	330	368	402	438	480	522	564
Leisure 9.5 mph	246	299	355	410	465	519	576	636	696	768	822	876
Racing	420	510	600	690	780	870	966	1,062	1,158	1,254	1,350	1,446
Canoeing or kayaking												
Leisure	108	132	156	180	204	228	253	276	300	324	348	372
Racing	258	312	366	420	474	534	590	642	696	750	804	858
Dance (vigorous aerobic)	330	402	474	546	618	690	744	798	852	906	950	1,014
Square	246	300	354	408	462	516	570	624	678	732	786	840
Digging trenches	360	438	516	594	642	750	828	906	996	1,086	1,176	1,266
Electrical work	144	174	204	234	270	300	330	360	390	420	450	480
Farming												
Cleaning stalls	336	408	480	552	624	696	768	840	912	984	1,056	1,128
Driving tractor	96	120	144	162	186	204	228	252	276	300	324	348
Feeding cattle	168	198	228	264	300	336	372	408	444	480	516	552
Shoveling grain	216	258	300	348	390	438	486	534	588	638	684	732
Fencing												
Moderate	174	216	258	300	342	378	420	462	504	546	588	630
Vigorous	378	438	522	582	684	762	846	930	1,014	1,098	1,182	1,266
Field hockey	330	402	474	546	618	690	762	834	906	978	1,050	1,122
Football (touch)	326	396	468	540	612	684	753	816	882	948	1,014	1,080
Forestry												
Ax chopping (fast)	732	894	1,050	1,212	1,374	1,530	1,692	2,010	2,208	2,406	2,604	2,862
Sawing by hand	300	366	432	498	564	630	696	762	828	894	960	1,026
Sawing (power)	192	228	264	306	648	390	426	462	498	540	582	624
Gardening												
Digging	312	378	444	516	582	648	720	792	864	936	1,008	1,080
Hedging	198	234	270	312	354	396	438	480	522	564	606	642

(Continues)

TABLE 6.1   Calories Expended per Hour for Various Physical Activities *(Continued)*

Activity	90	110	130	150	170	190	210	230	250	270	290	310
							kcal					
Mowing	276	336	396	456	516	576	636	396	756	816	876	936
Raking	132	162	198	222	252	276	306	336	366	396	426	456
Golf (walking)	216	258	300	348	390	438	486	534	588	636	684	726
Handball or racquetball												
Competitive	522	636	750	864	978	1,092	1,211	1,332	1,452	1,572	1,692	1,812
Horseback riding												
Walk	102	126	150	174	198	222	246	270	294	318	342	366
Sitting to trot	140	180	210	246	276	312	342	372	402	432	462	492
Posting to trot	222	276	330	374	432	486	534	582	630	678	726	774
Gallop	290	370	450	522	588	660	732	804	876	948	1,020	1,092
Horseshoes	138	168	198	228	258	288	318	348	378	408	438	468
Hiking (pack, 3 mph)	246	300	354	408	462	516	570	624	678	732	786	840
Ice hockey	354	438	522	600	684	762	846	930	1,014	1,098	1,182	1,356
Ice skating (9 mph)	210	276	342	384	432	486	534	582	630	678	726	774
Judo or karate	486	588	690	796	900	1,008	1,115	1,224	1,332	1,440	1,548	1,620
Jogging or running												
5 mph	348	432	516	594	612	750	828	906	984	1,062	1,140	1,218
6 mph	414	510	606	696	786	882	972	1,062	1,152	1,242	1,320	1,410
7 mph	504	588	640	798	906	1,008	1,116	1,224	1,332	1,440	1,548	1,638
8 mph	576	666	786	906	1,026	1,146	1,266	1,326	1,446	1,566	1,688	1,806
9 mph	630	738	876	1,068	1,146	1,278	1,410	1,542	1,674	1,806	1,932	2,058
Painting (inside)	84	102	120	138	156	174	192	210	228	246	264	294
Outside	198	234	312	354	396	438	480	522	564	606	648	690
Plastering	192	234	318	360	402	444	486	528	570	612	654	696
Rope jumping												
Slow	368	450	534	612	696	780	858	936	1,014	1,092	1,164	1,236
Fast	462	552	654	750	852	954	1,050	1,146	1,242	1,338	1,500	1,596
Scraping paint	162	192	222	285	294	324	348	396	432	468	504	549
Sedentary activities												
Lying down	54	66	78	90	102	114	126	138	150	162	179	186
Sitting	66	84	102	114	132	144	162	186	198	216	234	253
Standing	150	180	210	246	276	312	342	372	402	432	462	492
Skating												
In-line (13 mph)	564	654	744	858	972	1,086	1,200	1,314	1,428	1,542	1,656	1,770
Roller (9 mph)	242	276	330	384	432	486	534	582	630	678	726	774
Skiing (cross-country)												
4 mph	352	432	510	594	672	774	828	882	936	990	1,044	1,098
5 mph	412	504	600	690	786	882	972	1,062	1,152	1,242	1,332	1,416
Skiing (downhill)	380	432	510	594	672	750	828	906	984	1,062	1,140	1,218

Weight in Pounds

TABLE 6.1   **Calories Expended per Hour for Various Physical Activities** *(Continued)*

					Weight in Pounds							
	90	110	130	150	170	190	210	230	250	270	290	310
Activity						kcal						
Soccer or rugby	324	395	468	540	612	684	756	824	900	972	1,044	1,116
Squash (competitive)	384	504	624	690	786	882	972	1,062	1,152	1,242	1,332	1,410
Stair climbing and descending												
1 stair—25 trips/min	246	294	360	408	462	509	576	624	660	708	756	792
1 stair—30 trips/min	282	318	396	444	498	558	624	678	726	774	822	870
1 stair—35 trips/min	312	360	450	510	570	635	714	774	834	894	954	1,014
3 stairs—12 trips/min	294	342	426	486	540	599	678	732	786	840	894	948
3 stairs—15 trips/min	364	414	516	588	654	727	816	888	960	1,032	1,104	1,176
Stock clerk	132	162	192	222	252	276	306	336	366	396	426	456
Swimming												
Backstroke	420	510	600	690	780	870	966	1,062	1,164	1,260	1,356	1,452
Breastroke	404	486	576	660	750	934	927	1,020	1,113	1,206	1,299	1,392
Sidestroke	296	366	432	498	564	630	698	765	833	900	967	1,044
Crawl (slow)	306	693	486	522	612	660	732	804	876	948	1,020	1,092
Crawl (fast)	384	468	552	636	720	804	892	979	1,067	1,154	1,242	1,330
Table tennis	190	228	270	312	354	396	438	480	522	564	606	648
Tennis singles	276	330	384	444	504	564	626	686	746	806	866	926
Doubles	192	228	270	312	354	396	438	480	522	564	606	648
Typing (computer)	72	84	96	108	126	138	156	174	192	210	228	246
Volleyball	120	150	180	204	234	258	288	318	348	378	408	426
Walking												
3 mph	144	168	192	222	252	282	312	342	372	402	432	462
4 mph	212	246	288	336	378	430	468	516	558	600	642	684
5 mph	314	396	468	540	612	684	756	824	900	972	1,044	1,116
Wallpapering	120	144	198	222	246	276	306	336	366	396	426	456
Water-skiing	270	330	390	450	510	570	636	702	768	834	900	966
Weight training	274	340	408	468	534	594	660	732	798	864	930	996
Wrestling	462	558	990	768	870	972	1,074	1,176	1,278	1,380	1,482	1,524

Notes: The approximate figures in the table include resting energy expenditure (the kcal you would have expended during this period while at rest) and the kcal expended by the activity. The chart does not account for the additional caloric expenditure occurring from metabolism remaining above baseline for 20 minutes to several hours after exercise ceases (afterburn). Calculations are only approximate and include only the time you are actually performing the activity. Small differences do exist between males and females in kcal expended, but the difference is not significant in the total kcal expended for most activities.

Not all body weights are listed. Use the closest weight shown to determine number of kcal expended.

For optimum weight and fat loss, choose an activity that expends a minimum of 2,000 kcal per week in four to five workouts, or 400 to 500 kcal per exercise session.

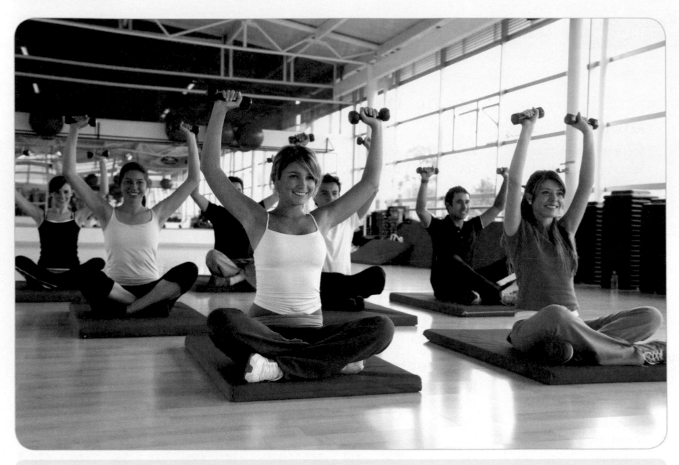

Social health benefits can be obtained by exercising with other people.

component. Social health benefits include increased so-cial support, a feeling of connection to others, decreased feelings of loneliness and depression, and motivation to maintain your exercise program. Joining a health club or exercising at the campus gym can produce these same benefits because you are exercising with others around you. Even people who engage in seemingly solitary physi-cal activities (such as running) see a benefit to being en-gaged with others. As a result, they often join running clubs or participate in races.

Design Your Personal Fitness Program

To design your exercise program, you need to recognize your preferences. Swimming laps is great for some peo-ple, whereas others find it too repetitious. Sports such as

basketball or tennis are great for some people, whereas others do not have enough skill to enjoy these sports. Take care to design a program that is consistent with your in-terests, skills, available time, access to facilities and equip-ment, and that costs an amount you can afford. This way, the likelihood of your continued participation in the pro-gram over time will greatly increase. The sections that follow offer guidelines to help you design your personal fitness program and to maintain that program once you start.

Include Exercises for All Components of Fitness

To be physically fit, your exercise program needs to include cardiorespiratory fitness activities, muscular strength and endurance training, flexibility stretches, and activities de-signed to improve body composition. To emphasize one

What I Need to Know

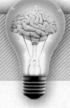

The Amount of Physical Activity You Need

In July 2011, the American College of Sports Medicine published guidelines recommending the type and amount of physical activity necessary to be healthy. On the basis of scientific evidence, the guideline included the following recommendations:

- Moderate-intensity cardiorespiratory exercise for 30 minutes or longer on at least 5 days a week for a total of at least 150 minutes per week.

- Vigorous-intensity exercise for 20 minutes or longer on at least 3 days a week for a total of at least 75 minutes per week.

- Weight-training exercises for each of the major muscle groups on 2 or 3 days a week.

- Neuromotor exercises involving balance, agility, and coordination on 2–3 days a week.

- Flexibility exercises for each of the major muscle-tendon groups of at least 60 seconds per exercise on at least 2 days a week.

ADAPTED FROM: Garber, C. E., Blissmer, B., Deschenes, M. R., Franklin, B. A., Lamonte, M. J., Lee, I-M., Nieman, D. C., and Swain, D. P. Quantity and quality of exercise for developing and maintaining cardiorespiratory, musculoskeletal, and neuromotor fitness in apparently healthy adults: Guidance for prescribing exercise. *Medicine & Science in Sports & Exercise* 43 (2011): 1334–1359.

component over another is to develop an unhealthy imbalance. For example, if you bike long distances, your cardiorespiratory fitness is probably excellent. However, your flexibility may be poor subjecting you to the risk of injury. Determine which physical activities are best for you by completing Health Check Up 6.5 (see Health Check Up 6.5 on the companion website). Once completed, place Health Check Up 6.5 in your Health Decision Portfolio.

Frequency, Intensity, and Duration

Next, you need to establish the frequency, intensity, and duration of the physical activities composing your program. Adults over 18 years of age need 30 minutes of physical activity on 5 or more days a week. Significant health benefits can be obtained by even a moderate amount of physical activity (such as brisk walking or raking leaves), although additional health benefits derive from greater amounts of physical activity (such as a 45-minute run). In fact, 30 to 60 minutes of physical activity broken into smaller segments of 10 to 15 minutes throughout the day also produces health benefits (President's Council on Physical Fitness and Sports, 2010). Physical activity that

produces health benefits usually entails perspiring and breathing heavily, but at a pace that still allows one to carry on a conversation.

Cardiorespiratory Fitness Exercises

Improvement of cardiorespiratory fitness requires prolonged physical activity—called **aerobic exercise**—that results in heavy breathing. Running, playing volleyball, dancing, walking, and swimming are all aerobic activities. During aerobic exercise, the body can provide all of its need for oxygen, allowing the activity to be sustained and continuous. In contrast, **anaerobic exercise**—such as

Aerobic exercise: exercise in which the body can provide all of its need for oxygen, allowing the activity to be sustained and continuous.

Anaerobic exercise: exercise that depletes oxygen over a short period of time—such as running a 100-yard dash or sprinting—and, therefore, cannot be sustained as long as aerobic exercise.

TABLE 6.2	**Recommended Moderate Physical Activities**

Even moderate physical activity can help improve your health. Here is a list of moderate physical activities and the duration they should be performed as recommended by the Surgeon General of the United States.

Activity	Duration
Washing and waxing a car	45–60 min
Washing windows or floors	45–60 min
Playing volleyball	45 min
Playing touch football	30–45 min
Gardening	30–45 min
Wheeling self in wheelchair	30–40 min
Walking 1¾ miles	In 35 min (20 min per mile)
Playing basketball (shooting baskets)	30 min
Bicycling 5 miles	In 30 min
Dancing fast (social)	30 min
Pushing a stroller 1½ miles	30 min
Raking leaves	30 min
Walking 2 miles	In 30 min (15 min per mile)
Doing water aerobics	30 min
Swimming laps	20 min
Playing wheelchair basketball	20 min
Playing basketball (playing a game)	15–20 min
Bicycling 4 miles	In 15 min
Jumping rope	15 min
Running 1½ miles	In 15 min (10 min per mile)
Shoveling snow	15 min
Stair walking	25 min

Note: The activities at the top of the list are less intense and therefore require a longer duration to produce benefits. The activities in the lower portion of the list are more intense and therefore require a shorter duration to produce benefits.

REPRODUCED FROM: U.S. Public Health Service. *Physical Activity and Health: A Report of the Surgeon General: Executive Summary*. Washington, DC: U.S. Department of Health and Human Services, 1996. http://www.cdc.gov/nccdphp/sgr/contents.htm

running a 100-yard dash or sprinting—depletes oxygen over a short period of time and, therefore, cannot be sustained as long as aerobic exercise. Table 6.2 lists moderate physical activities that can be incorporated into your fitness program to enhance cardiorespiratory fitness. One way to ensure your heart is beating fast enough to improve your cardiorespiratory fitness is to determine your target heart rate. Your **target heart rate** is how fast your heart should beat during exercise to improve your cardiorespiratory fitness. This is in contrast to your **resting heart rate**, which is how fast your heart beats when you are at rest.

Health Check Up 6.6 shows you how to calculate both these rates (see Health Check Up 6.6 on the companion website). After completing Health Check Up 6.6, place it in your Health Decision Portfolio.

Target heart rate: how fast the heart should beat during exercise to improve cardiorespiratory fitness.

Resting heart rate: how fast your heart beats when you are at rest.

Muscular Strength and Endurance Exercises

To improve muscular strength and endurance, you need to work muscle groups throughout your body (Cloe, 2010): *gluteals* (your butt), *quadriceps* (front of the thigh), *hamstrings* (back of the thigh), *hip adductors* (inner thigh) and *abductors* (outer thigh), *calf* (back of the lower leg), *lower back, abdominals, pectoralis major* (front of the upper chest), *rhomboids* (middle of the upper back between the shoulder blades), *trapezius* (upper portion of the back), *latissimus dorsi* (mid-back), *deltoids* (shoulder), *biceps* (front of the upper arm), and the *triceps* (back of the upper arm).

To weight train effectively, stick to some basic guidelines:

- Start with the large muscles before progressing to the smaller ones. This will allow you to lift heavier weights when you are less fatigued.

- Spend 1 to 2 seconds lifting the weight and 3 to 4 seconds lowering the weight. This avoids undue stress on the muscles and works them better by eliminating momentum. Do not jerk, bounce, or swing the weight.

- Perform two or three **sets** (successive periods of lifting without rest) of 8–12 **reps** (short for repetitions; the number of times the weight is lifted in each set). Start with lower weight and increase weight gradually until you can adhere to this guideline.

- As your muscles adapt to the weight over time (i.e., you can perform three sets of 12 reps each), increase the weight approximately 5–10%.

- Because muscle recovery takes 48 hours, do not lift more frequently than every other day. Alternatively, you can train one muscle group one day (e.g., your lower body) and another muscle group the next day (e.g., your upper body).

- Do not hold your breath. Breathe out as you lift the weight. This helps avoid excessive blood pressure during weight training.

Do not expect your body's appearance to change too quickly or you will be disappointed and tempted to give up weight training. Significant increases in muscle thickness take 4–6 weeks, although gains in strength occur sooner (Garzarella, Pollock, DeHoyos, and Takashi, 2000). This holds true for both men and women.

Flexibility Exercises

Never stretch a cold muscle. That can lead to injury. Instead, warm up the muscles by performing your program's cardiorespiratory activity for about 5 minutes, but at a lower intensity. Then, start each stretch slowly, holding the stretch for 10 to 30 seconds. Do not bounce into the stretch as that can cause injury. The stretch should not be painful. Stretch only as far as it is comfortable.

It is more important to stretch after exercising than before. Stretching afterward ensures that muscles are already warmed up and helps them recover from activity. Aside from stretching after exercise, stretching after a warm bath or shower, with the temperature in the muscles raised, is also good idea. See **FIG. 6.1 ▶** for flexibility exercises that stretch the upper body and **FIG. 6.2 ▶** for flexibility exercises that stretch the lower body.

Select Physical Activities That Work for You

Even if you start an exercise program, you will not continue with it if the activities you choose are not right for you. If you decide to swim regularly but you are a poor swimmer, you may get frustrated and eventually quit. If you decide to play soccer or softball but are not skilled at these sports, you may have difficulty maintaining your fitness program. If you decide to run but live where it gets extremely cold in the winter, you are likely to give up running during those months.

Furthermore, some activities involve certain characteristics that you may lack. If you are not very social, you would not want to select an intramural volleyball team as your form of exercise. Then again, you might purposefully do that to develop social skills. Some fitness activities

---

Sets: successive periods of lifting without rest.

Reps (repetitions): the number of lifts during each set.

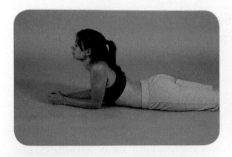

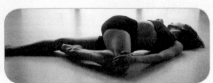

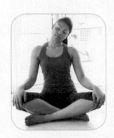

(a) Press-up

Stretches the lower back and abdominals. Lie face down with your arms under your face. Then, raise your upper body as you lean on your forearms. Hold for 30 seconds.

(b) Trunk twist

Stretches the lower back and sides. Lie on your side, straighten one leg, and bend the other knee on top of that leg. Extend the arm on the same side as the bent knee toward your foot, and extend the other arm out to the side. Then, push your bent knee down as you twist your body backward; all the while keeping upper body and shoulders touching the floor. Do one side and then alternate to the other.

(c) Head turns and tilts

Stretches the neck. Turn your head as far as it will go toward the right, and hold that stretch for a few seconds. Then, tilt your head toward the right and hold that stretch for a few seconds. Next, turn and tilt in the same manner to the left.

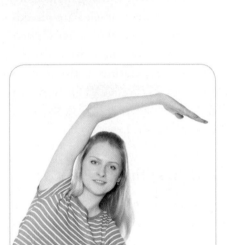

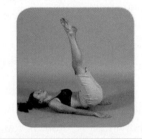

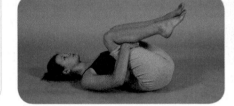

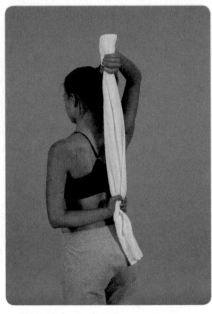

(d) Lateral stretch

Stretches the trunk. Stand with your feet spread at shoulder width, knees bent, and place one hand on your hip. Then raise the other arm over your head, as you bend toward the other side. Do one side and then alternate to the other.

(e) Double knee to chest

Stretches the lower back and hips. Lie on your back and straighten your legs. Hold the back of your thighs and pull your knees toward your chest. Hold for a few seconds and then extend your legs up while straightening your knees. After a few seconds, return to the previous position with the knees bent toward your chest. After a few seconds, return to your original position with your legs straight out.

(f) Triceps stretch

Stretches the upper arms. While holding a towel with one hand, throw it over your back. Then grab the lower part of the towel with the other hand, reaching as far up the towel as you can. Attempt to have your hands touch each other. Do one arm and then alternate to the other.

FIGURE 6.1   Upper body stretches.

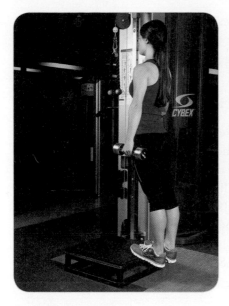

(a) Lower leg stretch

Stretches the Achilles tendon. While holding onto a railing, stand with the front half of your foot on a step. Raise as high up on your toes as you can. Hold for 30 seconds. Do one foot and then alternate to the other.

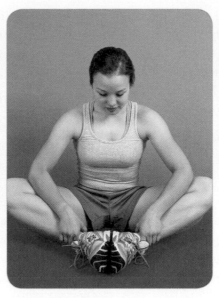

(b) Sole stretch

Stretches the inner thighs and hips. While seated, place the souls of your feet together while pushing your knees toward the floor. Hold for 30 seconds.

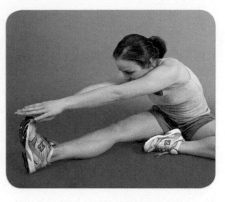

(c) Modified hurdler stretch

Stretches the back of the thighs. Sit with one leg straight out and the other leg bent with the foot near the body. Then reach as far as you can toward the soul of the straight leg. Do one thigh and then alternate to the other.

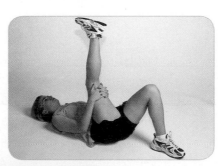

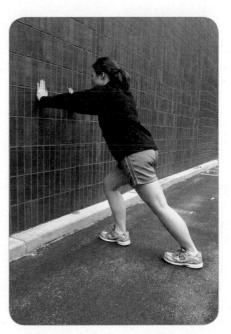

(d) Alternate leg stretch

Stretches the back of the thighs, hips, knees, ankles, and buttocks. While lying on your back, place your hand behind the lower thigh of one leg and pull that leg toward your head with the knee bent. Hold for a few seconds. Then straighten that knee and raise the leg straight up. Hold that position for a few seconds. Next, bend the knee once again and by pulling on your toes, try to straighten the leg. Do one leg and then alternate to the other.

(e) Calf stretch

Stretches the calf. Stand with your hands on a wall, with elbows straight. With one knee bent slightly, place the other foot flat on the floor and a few feet back. Make sure the knee is straight. Hold for 30 seconds. Then bend the knee with the foot remaining flat on the floor. Hold for 30 seconds. Do one calf and then alternate to the other.

FIGURE 6.2   Lower body stretches.

involve competition and you may abhor competition. To determine which physical activities are best for you, complete Health Check Up 6.6 (see Health Check Up 6.6 on the companion website). Once completed, place Health Check Up 6.6 in your Health Decision Portfolio.

Incorporate Exercise into Your Daily Life

Exercise does not have to be tedious or time consuming. You can build it into your normal everyday activities. Walk up or down stairs instead of taking an elevator. Get off the bus or the train a stop before you normally would and walk the rest of the way to your destination. Stretch at your desk as a break from work or study. Walk instead of taking the car. In fact, walking is an excellent fitness activity. It requires no special skill and it can be incorporated into your daily routine. Table 6.3 will help you develop a walking program.

Schedule Exercise

If you want to exercise regularly, schedule it into your routine. You are more likely to engage in physical activity if it is at the same time and on the same days each week. That way, you will know not to plan any other activities during that time. If you just exercise when you feel like it, you are more likely either to forget or to decide to refrain from exercising when you feel like doing something else. You can make fitness a priority by scheduling exercise first and working other activities around it.

TABLE 6.3	Guidelines for Developing a Walking Program

Walking regularly can help you develop physical fitness. However, to prevent injury, the walking program should start at a low level and increase in intensity gradually. This table presents a walking program that meets these criteria.

Week	Warm-Up	Target Zone Exercising	Cool-Down	Total Time
Week 1				
Session A	Walk 5 min	5-min brisk walk	5-min slow walk	15 min
Session B	Walk 5 min	5-min brisk walk	5-min slow walk	15 min
Session C	Walk 5 min	5-min brisk walk	5-min slow walk	15 min
Week 2	Walk 5 min	7-min brisk walk	Walk 5 min	17 min
Week 3	Walk 5 min	9-min brisk walk	Walk 5 min	19 min
Week 4	Walk 5 min	11-min brisk walk	Walk 5 min	21 min
Week 5	Walk 5 min	13-min brisk walk	Walk 5 min	23 min
Week 6	Walk 5 min	15-min brisk walk	Walk 5 min	25 min
Week 7	Walk 5 min	18-min brisk walk	Walk 5 min	28 min
Week 8	Walk 5 min	20-min brisk walk	Walk 5 min	30 min
Week 9	Walk 5 min	23-min brisk walk	Walk 5 min	33 min
Week 10	Walk 5 min	26-min brisk walk	Walk 5 min	36 min
Week 11	Walk 5 min	28-min brisk walk	Walk 5 min	38 min
Week 12	Walk 5 min	30-min brisk walk	Walk 5 min	40 min
Week 13 and on	Check your pulse periodically to see whether you are exercising within your target zone. As you become more fit, try exercising within the upper range of your target zone. Gradually increase your brisk walking time to 30 to 60 min three or four times a week. Remember that your goal is to gain the benefits you are seeking and to enjoy the activity.			

REPRODUCED FROM: The National Heart Lung and Blood Institute, Your Guide to Lowering High Blood Pressure. http://www.nhlbi.nih.gov/hbp/prevent/p_active/walk.htm

What I Need to Know

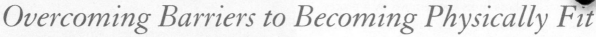

Overcoming Barriers to Becoming Physically Fit

Researchers have studied barriers that interfere with people being physically active. Among these barriers are cost, time, access to convenient facilities, and high crime rates and unsafe environments. Factors that affect your health behavior include financial, psychological, social, and environmental barriers.

1. Describe a health behavior you would like to adopt or an unhealthy behavior you would like to give up.

    _____

    _____

2. Identify the barriers that make it more difficult for you to make this health behavior change.

    (A) Financial barriers, such as cost, time, or inconvenience:

    (i) _____

    (ii) _____

    (iii) _____

    (B) Psychological barriers, such as embarrassment or fear of failure:

    (i) _____

    (ii) _____

    (iii) _____

    (C) Social barriers, such as peer pressure:

    (i) _____

    (ii) _____

    (iii) _____

    (D) Environmental barriers, such as fast food restaurants being convenient:

    (i) _____

    (ii) _____

    (iii) _____

3. For each of the 12 barriers listed above, identify a strategy that would be successful in helping you behave more healthfully. (Note that use of these strategies is sort of like "chaining.")

    (A) Strategies to remove financial barriers:

    (i) _____

    (ii) _____

    (iii) _____

    (B) Strategies to remove psychological barriers:

    (i) _____

    (ii) _____

    (iii) _____

    (C) Strategies to remove social barriers:

    (i) _____

    (ii) _____

    (iii) _____

    (D) Strategies to remove environmental barriers:

    (i) _____

    (ii) _____

    (iii) _____

You can now formulate a plan using the strategies listed above to take charge of your health behavior.

ADAPTED FROM: President's Council on Physical Fitness and Sports. Physical activity facts. *Resources*. 2010. Available at: http://www.fitness.gov/resources_factsheet.htm; Adapted from: Seefeldt, V., Malina, R. M., and Clark, M. A. Factors affecting levels of physical activity in adults. *Sports Medicine* 32 (2002): 143–168.

Use the Behavioral Strategy of Chaining

A chain has many links, and so does behavior. Consider exercise. You need to buy the right clothing, dress in that clothing, and travel to a place to exercise (e.g., a track or gym). The more of those links you remove, by a process called "chaining," the more likely you are to exercise. **Chaining** is a behavior change strategy whereby obstacles (links of the chain) to achieving a particular behavior are removed, making a positive outcome more likely. If you lay out your exercise clothing (shorts, shirt, shoes, etc.) before you go to class, you avoid having to search for that clothing when you get home—in other words, you remove that link. Better yet, if you wear that clothing to class, you do not even have to go home to change. If you join a health club within walking distance of your classes, you eliminate the link of having to travel very far to get to the gym. The idea is to make exercising as easy as possible. Chaining can help you do that.

Evaluate Health and Fitness Clubs

You are probably fortunate in that your campus has fitness facilities. Most likely, they are free for you to use. When you graduate, however, to maintain a lifetime of fitness you may consider joining a health and fitness club. There are many choices when it comes to such clubs, and deciding which one is best for you can be confusing. To spend your money wisely, you should evaluate any club you are thinking of joining. The American College of Sports Medicine (2006) publishes standards for health and fitness clubs. These standards pertain to the equipment available, how use of that equipment is supervised, the quality of the relationship between the staff and clients, and safety procedures in case of accidents or emergencies. Health Check Up 6.7 will help you evaluate the club(s) you are considering to join (see Health Check Up 6.7 on the companion website). Once completed, place Health Check Up 6.7 in your Health Decision Portfolio.

Evaluate Home Exercise Equipment

Some people find it more convenient to exercise at home than at the club. Others prefer to work out at home because they are embarrassed to have others watch them exercise. For these reasons and more, many people

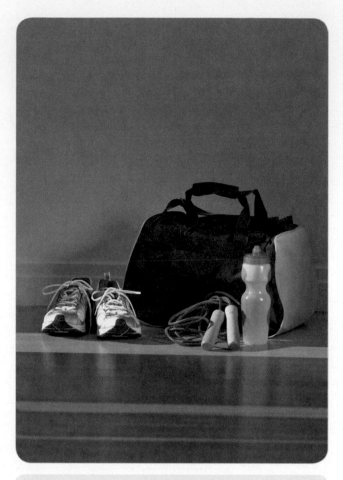

Preparation beforehand by laying out clothing is one way to make it easier to be physically active. Such preparation reduces the links in the chain of activities necessary to engage in exercise.

purchase home exercise equipment such as a stationary bike, weights, a treadmill, or other aids to being physically fit. Because it can be quite expensive, you should carefully evaluate exercise equipment before making a purchase. The Federal Trade Commission offers this advice when making an evaluation: Evaluate advertising

Chaining: a behavior change strategy that considers the many obstacles to performing a behavior as links in a chain; decreasing the number of links makes the behavior easier to do and more likely to occur.

claims for fitness products carefully. Be skeptical of claims that you will lose several pounds, inches, or pant sizes in a short time (e.g., "7 inches in 7 days" or "3 dress sizes in 1 month"). Even when the use of exercise equipment is combined with dietary changes, it is virtually impossible for most consumers to achieve such major changes in appearance in a few days or weeks.

The Federal Trade Commission (2009) advises consumers to:

■ Ignore claims that an exercise machine or device can provide long-lasting, easy, "no-sweat" results in a short time. These claims are false: You cannot get the benefits of exercise unless you exercise regularly over a long period of time.

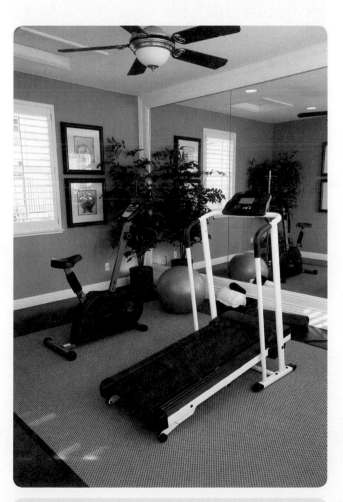

When choosing home health equipment, adhere to the guidelines provided by the Federal Trade Commission.

■ Question claims that a product can burn fat off a particular part of the body; for example, the buttocks, hips, or stomach. Achievement of a major change in your appearance requires sensible eating and regular exercise that works the whole body.

■ Read the ad's fine print. The advertised results may be based on more than just use of a machine; they also may be based on restriction of calories.

■ Be skeptical of testimonials and before-and-after pictures from *satisfied* customers. Their experiences may not be typical. Just because one person had success with the equipment does not mean you will, too.

■ Do the calculations when you read statements like "three easy payments of ... " or "only $49.95 a month." The advertised cost may not include shipping and handling fees, sales tax, and delivery and set-up fees. Find out the details before you order.

■ Get details on warranties, guarantees, and return policies. A "30-day money-back guarantee" may not sound as good if you have to pay shipping on a bulky piece of equipment you want to "return to sender."

■ Check out the company's customer and support services. Call the advertised toll-free numbers to get an idea of how easy it is to reach a company representative and how helpful he or she is.

Finalize Your Personal Fitness Program

Now that you know the essential components of an effective personal fitness program, you can apply this knowledge. Complete Health Check Up 6.8 to design an exercise program that is just right for you (see Health Check Up 6.8 on the companion website). After completing Health Check Up 6.8, place it in your Health Decision Portfolio.

Maintain Your Exercise Program

Starting an exercise program is the first step to becoming physically fit. Maintaining that program over time is the next step. Fortunately, there are several effective techniques you can use to continue your exercise program once you start it.

Use Social Support

When you get the support of others, you are more likely to maintain your exercise program. That support can take many forms. Perhaps you exercise with a friend or in a group. In that case, you do not want to let other people down by not showing up. Perhaps a family member is paying for your health and fitness club membership. To not work out would make you feel guilty and selfish. Or, perhaps your family is so proud of you for exercising that they brag about you to other relatives and friends. To revert back to a sedentary lifestyle would let your family down and deprive you of their feelings of pride. One strategy, then, to maintain your exercise program is to enlist the support of other people.

Develop a Contract

Another technique to help you maintain your workouts is to write a contract in which you agree to exercise regularly. The contract should include a *specific* behavior and a *date* by when the behavior will be evaluated. See the Applying Behavior Change Theory feature My Health Commitment, a behavioral change contract, on the companion website. Use this contract to determine and state your fitness-related goal and commit to a timetable for reaching it. If you are successful, reward yourself as specified in the contract. If you are not, make whatever adjustments are necessary and form a new contract. Once completed, place the Applying Behavior Change Theory feature in your Health Decision Portfolio.

Use Reminder Systems

There are effective strategies you can use to remind and encourage yourself to be physically active. A simple, low-tech way is to put notes in places where you are sure to see them—bathroom mirrors or refrigerators work well. Or, you could use a little technology—program a text message to be sent to you an hour or so before your regular routine or ask a friend to call or text you a reminder message.

Keep a Journal

Some people keep a detailed journal that includes the days on which they exercised, the specific physical activity they

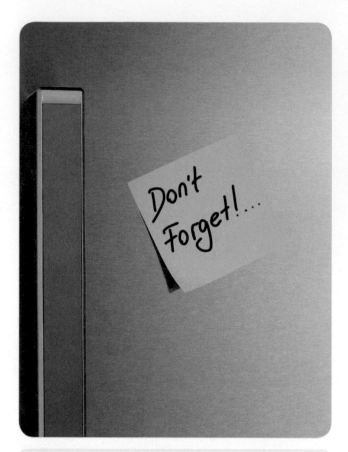

A note placed on a refrigerator or on a bathroom mirror can serve as a reminder to exercise.

performed, the intensity and duration of that activity, the weather (if the activity was performed outdoors), and their feelings or body sensations during and after the activity. This level of detail, which they read periodically, reinforces their exercise behavior and helps them maintain their workout program.

Such a detailed journal, however, may not be necessary. For example, some runners and walkers only keep a record of their mileage. They can then add up their mileage and plot it on a map showing how far they have traveled over time. You can keep a journal to record any details in which you are interested; for example, your resting heart rate, the amount of weight you are lifting, or notes about any friends or people you meet during exercise (especially if you are interested in using exercise to make friends). Noting changes over time will help motivate you to maintain your exercise program.

Make It Fun

I tried downhill skiing once. Being an athlete, I thought I would try an advanced slope. Getting a little behind on each curve, I eventually saw a forest of trees approaching that I would not be able to avoid. As my heart started racing, I did the first thing that came to mind—I sat on my rear end and stopped myself just short of a catastrophe. I spent the rest of the day in the lodge cowering behind a hot drink. Skiing was just not fun for me, so I never tried it again.

If you do not enjoy the physical activity, you will likely not maintain it over time. Making the activity fun is important and can be accomplished in many ways; here are a few suggestions:

- Spice up a more monotonous routine by listening to your favorite music.

- Make exercise a social event by using a gaming console to play a virtual sport with friends.

- Satisfy your competitive spirit by finding a sport in which you have talent and can demonstrate your skill in competition.

- Focus on the enjoyable aspects of the activity (e.g., paying attention to the sounds of the birds and the wind rustling through the leaves when running). If you enjoy what you are doing, you are more likely to continue doing it. Health Check Up 6.9 helps you strategize ways to maintain your exercise program (see Health Check Up 6.9 on the companion website). After completing Health Check Up 6.9, place it in your Health Decision Portfolio.

Avoid Injuries

More than 10,000 people receive treatment in the nation's emergency departments each day for injuries sustained in sports, recreation, or exercise activities. At least one of every five emergency department visits for an injury results from participation in sports or recreation, and injuries are a leading reason people cease participation in beneficial physical activity (Centers for Disease Control and Prevention, 2006). If you can prevent fitness injuries, you are more likely to maintain your exercise program and be physically fit.

Common Fitness Injuries

Injuries commonly experienced by physically active people include ankle sprain; charley horse; tennis elbow; fractured bones; hamstring and quadriceps muscle pulls; knee ligament, tendon, and cartilage problems; shin splints; tendonitis; and muscle soreness and cramps. The causes and treatments of these and other common fitness injuries are presented in Table 6.4.

Strategies for Injury Prevention

When you exercise, experts recommend that you follow these tips (American Academy of Orthopaedic Surgeons, 2007; American College of Emergency Physicians, 2010):

- Always wear appropriate safety gear. If you bike, always wear a bike helmet. Wear the appropriate shoes for each sport.

- Warm up before exercising. This could be a moderate activity such as walking at your normal pace while emphasizing your arm movements.

- Drink a sufficient amount of water before, during, and after your routine.

- Always exercise at a comfortable fitness level.

- Exercise for at least 30 minutes a day. You can break this into shorter periods of 10 or 15 minutes during the day.

- Follow the 10% rule. Never increase your program (i.e., walking or running distance or amount of weight lifted) more than 10% a week.

- Try not to do the exact same routine 2 days in a row; for example, on successive days you might walk, swim, play tennis, and then lift weights. This works different muscles and keeps exercise more interesting.

- When working out with exercise equipment, read instructions carefully, and, if needed, ask a qualified person to help you. Check treadmills or other exercise equipment to be sure they are in good working order.

TABLE 6.4 **Common Injuries: Causes and Treatments**

Injury	Cause	Treatment
Ankle sprain	Twisting, stepping on someone's foot. Exacerbated by poor flexibility.	RICE (Rest, Ice, Compression, and Elevation). See a healthcare provider if swelling or pain persists for 3 days or if pain prevents walking.
Charley horse (thigh bruise)	A blow to the relaxed thigh.	RICE. See a healthcare provider if pain or discoloration does not disappear after a few days or if numbness, weakness, or tingling occurs.
Tennis or pitcher's elbow	Twisting of the arm.	Apply ice after exercise. See a healthcare provider if pain persists after several weeks.
Fractures (broken bone)	A blow to the bone.	Immobilize the body part. Apply ice immediately to decrease swelling, compress the area with a compression bandage, and elevate the body part. See a healthcare provider as soon as possible.
Hamstring pulls (strains of the muscle group in the upper back of the leg)	Stretching the muscle. Exacerbated by poor flexibility.	RICE. See a healthcare provider if severe swelling or discoloration occurs, if pain persists after 10 to 15 days of self-treatment, or if numbness, tingling, or weakness occurs.
Quadriceps pulls (strains of the muscle group in the upper front of the leg)	Overstretching the muscle. Exacerbated by poor flexibility.	RICE. See a healthcare provider if severe swelling or discoloration occurs, if pain persists after 10 to 15 days of self-treatment, or if numbness, tingling, or weakness occurs.
Knee cartilage tears	Long-term wear and tear.	If a minor tear, aspirin, ibuprofen, and strengthening and flexibility exercises might help. If not, surgery may be needed. A healthcare provider should be consulted to diagnose the extent of the injury.
Knee ligament tears and tendon ruptures	Movement of the joint through too large a range of motion. Exacerbated by poor flexibility.	A medical care provider should be consulted to diagnose the injury. Surgery is needed to repair the ligament or to reattach the tendon.
Shin splints (inflammation of the large bone in the lower leg)	Overuse, exercising on hard surfaces.	RICE for several days and then apply heat, refrain from exercising on hard surfaces, cut back on the intensity and duration of exercise, use stretching exercises, wear well-fitted shoes. See a healthcare provider if pain persists for more than 3 weeks or if the injury reoccurs.
Tendonitis (inflammation of a tendon such as the Achilles tendon)	Overuse of the body part.	RICE. Stretching exercises. Exercise lightly until pain disappears.
Blisters	Friction causing the top skin layer to separate from the second layer.	Apply antibiotic salve if blister breaks. For blisters on the feet, use clean socks, apply petroleum jelly to the blister to decrease friction, and wear comfortably fitting shoes. See a healthcare provider if pain occurs under the arms or in the groin or if redness occurs in the involved limb, as these are signs of infection.

TABLE 6.4	Common Injuries: Causes and Treatments *(Continued)*	
Injury	**Cause**	**Treatment**
Stress fracture (a small crack in the bone's surface)	Overuse or exercise at too intense a level.	Cut back on workouts, exercise on soft surfaces, rest, and ensure that proper footwear is used. See a healthcare provider if night pains occur or if pain increases with activity.
Nosebleed	Blow to the nose.	While seated and with the head tilted forward, squeeze the nose between the thumb and forefinger for 5 to 10 minutes. Do not lie down or lean the head backwards.
Groin strain	Running, jumping, or twisting. Exacerbated by poor flexibility.	RICE
Hernia (a body organ—usually the intestine—protruding through a tear in the abdominal wall)	Lifting a heavy object with improper form, such as might occur during weight training.	A healthcare provider should be consulted to determine whether surgery is needed to repair the tear in the abdominal wall.
Muscle soreness	Warming up improperly, doing too much too soon, lack of flexibility.	Increase flexibility exercises, cut back on workouts, warm up and cool down properly.
Muscle cramps	Fatigue, tightness of muscle, or fluid imbalance (salt or potassium).	Stretch the muscle, drink water or a sports drink, rub the area to increase blood flow.

If you are new to weight training, make sure you get proper information before you begin.

- Stop exercising if you experience severe pain or swelling. Discomfort that persists should always be evaluated.

- Stop exercising if you experience dizziness, shortness of breath, irregular heartbeat, or increased fatigue. Consult with your healthcare provider if these symptoms occur.

- Complete Health Check Up 6.10 to plan ways to prevent exercise injuries. Once completed, place Health Check Up 6.10 in your Health Decision Portfolio (see Health Check Up 6.10 on the companion website).

Warm Up

When you begin to exercise, muscles need oxygen to contract. Your heart rate, blood flow, cardiac output, and breathing rate increase to supply this increased need for oxygen to working muscles. In addition, your blood temperature increases, raising the temperature of the muscles. A warm-up before exercise is needed to ensure these changes occur gradually. Specifically, a warm-up leads to efficient calorie burning by increasing your core body temperature, produces faster and more forceful muscle contractions, prevents injuries by improving the elasticity of your muscles, prevents the buildup of lactic acid in the blood, and improves joint range of motion (American Council on Exercise, 2010c).

The warm-up consists of two phases. The *aerobic phase* warms up muscles to be used during the exercise. It involves performing the same activity to be performed during the exercise but at a lower intensity. For example, if you are going to run, the aerobic phase might consist of a slow jog. The *flexibility phase*, conducted after the aerobic warm-up, involves stretching the muscles to be used during the exercise.

Cool Down and Stretch

After exercise, a cool-down is needed to get the blood that has been pooled in the muscles back to the heart. Without a cool-down, you might feel dizzy because of low blood pressure. To prevent this sensation, a slow walk or jog is recommended. In addition, stretching of fatigued muscles can prevent muscle spasms.

When your muscles are tight, you are more likely to become injured. This is because your range of motion is limited, and when you move beyond that range, you may tear tendons or ligaments or develop sprains. Stretching exercises increase flexibility and help you prevent exercise injuries. Figures 6.1 and 6.2 presented earlier in this chapter describe excellent stretching exercises.

Replace Fluids

Failure to drink enough water during exercise can lead to **dehydration**, which can cause nausea, diarrhea, and weakness. Drinking too much water, however, can lead to **hyponatremia**, or low blood sodium levels. Hyponatremia can result in nausea, disorientation, muscle weakness, coma, or death. Recognizing these threats, the International Marathon Medical Director's Association (IMMDA) in 2006 revised its guidelines for fluid replenishment before, during, and after exercise. The International Marathon Medical Director's Association (2006) recommends that exercisers drink when thirsty and not force fluid replacement. In other words, if you are not thirsty, refrain from drinking. The IMMDA also advises drinking of a sports drink for a vigorous workout longer than 30 minutes. Sports drinks contain added carbohydrates that are absorbed by the body 30% faster than water and provide energy. They also contain electrolytes—sodium and potassium—that speed absorption of fluids and help maintain healthy blood sodium levels (Bieler, 2006).

Avoid Overuse

Too much of a good thing is too much of a good thing. You wouldn't take more than the recommended dosage of a medication prescribed by your physician, just as you shouldn't engage in more exercise than is recommended.

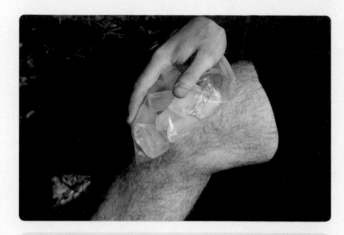

Many exercise injuries can be self-treated by resting, icing, compressing, and elevating the injured body part.

To do so subjects you to *overuse syndrome* in which symptoms of fatigue, muscle strain, joint soreness, and frequent illness can occur. The best way to prevent overuse syndrome is to follow your exercise plan and listen to your body. If any of the above symptoms occur, adjust your exercise until you are feeling better. Remember not to overdo it.

Treat Injuries That Do Occur

If you are physically active, inevitably injuries will occur. However, if the precautions discussed earlier are taken, injuries will be kept to a minimum and will be less severe. When injuries do occur, there are several self-help steps you can take to recover faster. However, it is also important to recognize situations that require the help of a healthcare provider.

RICE

Some injuries can be self-treated. These include a charley horse (a bruise to the thigh muscle), muscle strains

Dehydration: too little water/fluid in the body, which can cause nausea, diarrhea, and weakness.

Hyponatremia: drinking too much water resulting in low blood sodium levels, which can lead to nausea, disorientation, muscle weakness, coma, or death.

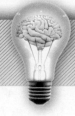

What I Need to Know

Exercising in Hot and Cold Weather

Exercising in cold or hot weather presents certain risks. In cold weather, there is the risk of frostbite; in hot weather, there is the risk of heat exhaustion or heat stroke. To prevent injury in hot or cold weather, follow the guidelines listed below.

Exercising in Cold Weather	Exercising in Hot Weather
Do not underdress or overdress. Dress in layers so you can remove clothing if you get too warm.	Dress in layers so you can remove clothing if you get too warm.
Avoid nylon clothing because it prevents air from passing over the skin and evaporating to cool the skin.	Avoid nylon clothing because it prevents air from passing over the skin and evaporating to cool the skin.
Wear sunblock to protect the skin from the sun. Any exposed skin—such as your nose, fingers, or ears—should be covered in this way.	Wear sunblock to protect the skin from the sun. Any exposed skin—such as your face, ears, arms, legs, chest, or back—should be protected.
Listen to the weather report before exercising. If the temperature or the windchill factor is too low, avoid exercising outdoors.	Listen to the weather report before exercising. If the temperature is above 90°F and the humidity is above 70%, avoid vigorous exercise outdoors.
Warm up longer than usual and do not begin your exercise program until you have started to perspire.	Warm up for a shorter time than usual.
Protect the head, ears, nose, fingers, and toes. Gloves will protect the fingers. Warm socks will protect the toes. A scarf can protect the nose. A warm hat will keep heat in.	Because the body loses a considerable amount of heat through the head, if you wear a hat, make sure it is lightweight, light-colored, and ideally made of ultraviolet (UV)-blocking material. If you do not wear a hat, a sun visor with a brim will protect the face from the sun while allowing for heat to be dissipated through the head. However, make sure to use sunscreen if your hair is thinning.
Acclimate to the cold by starting with short workouts, then gradually increasing the duration and intensity of your workouts as you get used to the cold.	Acclimate to the heat and humidity by starting with short workouts, then gradually increasing the duration and intensity of your workouts as you get used to the heat.
Drink cold water when thirsty to replenish fluids lost.	Drink cold water when thirsty to replenish fluid loss and prevent heat stroke or other injuries. If exercising intensely for more than 30 minutes, drink a sports drink to replenish sodium and potassium.

Myths *and* Facts

About Physical Fitness

MYTH	FACT
If I participate in aerobic exercise frequently and my resting heart rate is low, I am physically fit.	Physical fitness involves more than just cardiorespiratory fitness. Although your resting heart rate may be low, your muscular strength, muscular endurance, or flexibility may indicate you are unfit.
To become physically fit and avoid or postpone such illnesses as heart disease and stroke, I need to work out vigorously every day.	Research indicates that you can be healthier even if you work out at a moderate rate most days a week. Activities such as biking to class, dancing, shoveling snow, and walking stairs are all examples of moderate physical activities.
To lose a lot of weight by exercising, you need to perspire a lot.	Your weight loss is determined by the number of calories you take in compared to the number of calories you expend. The amount of sweat you produce will not significantly affect your weight, and, if you perspire too much without replenishing lost fluids, it could result in injury.
All popular health and fitness clubs are pretty much the same.	Health and fitness clubs may vary significantly. They may differ in the qualifications of the staff, the equipment available, the average wait time to use the equipment, hours of operation, distance from where you live, and other important factors you should consider before deciding which club is right for you.
If injured, you need to stop exercising and see a healthcare provider.	Many exercise injuries can be self-treated by resting, icing, compressing, and elevating the injured area. Consult Table 6.4 for more guidance. When one part of the body is injured, other parts can still be exercised. For example, if you pull a hamstring muscle, you can still exercise your upper body by using an arm bike (a bicycle ergometer) that does not require the use of your legs.

(such as a hamstring pull), tendonitis (inflammation of a tendon), and ankle sprains. To treat these injuries, use **RICE**: rest, ice, compression, and elevation. *Rest* the injured body part until it is no longer painful. *Ice* the body part for approximately 20 minutes throughout the day to prevent swelling. Use a *compression* bandage, such as an Ace bandage, to prevent swelling and to support the body part. And, *elevate* the body part to facilitate blood flow, which will remove excess fluids and reduce swelling.

When to Seek Medical Attention

Some injuries require the attention of a healthcare provider. These include ruptured tendons, torn ligaments, broken bones, and hernias (in which part of the intestine protrudes through a tear in the abdominal wall). If these injuries are suspected, a medical examination (including x-ray or MRI) is advised to diagnose the injury and determine the best course of action. Treatment may include immobilization of the body part (e.g., placing it in a cast)

or surgical repair of the injured tissue (such as knee surgery to repair torn cartilage or a ruptured tendon).

Physical Therapy

A healthcare provider may recommend physical therapy to help you recover from injury. One of the goals of physical therapy is to strengthen the muscles around the injured area to provide support during movement. Another goal is to increase flexibility around the injured area to make movement easier and to prevent injury once you return to exercise. In addition, physical therapy can help improve balance to make exercise more efficient, thereby preventing injury.

> **RICE:** self-treatment for injury that includes rest, ice, compression, and elevation of the injured body part.

SUMMARY

To help you make healthy decisions when becoming physically fit and to maintain that level of fitness, a summary of this chapter is provided.

- Physical fitness is the ability to meet the demand of everyday life with energy remaining to participate in leisure and recreational activities. It is composed of cardiorespiratory fitness, muscular strength and endurance, and flexibility.

- Muscular strength is the force the muscle can contract, or the most amount of weight that can be lifted one time. Muscular endurance is the ability of the muscle to contract repeatedly or for a sustained period of time.

- Flexibility refers to the range of motion around a joint. Flexibility improves posture, increases relaxation, releases muscle tension and soreness, and reduces the risk of injury.

- Body composition is the amount of body fat compared to other body components, which are referred to as lean body mass.

- The physical benefits of being fit include reduced risk of development of heart disease, stroke, type 2 diabetes, and certain cancers. Being fit is associated with lower blood pressure and serum cholesterol, as well as lower weight.

- The psychological benefits of being fit include reduced feelings of depression and anxiety and an increased self-esteem. These benefits may be a result of brain neurotransmitters being produced that provide a sense of euphoria and well-being.

- The sociological benefits of being fit include increased social support, feeling connected to others, decreased feelings of loneliness and depression, and motivation to maintain the exercise program.

- When designing an exercise program, include activities for all components of physical fitness, exercise for 30 minutes on 5 or more days a week, and maintain your target heart rate. Include activities that you enjoy and that can fit into your schedule.

- Effective weight training starts with the larger muscles and progresses to the smaller ones, spends 2 seconds on lifting the weight and 3–4 seconds on lowering the weight, involves two or three sets of 8–12 repetitions for each set, increases the weight periodically but no more than 5–10% at a time, does not use the same muscles to lift 2 days in a row, and involves exhaling during the lifting phase.

- Exercise can be incorporated into your daily routine. For example, you can walk the stairs rather than take the elevator.

- For an exercise program to be effective, it should be scheduled and not left to chance, and chaining should be used to encourage exercise by making it more convenient to do.

- Several factors should be considered before choosing a health club to join: the equipment available, how the use of that equipment is supervised, the quality of staff–clients relationships, and safety procedures.

- When purchasing home exercise equipment, be skeptical of advertisements that promise unrealistic results, question claims that fat can be burned off of a particular body part, read the ad's fine print, be skeptical of testimonials, get details about warranties, and check out the company's customer support services.

- To maintain an exercise program, use social support, develop an exercise behavioral contract, use reminder systems, keep a journal, and make it fun.

- To avoid exercise injuries, wear appropriate safety gear, warm up before exercising and cool down afterward, drink water when thirsty, never increase the intensity of the exercise by more than 10%.

- To self-treat injury, use RICE: rest, ice, compression, and elevate the injured body part. Medical attention should be sought when the extent of the injury is unclear, when tendon or ligament ruptures or broken bones occur, and when symptoms persist.

REFERENCES

American Academy of Orthopaedic Surgeons. *Safe Exercise*. 2007. Available at: http://orthoinfo.aaos.org/topic.cfm?topic=A00418.

American College of Emergency Physicians. *Exercising Proper Care While Working Out*. 2010. Available at: http://www.acep.org/patients.aspx?id=26170.

American College of Sports Medicine. *ACSM's Health/Fitness Facility Standards and Guidelines*, 3rd ed. Indianapolis, IN: American College of Sports Medicine, 2006.

American Council on Exercise. Don't deprive yourself of the rewards of exercise. *Fit Facts*. 2010a. Available at: http://www.acefitness.org/fitfacts/fitfacts_display.aspx?itemid=2615.

American Council on Exercise. Flexible benefits. *Fit Facts*. 2010b. Available at: http://www.acefitness.org/fitfacts.

American Council on Exercise. Warm up to work out. *Fit Facts*. 2010c. Available at: http://www.acefitness.org/fitfacts/fitfacts_display.aspx?itemid=2629.

American Council on Exercise. *Strength Training Benefits More Than Muscles*. 2010d. Available at: http://www.acefitness.org/healthandfitnesstips/healthandfitnesstips_display.aspx?itemid=105.

Bieler, K. W. What to drink when: Liquid assets. *Runner's World* 41 (2006): 7174.

Centers for Disease Control and Prevention. *Preventing Injuries in Sports, Recreation, and Exercise*. 2006. Available at: http://www.cdc.gov/ncipc/pub-res/research_agenda/05_sports.htm.

Cloe, R. Strength training basics. *The Fitness Jumpsite*. 2010. Available at: http://www.primusweb.com/fitnesspartner/activity/trainbasics.htm.

Federal Trade Commission. Pump fiction: Tips for buying exercise equipment. *FTC Consumer Alert*. 2009. Available at: http://www.ftc.gov/bcp/edu/pubs/consumer/products/pro10.shtm.

Garzarella, L., Pollock, M. L., DeHoyos, D. V., and Takashi, A. Time course for strength and muscle thickness changes following upper and lower body resistance training in men and women. *Journal of Applied Physiology* 81 (2000): 174–180.

Greenberg, J. S., Dintiman, G. B., and Oakes, B. M. *Physical Fitness and Wellness*, 3rd ed. Champaign, IL: Human Kinetics, 2004.

International Marathon Medical Directors Association. *Revised Fluid Recommendations for Runners and Walkers*. London: International Marathon Medical Directors Association, 2006. Available at: http://www.aims-association.org/guidelines_fluid_replacement.htm.

President's Council on Physical Fitness and Sports. Physical activity facts. *Resources*. 2010. Available at: http://www.fitness.gov/resources_factsheet.htm.

INTERNET RESOURCES

President's Council on Physical Fitness and Sports
http://www.fitness.gov/

American Alliance for Health, Physical Education, Recreation and Dance
http://www.aahperd.org/

American College of Sports Medicine
http://www.acsm.org/

American Council for Fitness and Nutrition
www.sourcewatch.org/index.php?title=American_Council_for_Fitness_and_Nutrition

Medicine and Science in Sports and Exercise
http://www.ms-se.com/pt/re/msse/home.htm

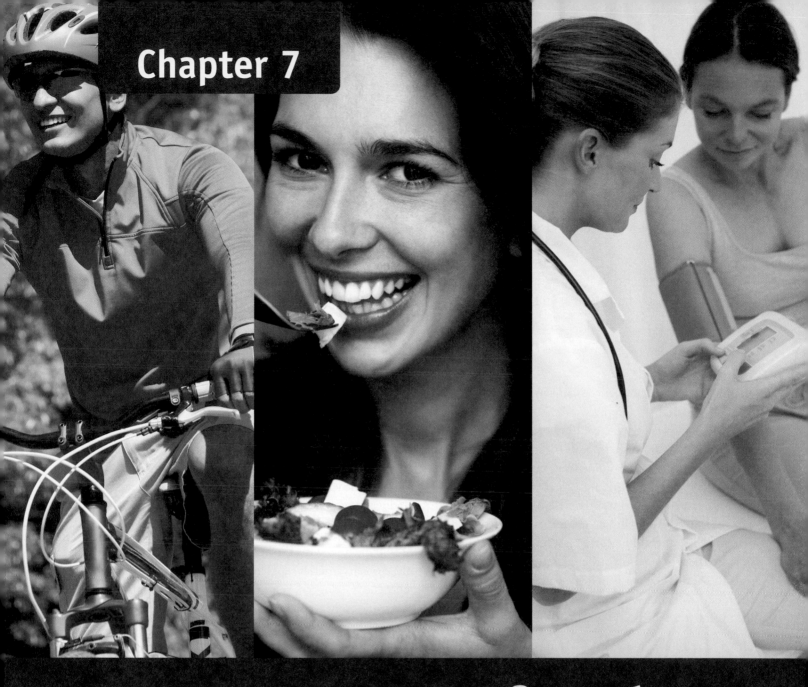

Chapter 7

Preventing Lifestyle Diseases

 Access Health Check Ups and Health Behavior Change activities on the Companion Website:
go.jblearning.com/Empowering.

Learning Objectives

- Discuss the risk factors associated with heart disease and describe how to prevent development of heart disease.

- Discuss the risk factors associated with stroke and describe how to prevent stroke.

- Discuss the risk factors associated with cancer and describe how to prevent cancer.

- Discuss the risk factors associated with diabetes and describe how to prevent diabetes.

- Summarize the factors common to lifestyle diseases and explain how to prevent lifestyle diseases by controlling these risk factors.

As I kept my father company in his hospital room the night before he was scheduled for coronary bypass surgery, I could not help but reflect on what brought him to that point. It did not take long to make a list. His diet contained too much saturated fat, he did not engage in regular physical activity, he smoked cigarettes and a pipe, he was diabetic, and he experienced a great deal of stress in his job in New York City's garment district. Not only did he suffer as a result of his lifestyle, but also the whole family suffered with and for him. The purpose of this chapter is to help you prevent your family from experiencing what my family experienced and to help you live a longer and healthier life.

Heart disease is but one disease that results from health behaviors within an individual's control. We call these **lifestyle diseases**. Other examples of common lifestyle diseases are stroke, cancer, and diabetes. Sexually transmitted diseases (discussed later in this text) are also diseases that result from health behavior decisions. In this chapter, prevalent lifestyle diseases are discussed with advice on how you can prevent them from occurring or at least postpone their occurrence for as long as possible.

Heart Disease

The circulatory system is composed of arteries, capillaries, and veins. **Arteries** are large blood vessels that transport the blood away from the heart, supplying oxygen and nutrients to organs and tissues of the body. **Capillaries** are smaller blood vessels that transport oxygen- and nutrient-rich blood from the arteries to all cells of the body; they also transport blood back from body cells to veins. **Veins** are blood vessels that return blood to the heart after oxygen and nutrients have been exchanged for carbon dioxide and waste products in the cells.

Without oxygen and nutrients, body organs and tissues would die. Likewise, the heart muscle itself would die. If the coronary arteries supplying the heart with oxygen and nutrients are clogged, heart tissue will die. If enough heart tissue dies, a heart attack can occur, which may result in death. Clogged arteries happen as a result of several factors, termed *risk factors*.

Lifestyle diseases: diseases that result from health behaviors people adopt or do not adopt.

Arteries: large blood vessels that leave the heart to supply oxygen and nutrients to organs and tissues of the body.

Capillaries: small blood vessels that transport oxygen and nutrients from the arteries to all cells of the body and from body cells to veins.

Veins: blood vessels that return blood to the heart after oxygen and nutrients are exchanged for carbon dioxide and waste products.

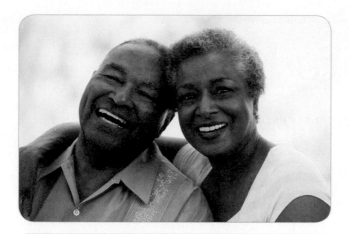

Males over 45 years old, females over 55 years old, and anyone who has a close family member who developed heart disease are at risk of development of heart disease themselves.

Risk Factors You Cannot Change

There are certain risk factors for heart disease over which you have no control. Still, recognition of these risk factors may provide added incentive to manage those risk factors over which you *do* have control. The risk factors you cannot control include:

- *Family history:* If your father or brother was diagnosed with heart disease before age 55 or if your mother or sister was diagnosed with heart disease before age 65, you are in a higher risk group.

- *Age:* If you are a male and older than age 45, you are in a higher-risk group than younger men. And, if you are a female older than age 55, you, too, are in a higher-risk group.

Risk Factors You Can Change

There are several additional risk factors associated with coronary heart disease. The more of these risk factors you have, the greater the likelihood that you will develop heart disease. The good news, however, is that you can control these risk factors either by a change in lifestyle and/or with medication.

High Blood Cholesterol

Cholesterol is a waxy, fat-like substance found in the membranes of cells in all parts of the body. The body uses cholesterol to make hormones, bile acids, vitamin D, and other substances. Cholesterol circulates in the bloodstream but cannot travel by itself. As with oil and water, cholesterol (which is fatty) and blood (which is watery) do not mix. So cholesterol travels in packages called *lipoproteins*, which have fat (lipid) inside and protein outside. Two main kinds of lipoproteins carry cholesterol in the blood:

- *Low-density lipoprotein* (LDL): Also called *bad* cholesterol because it carries cholesterol to tissues, including the arteries. Most of the cholesterol in the blood is the LDL form. The higher the level of LDL in the blood, the greater your risk for heart disease.

- *High-density lipoprotein* (HDL): Also called *good* cholesterol because it takes cholesterol from tissues to the liver, which removes it from the body. A low level of HDL increases your risk for heart disease. A high level of HDL decreases your risk for heart disease.

If there is too much cholesterol in the blood, some of the excess can become trapped in artery walls. Over time, this excess builds up and is called *plaque*. The plaque can narrow the blood vessels and make them less flexible, a condition called *atherosclerosis*, or *hardening of the arteries*. This process can happen to blood vessels anywhere in the body, including those of the heart. If the coronary arteries become partly blocked by plaque, then the blood may not be able to bring enough oxygen and nutrients to the heart muscle. This can cause chest pain, or **angina**. Some cholesterol-rich plaques are unstable. That is, they have a

Cholesterol: a waxy, fat-like substance found in the membranes of cells in all parts of the body that is used to make hormones, bile acids, vitamin D, and other substances.

Angina: chest pain resulting from coronary arteries not being able to bring enough oxygen and nutrients to the heart muscle because they are partly blocked by plaque.

What I Need to Know

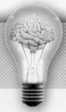

Blood Cholesterol Classifications

Total Cholesterol	
Less than 200 mg/dL	Desirable
200–239 mg/dL	Borderline high
240 mg/dL and above	High
LDL Cholesterol	
Less than 100 mg/dL	Optimal (ideal)
100–129 mg/dL	Near optimal/above optimal
130–159 mg/dL	Borderline high
160–189 mg/dL	High
190 mg/dL and above	Very high
HDL Cholesterol	
Less than 40 mg/dL	Major heart disease risk factor
60 mg/dL and above	Gives some protection against heart disease.

Note: mg = milligram (0.001 gram); dL = deciliter (0.1 liter).

Source: National Heart, Lung, and Blood Institute. High Blood Cholesterol: What You Need To Know. 2005. Available at: http://www.nhlbi.nih.gov/health/public/heart/chol/wyntk.htm

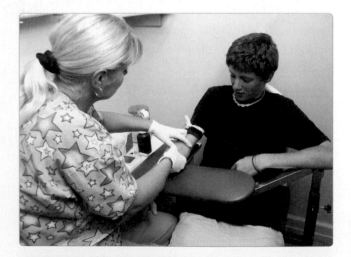

Everyone should periodically have their blood chemistry tested to determine if their cholesterol levels place them at risk for development of heart disease.

thin covering and can burst, releasing cholesterol and fat into the bloodstream. The release can cause a blood clot to form over the plaque, blocking blood flow through the artery and causing a heart attack.

What Affects Cholesterol Levels?

Various factors can cause unhealthy cholesterol levels. Some of the factors cannot be changed; for example, *heredity* partially determines HDL levels, and *age* affects total cholesterol levels. Cholesterol begins to rise around age 20 and continues to go up until about age 60 or 65. Before age 50, men's total cholesterol levels tend to be higher than those of women the same age. However, after age 50, women's total cholesterol levels tend to be higher than those of men. This is because women's LDL levels often rise after menopause.

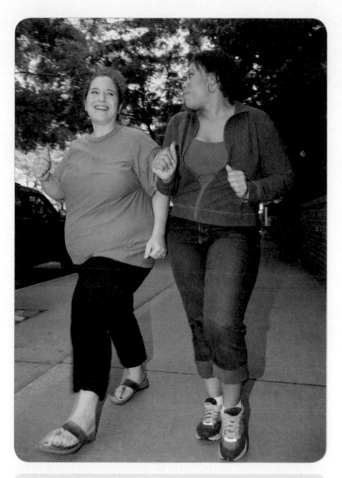

Being overweight places one at risk for heart disease. Exercise can help control weight and improve blood chemistry related to heart disease risk.

Overweight/Obesity

Excess weight tends to increase LDL levels while lowering HDL levels. Also, it typically increases fatty substances in the blood called **triglycerides**. Loss of extra pounds can help lower LDL and triglyceride levels while raising HDL levels.

Physical Inactivity

Being physically inactive contributes to overweight and can raise LDL levels and lower HDL levels. Regular physical activity can raise HDL levels and lower triglyceride levels and can help with weight loss (and in that way help lower LDL levels and reduce the risk of heart disease).

Diabetes

Recent estimates predict up to a third of Americans born today will develop diabetes in their lifetimes. One of the most serious health issues facing diabetes patients is heart disease. Heart disease and stroke affect diabetics more than twice as often as people without diabetes. Some experts argue that diabetes is now the largest cause of heart disease in the United States (Cagan, 2010).

Tobacco Use

You may be surprised to learn that tobacco use causes more deaths per year from heart disease than from lung cancer. One of the reasons is that tobacco use increases blood pressure and blood-clotting tendencies. In fact, the risk of smokers for development of heart disease is two to four times greater than that of nonsmokers. Further evidence of the connection between tobacco use and heart disease comes from studies showing that coronary heart disease is substantially reduced within 1 to 2 years of smoking cessation. The risk of stroke also decreases steadily after stopping the use of tobacco (American Dental Hygienists' Association, 2010).

Although we cannot change our heredity or age, there are lifestyle changes we can make to improve our cholesterol levels. These choices include appropriate diet, sufficient exercise, and medication if needed.

Diet

Three nutrients in the diet make LDL levels rise and thus increase risk of heart disease:

- *Saturated fat*, a type of fat found mostly in foods that come from animals.

- *Trans fat*, found mostly in foods made with hydrogenated oils and fats, such as stick margarine, crackers, and french fries.

- *Cholesterol*, which comes only from animal products.

Triglycerides: fatty substances in the blood and in food that lower HDL and are related to the development of coronary heart disease.

What I Need to Know

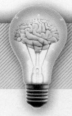

What Are Triglycerides?

Triglycerides, which are produced in the liver, are a type of fat found in the blood and in food. Causes of raised triglycerides are overweight/obesity, physical inactivity, cigarette smoking, excess alcohol intake, and diets very high in carbohydrates (contributing 60% or more of total calories). Triglyceride levels that are borderline high (150–199 mg/dL) or high (200–499 mg/dL) may increase the risk for heart disease. Levels of 500 mg/dL or higher need to be lowered with medica-tion to prevent the pancreas from becoming inflamed. To keep your own blood triglyceride levels in check: control your weight, be physically active, don't smoke, limit alcohol intake, and limit simple sugars and sugar-sweetened beverages.

REPRODUCED FROM: National Heart, Lung, and Blood Institute. *Your Guide to Lowering Your Cholesterol With TLC: Therapeutic Lifestyle Changes.* Washington, DC: National Heart, Lung, and Blood Institute, 2005.

Complete Health Check Up 7.1 to determine your risk of having a heart attack sometime within the next 10 years (see Health Check Up 7.1 on the companion website). Once completed, place Health Check Up 7.1 in your Health Decision Portfolio.

Stroke

Stroke is another circulatory disorder; stroke occurs when a portion of the brain is deprived of the flow of oxygenated blood. Without oxygenated blood, brain cells start to die after a few minutes. The brain can be deprived of blood because of a blockage of the blood vessels supplying the brain (*ischemic stroke*) or a rupture of those blood vessels (*hemorrhagic stroke*). For example, if a blood clot breaks away from plaque buildup in a carotid (neck) artery and travels to and lodges in an artery in the brain, the clot can block blood flow to part of the brain (an ischemic stroke) causing brain tissue death. Or, an artery in the brain may rupture and leak blood (hemorrhagic stroke). The pressure from the leaked blood damages brain cells. **FIG. 7.1 ▶** and **FIG. 7.2 ▶** depict the two different types of stroke.

Symptoms

If brain cells die or are damaged because of a stroke, symptoms occur in the parts of the body that these brain cells control. Examples of stroke symptoms include sudden weakness; paralysis or numbness of the face, arms, or legs; trouble speaking or understanding speech; and trouble seeing. A stroke can cause lasting brain damage, long-term disability, or even death.

Causes of Stroke

One of the causes of stroke is atherosclerosis. **Atherosclerosis** is a disease in which a fatty substance called *plaque* builds up on the inner walls of the arteries. Plaque hardens

Stroke: when the brain is deprived of blood because of a blockage of the blood vessels supplying the brain or a rupture of those blood vessels.

Atherosclerosis: when plaque narrows coronary blood vessels and makes them less flexible; also called hardening of the arteries.

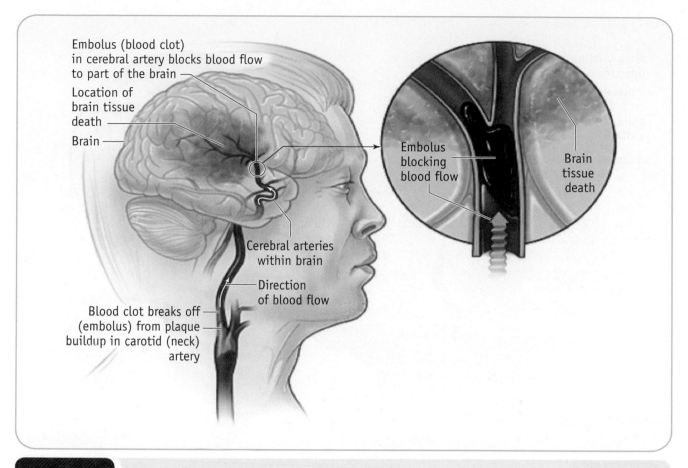

Embolus (blood clot) in cerebral artery blocks blood flow to part of the brain

Location of brain tissue death

Brain

Cerebral arteries within brain

Direction of blood flow

Blood clot breaks off (embolus) from plaque buildup in carotid (neck) artery

Embolus blocking blood flow

Brain tissue death

FIGURE 7.1 Ischemic stroke.

REPRODUCED FROM: *Diseases and Conditions Index*. Stroke. National Heart, Lung, and Blood Institute. 2011. Available at: http://www.nhlbi.nih.gov/health/dci/Diseases/stroke/stroke_what.html.

and narrows the arteries, which limits the flow of blood to tissues and organs such as the heart and brain. Plaque in an artery can rupture and form blood clots (*embolisms*), which can partly or completely block an artery. If this occurs in the carotid arteries supplying the brain, the result is an ischemic stroke.

Another cause of stroke is high blood pressure that leads to sudden bleeding in the brain causing a hemorrhagic stroke. The bleeding causes swelling of the brain and increased pressure in the skull, damaging brain cells and tissues.

Risk Factors

Risk factors related to stroke include (*Diseases and Conditions Index*, 2011):

- *High blood pressure.* High blood pressure is the main risk factor for stroke. Blood pressure is considered high if systolic blood pressure stays at or above 140/90 mmHg over time.

- *Smoking.* Smoking can damage blood vessels and raise blood pressure. Smoking also may reduce the amount of oxygen that reaches the body's tissues.

157

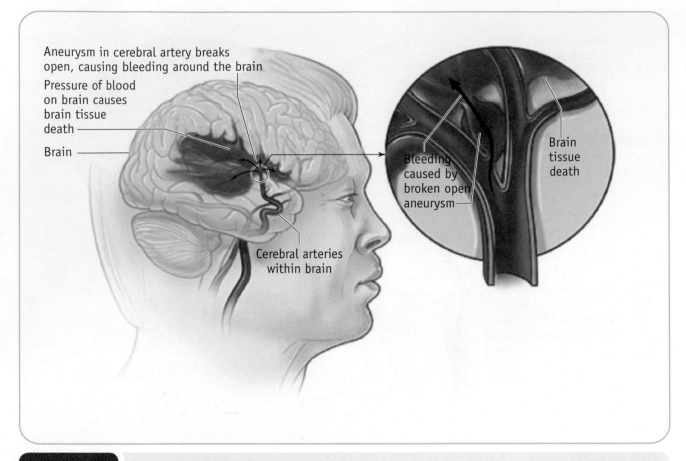

FIGURE 7.2 Hemorrhagic stroke.
REPRODUCED FROM: *Diseases and Conditions Index*. Stroke. National Heart, Lung, and Blood Institute. 2011. Available at: http://www.nhlbi.nih.gov/health/dci/Diseases/stroke/stroke_what.html.

Exposure to secondhand smoke also can damage the blood vessels.

- *Diabetes.* Diabetes is a disease in which the blood sugar level is high because the body does not make enough insulin or does not use insulin properly. Insulin is a hormone that helps move sugar from the blood into cells, where it is used for energy.

- *Heart disease.* Coronary heart disease can cause blood clots that can lead to a stroke.

- *Brain aneurysms.* Aneurysms are balloon-like bulges in an artery that can stretch and burst.

- *Age and gender.* The risk of stroke increases as one gets older. At younger ages, men are more likely than women to have strokes. However, women are more likely to die from strokes. Women who take birth control pills also are at slightly higher risk of stroke. How birth control pills cause strokes is not completely understood, but it is suspected that the increased risks of blood clots and high blood pressure associated with oral contraceptives are factors (Increased stroke risk from birth control pills, review finds, 2009).

- *Race and ethnicity.* Strokes occur more often in African American, Alaska Native, and American Indian adults than in white, Hispanic, or Asian American adults.

- *Personal or family history of stroke.* Having a stroke increases the risk for another one. A person's risk of having a repeat stroke is the highest right after a stroke. A family history of stroke also increases the risk of stroke.

Estimated New Cases*

Male	Female	Male	Female
Prostate	Breast	Lung & bronchus	Lung & bronchus
241,740 (29%)	226,870 (29%)	87,750 (29%)	72,590 (26%)
Lung & bronchus	Lung & bronchus	Prostate	Breast
116,470 (14%)	109,690 (14%)	28,170 (9%)	39,510 (14%)
Colon & rectum	Colon & rectum	Colon & rectum	Colon & rectum
73,420 (9%)	70,040 (9%)	26,470 (9%)	25,220 (9%)
Urinary bladder	Uterine corpus	Pancreas	Pancreas
55,600 (7%)	47,130 (6%)	18,850 (6%)	18,540 (7%)
Melanoma of the skin	Thyroid	Liver & intrahepatic bile duct	Ovary
44,250 (5%)	43,210 (5%)	13,980 (5%)	15,500 (6%)
Kidney & renal pelvis	Melanoma of the skin	Leukemia	Leukemia
40,250 (5%)	32,000 (4%)	13,500 (4%)	10,040 (4%)
Non-Hodgkin lymphoma	Non-Hodgkin lymphoma	Esophagus	Non-Hodgkin lymphoma
38,160 (4%)	31,970 (4%)	12,040 (4%)	8,620 (3%)
Oral cavity & pharynx	Kidney & renal pelvis	Urinary bladder	Uterine corpus
28,540 (3%)	24,520 (3%)	10,510 (3%)	8,010 (3%)
Leukemia	Ovary	Non-Hodgkin lymphoma	Liver & intrahepatic bile duct
26,830 (3%)	22,280 (3%)	10,320 (3%)	6,570 (2%)
Pancreas	Pancreas	Kidney & renal pelvis	Brain & other nervous system
22,090 (3%)	21,830 (3%)	8,650 (3%)	5,980 (2%)
All sites	All sites	All sites	All sites
848,170 (100%)	790,740 (100%)	301,820 (100%)	275,370 (100%)

Estimated Deaths

*Excludes basal and squamous cell skin cancers and in situ carcinoma except urinary bladder.

FIGURE 7.3 Leading sites of new cancer cases and deaths: 2010 estimates.
REPRODUCED FROM: American Cancer Society. *Cancer Facts and Figures 2012.* Atlanta, GA: American Cancer Society, 2012.

Other risk factors associated with stroke include alcohol and illegal drug use, high blood cholesterol levels, lack of physical activity, an unhealthy diet, obesity, stress, and depression.

Cancer

Cancer is the uncontrolled growth of abnormal cells in the body (called *malignant* cells). Normal cells multiply when the body needs them and die when the body does not need them. Cancer appears to occur when the growth of cells in the body is out of control and cells divide too quickly. It can also occur when cells fail to die. The three most common cancers for men in the United States are prostate cancer, lung cancer, and colon cancer. For women in the United States, the three most common cancers are

breast cancer, colon cancer, and lung cancer. **FIG. 7.3** lists new cases of cancer and cancer deaths for 2010. Complete Health Check Up 7.2 to determine your risk of developing cancer. Once completed, place Health Check Up 7.2 in your Health Decision Portfolio.

Symptoms

Symptoms of cancer depend on the type and location of the cancer. For example, lung cancer can cause coughing, shortness of breath, or chest pain. Colon cancer often causes diarrhea, constipation, and blood in the stool.

Cancer: uncontrolled growth of abnormal cells in the body (called *malignant* cells) that can result in disability or death.

However, some cancers may not have any symptoms at all until a late stage of development of the cancer. The following symptoms often occur with most cancers: chills, fatigue, fever, loss of appetite, night sweats, and weight loss.

Types of Cancer

Cancer can occur in many different parts of the body. Although prevention and treatment may be similar, cancer at different sites and at different stages has variations. **Staging** is a determination of the extent of a cancer in the body based on the size of the tumor, whether lymph nodes contain cancer, and whether the cancer has spread from the original site to other parts of the body. Stage 1 cancers are localized, and higher-stage cancers are progressively more spread throughout the body. Later-stage cancers are generally more difficult to treat and result in more deaths. Different types of cancers are discussed in the following sections.

Lung Cancer

Lung cancer results in more deaths than any other cancer in men and women. In 2010, approximately 28% of all cancer deaths were from lung cancer (American Cancer Society, 2010). Since 1987, more women have died of lung cancer than of breast cancer.

Symptoms

Symptoms of lung cancer include persistent cough, sputum consisting of blood, chest pain, voice change, and recurrent pneumonia or bronchitis.

Risk Factors

Cigarette smoking causes most lung cancer. Chewing tobacco and cigar or pipe smoking are also risk factors. Occupational exposure such as working in coal mines increases risk, as does environmental exposure to secondhand smoke, radon, asbestos, certain metals, radiation, and air pollution. A history of tuberculosis is another risk factor.

Treatment

Depending on the type and stage of the lung cancer, treatment consists of surgery, radiation therapy, chemotherapy, and cancer-fighting medication. Because there is no screening test for lung cancer, it is often diagnosed after it has spread. Therefore, treatment usually involves radiation and chemotherapy in conjunction with surgery. Lung cancer patients will often experience remission, a period of time they are cancer-free. However, the cancer is apt to return. The 1-year survival rate is 42%, but the 5-year survival rate is only 16%. (The 5-year survival rate is 53% for patients whose cancer is localized; however, only 15% of patients are diagnosed at this stage.)

Colorectal Cancer

Colorectal, or colon, cancer is cancer that starts in the large intestine (colon) or the rectum (end of the colon). In the United States in 2010, there were 142,570 new cases of colorectal cancer diagnosed and 51,370 deaths attributed to colon cancer.

Symptoms

Many cases of colon cancer have no symptoms. When symptoms do occur, they may include abdominal pain and tenderness in the lower abdomen, blood in the stool, diarrhea, constipation, or other change in bowel habits, narrow stools, and weight loss with no known reason. Because colon cancer is usually asymptomatic, it is recommended that individuals 50 years and older periodically be screened—usually every 10 years—for colon cancer by a *colonoscopy*. Colonoscopy is a screening exam that lets a doctor look at the inside of the entire colon for polyps or signs of cancer. Polyps are small growths that over time can become cancer. During a colonoscopy, a thin, flexible, hollow, lighted tube containing a tiny video camera is gently eased inside the colon and sends pictures to a video display screen. Patients are usually given medicine to help them relax and sleep during the 30-minute exam. If polyps are detected, they are removed.

Staging: determination of the extent of a cancer in the body based on the size of the tumor, whether lymph nodes contain cancer, and whether the cancer has spread from the original site to other parts of the body.

Risk Factors

Those at higher risk of development of colon cancer are (National Center for Biotechnology Information, 2010):

- Older than 60 years of age

- African American or of eastern European descent

- Eat a diet high in red or processed meats

- Have cancer elsewhere in the body

- Have colorectal polyps

- Have inflammatory bowel disease (Crohn's disease or ulcerative colitis)

- Have a family history of colon cancer

- Have a personal history of breast cancer

- Smoke cigarettes

- Drink alcohol

Treatment

Treatment depends partly on the stage of the cancer and may include surgery to remove cancerous cells, chemotherapy to kill cancerous cells, and radiation therapy to destroy cancerous tissue. Colon cancer is a treatable disease if caught early. The 5-year survival rate is 74% for stage 1 colon cancer, between 37% and 67% for stage 2, 28–73% for stage 3, and 6% for stage 4. If the colon cancer does not recur within 5 years, then patients are considered cured. Stage 1, 2, and 3 cancers are considered potentially curable. In most cases, stage 4 cancer is not considered curable, although there are exceptions (American Cancer Society, 2011b).

Skin Cancer

Skin cancer is the most common of all cancers. It accounts for nearly half of all cancers in the United States. In 2011, there were more than 2 million cases of non-melanoma skin cancer diagnosed and 123,590 cases of melanoma skin cancer (the most deadly type of skin cancer). In 2011, 11,790 deaths occurred as a result of melanoma. One American dies of melanoma almost every hour (American Academy of Dermatology, 2011).

Symptoms

Signs of skin cancer include (American Cancer Society, 2011c):

- Any change on the skin, especially in the size or color of a mole or other darkly pigmented growth or spot, or a new growth.

- Scaliness, oozing, bleeding, or change in the appearance of a bump or nodule.

- The spread of pigmentation beyond its border such as dark coloring that spreads past the edge of a mole or mark.

- A change in sensation, itchiness, tenderness, or pain.

Risk Factors

Risk factors for the development of skin cancer include:

- Unprotected and/or excessive exposure to ultraviolet (UV) radiation.

- Fair complexion.

- Occupational exposures to coal tar, pitch, creosote, arsenic compounds, or radium.

- Family history.

- Multiple or atypical moles.

- Severe sunburns as a child.

Prevention

The best ways to lower the risk of development of skin cancer involve avoidance of intense sunlight for long periods of time and use of sun safety practices. In particular (American Cancer Society, 2011c):

- Avoid the sun between 10 a.m. and 4 p.m.

- Seek shade: Look for shade, especially in the middle of the day when the sun's rays are strongest. Practice the shadow rule: If your shadow is shorter than you, the sun's rays are at their strongest.

- Cover up with protective clothing to guard as much skin as possible when you are out in the sun. Choose comfortable clothes made of tightly woven fabrics that you cannot see through when held up to a light.

- Use sunscreen and lip balm with a sun protection factor (SPF) of 15 or higher. Apply a generous amount of sunscreen (about a palmful) and reapply after swimming, toweling dry, or perspiring. Use sunscreen even on hazy or overcast days.

- Cover your head with a wide-brimmed hat, shading your face, ears, and neck. If you choose a baseball cap, remember to protect your ears and neck with sunscreen.

- Wear sunglasses with 99–100% UV absorption to provide optimal protection for the eyes and the surrounding skin.

- Follow these practices to protect your skin even on cloudy or overcast days. UV rays travel through clouds.

- Avoid other sources of UV light. Tanning beds and sun lamps are dangerous because they can damage your skin.

Treatment

Treatment for skin cancer may involve surgery to remove the cancerous tissue, radiation therapy, which uses x-rays or other types of radiation to kill cancer cells or keep them from growing, chemotherapy, which uses drugs to stop the growth of cancer cells either by killing them or by stopping them from dividing, and photodynamic therapy, which uses a drug and laser light to kill cancer cells. The 5-year survival rate for melanoma is 91%. Approximately 84% of melanomas are diagnosed at a localized stage where the 5-year survival rate is 98%. Five-year survival rates for cancers that have metastasized to the region of the original cancer or to a distant site are 62% and 15%, respectively (American Academy of Dermatology, 2011).

Breast Cancer

More than 200,000 new cases of breast cancer occurred among women in 2010 and almost 2,000 among men. Furthermore, in 2010, more than 40,000 women and almost 400 men died of breast cancer (American Cancer Society, 2010).

Symptoms

Large tumors of the breast may be able to be felt or be painful. However, breast cancer is most often diagnosed by a mammogram (an x-ray of the breast) before it is felt by the patient or a physician. Other less common breast symptoms include thickening, swelling, tenderness, skin irritation, redness, scaliness, or nipple abnormalities such as discharge.

Risk Factors

There are several risk factors for breast cancer that cannot be modified. These include a family history of breast cancer and inherited mutations in certain genes (BRCA1 and BRCA2). These mutations are associated with 5–10%

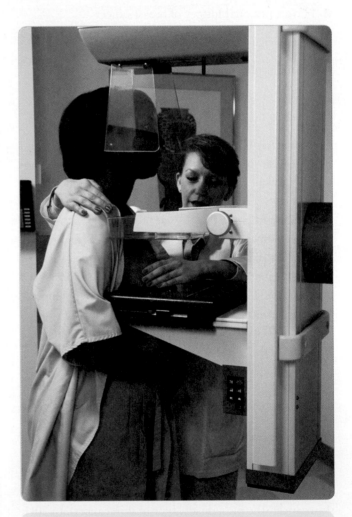

Mammography can identify breast tumors before they can be felt by either the patient or the physician.

of all breast cancer cases, although they appear in only 1% of the population. For this reason, absent a family history of breast cancer, widespread screening for these mutations is not recommended. Other risk factors are menstrual periods that start early or end late in life; never having given birth to children; and giving birth to one's first child after age 30.

Modifiable risk factors include being overweight or obese, physical inactivity, consumption of one or more alcoholic drinks a day, use of oral contraceptives, and use of estrogen and progestin (formerly called hormone replacement therapy). Behaviors that are associated with lower risk of breast cancer include breastfeeding, moderate or vigorous physical activity, and maintaining a healthy weight.

Treatment

Early detection is key in treatment of breast cancer. Because mammography is one of the most effective ways of detecting breast cancer early, mammograms are recommended for all women, although recommendations for when to start screening and how often to be screened differ among medical organizations.

Depending on the size of the tumor and its stage of development, treatment might consist of lumpectomy (surgical removal of the tumor), mastectomy (surgical removal of the breast), radiation therapy, chemotherapy, or hormone therapy (such as tamoxifen). Studies have found that survival rates are similar between lumpectomy plus radiation and mastectomy when the cancer has not spread, thereby sparing many women the trauma of losing a breast to surgery. Five-year survival rates vary by the stage of the cancer: stage 1 is 88%, stage 2 ranges from 74% to 81%, stage 3 ranges from 41% to 67%, and stage 4 is 15% (American Cancer Society, 2011a).

Cervical Cancer

Just over 12,000 new cases of cancer of the cervix were diagnosed in 2010, with 4,210 deaths.

Symptoms

The most common symptom of cervical cancer is abnormal vaginal bleeding. Other symptoms include bleeding after menopause and vaginal discharge. The most prevalent cause of cervical cancer is infection by the human papillomavirus (HPV), which is most commonly acquired by sexual activity with an infected partner.

Risk Factors

Risk factors for cervical cancer include having multiple sexual partners, suppressed immune system function, having multiple childbirths, cigarette smoking, and use of oral contraceptives.

Prevention

Two vaccines to prevent the most common forms of HPV infections have been approved by the Food and Drug Administration: Gardasil and Cervarix. Screening consists of a Pap test in which small samples of cells are taken from the cervix and then examined under a microscope. Early detection provided by the Pap test allows for more effective and less invasive treatment.

Treatment

Treatment of cervical cancer may include the destruction of precancerous tissue by electrical current (electrocoagulation) or extreme cold (cryotherapy), by laser, or by surgery. Full-blown cervical cancer is often treated by surgery, radiation, or chemotherapy. The 1-year survival rate is 87%, and the 5-year survival rate is 71%.

Endometrial Cancer

In 2010, almost 44,000 new cases of cancer of the uterus were diagnosed, with almost 8,000 deaths. Most cancers of the uterus occur in the inner lining, called the endometrium.

Symptoms

Symptoms of endometrial cancer include uterine bleeding or spotting, pain during urination, pain during sexual intercourse, and pain in the abdomen.

Risk Factors

An increased estrogen level is the major risk factor for endometrial cancer. Estrogen levels are increased by being overweight or obese, never giving birth, experiencing late menopause, and the presence of ovarian cysts. Estrogen levels are also artificially increased by menopausal estrogen therapy (historically referred to as hormone replacement therapy). Additional risk factors are infertility and diabetes. A history of pregnancy and the use of oral contraceptives (both of which raise progesterone levels, but suppress estrogen) provide protection against endometrial cancer.

Treatment

Depending on the stage at which the endometrial cancer is diagnosed, treatment may entail surgery, radiation, hormone therapy, or chemotherapy. The 1-year survival rate is 92%, and the 5-year survival rate is 83%.

Prostate Cancer

With the exception of skin cancer, prostate cancer is the most frequently diagnosed cancer in men. It is estimated that one in six men will be diagnosed with cancer of the prostate during his lifetime, with 1 in 36 dying from it.

Symptoms

Symptoms of prostate cancer include weak or interrupted urine flow, inability to urinate, difficulty starting or stopping urine flow, blood in the urine, frequent urination especially at night, and pain or burning when urinating. Because many of these symptoms also occur when the prostate is enlarged but not cancerous, screening is advised. Screening consists of a digital examination of the prostate and a blood test for prostate specific antigen (PSA).

Risk Factors

The older the man, the more prone he is to develop prostate cancer and the more likely he is to die of it. Men aged 70–74 have the highest incidence rate. Race and ethnicity are also risk factors. African-American men have a higher incidence and are more likely to die of prostate cancer than white men. In contrast, the rates of other racial and ethnic groups are lower than those of both whites and African Americans. Education is also related to prostate

cancer risk: the lower the education level of patients, the higher their *death rate* from prostate cancer. However, the *incidence rate* is higher for men with more education. These findings are most likely due to more highly educated men acquiring regular screenings and, therefore, being more likely to have their cancer diagnosed. This conclusion is supported by the finding that less educated men are diagnosed at later stages of cancer than are more educated men. Men with less education are more likely to be without health insurance, thereby lessening their chances of regular screenings; this means more late-stage diagnoses and worse outcomes (higher death rates) among this group.

Family history is another risk factor for prostate cancer. Men with a father or brother who developed prostate cancer are two to three times more likely to develop prostate cancer than are men without this family history. When two or more close relatives have prostate cancer, the risk of a man developing the disease increases three to five times.

Although the data are not conclusive, medical experts recommend eating nutritiously to prevent prostate cancer. Specifically, it is recommended that one's daily diet consist of five servings of fruits and vegetables, a minimum of red meat, and only three servings of dairy products. Maintenance of a healthy weight is also recommended.

Treatment

Some cancers are slow growing, whereas others are faster growing. Prostate cancer tends to grow slowly. The expected progression of the cancer is considered when treatment is chosen, as is the patient's age. For an older patient with a slow-growing prostate cancer and with 10 years or so of natural life span remaining, treatment will be less aggressive. Given these considerations, treatment may include *active surveillance* (monitoring the development of the cancer with the intent of further treatment if necessary); surgical removal of the prostate and nearby tissue; radiation; or hormonal therapy. Survival rates are quite high due to the slowly progressing nature of prostate cancer. Almost half of male cancer survivors in the United States are prostate cancer survivors.

What I Need to Know

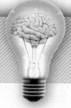

The Controversy Regarding PSA Screening

Whether men should be screened for prostate cancer with a PSA blood test is somewhat controversial. In 2008, the U.S. Preventive Services Task Force, which evaluates medical screenings and makes recommendations regarding those screenings, published new guidelines for use of the PSA test. It states that men age 75 years and older should not be screened for PSA because the length of time one is expected to survive with prostate cancer is greater than 10 years, and a 75-year-old man's average life expectancy is only another 10 years. Men older than 75 should not be subjected to the test, as it could lead to other medical procedures.

For men younger than 75 years, the task force states, "Current evidence is insufficient to assess the balance of benefits and harms of screening." The "harms" referred to relate to unnecessary medical screenings. The reasoning behind these recommendations pertains to the lack of evidence of the validity of PSA screening when a cutoff score of 4.0 ng/mL (nanograms per milliliter) is used, as was standard practice. To respond to the lack of sensitivity of the screening at a score of 4.0 ng/mL, a lower score of 2.5 ng/mL has increasingly been used. However, lowering the score leads to more false positives and, therefore, subjects men to more unnecessary biopsies and other medical procedures. Other evidence that affects this controversy includes two recent large-scale, long-term studies concluding that PSA screening does not affect the prostate cancer death rate (Andriole et al., 2009; Schroder et al., 2009). The researchers found that the rate of death from prostate cancer was very low and did not differ significantly between a group of men who were screened and a group of men who were not.

Recognizing the controversy and lack of clear guidance, most major medical organizations recommend that clinicians discuss the potential benefits and known harms of PSA screening with their patients and consider the preferences of their patients rather than routinely ordering PSA screening. Among these organizations are the American Academy of Family Physicians, American College of Physicians, American College of Preventive Medicine, and American Medical Association. In contrast, the American Urological Association and the American Cancer Society recommend digital rectal examinations and PSA screening for men annually beginning at age 50.

Testicular Cancer

Testicular cancer is cancer that develops in the testicles, the male reproductive glands located in the scrotum. The exact cause of testicular cancer is unknown. Because testicular cancer is the most common form of cancer in men between the ages of 15 and 35, it is of specific concern for college-age males. White men are more likely than African-American and Asian-American men to develop testicular cancer.

Symptoms

Often there are no symptoms of testicular cancer. However, symptoms that may occur include discomfort or pain in a testicle, a feeling of heaviness in the scrotum, pain in the back or lower abdomen, enlargement of a testicle or a change in the way it feels, excess development of breast tissue, and a lump or swelling in either testicle.

A physical examination is the typical way testicular cancer is identified. The exam reveals a lump in one of the

TABLE 7.1 Cancer Screening Guidelines

Cancer Site	Population	Test or Procedure	Frequency
Breast	Women, age 20+	Breast self-examination (BSE)	It is acceptable for women to choose not to do BSE or to do BSE regularly (monthly) or irregularly. Beginning in their early 20s, women should be told about the benefits and limitations of BSE. Whether a woman ever performs BSE, the importance of prompt reporting of any new breast symptoms to a health professional should be emphasized. Women who choose to do BSE should receive instruction and have their technique reviewed on the occasion of a periodic health examination.
		Clinical breast examination (CBE)	For women in their 20s and 30s, it is recommended that CBE be part of a periodic health examination, preferably at least every 3 years. Asymptomatic woman age 40 and older should continue to receive a CBE as part of a periodic health examination, preferably annually.
		Mammography	Begin annual mammography at age 40.*
Cervix†	Women, age 21+	Pap test HPV DNA test	Cervical cancer screening should begin approximately 3 years after a woman begins having vaginal intercourse, but no later than 21 years of age. Screening should be done every year with conventional Pap tests or every 2 years using liquid-based Pap tests. At or after age 30, women who have had 3 normal test results in a row may undergo screening every 2 to 3 years with cervical cytology (either conventional or liquid-based Pap test) alone, or every 3 years with an HPV DNA test plus cervical cytology. Women 70 years of age and older who have had 3 or more normal Pap tests and no abnormal Pap tests in the past 10 years and women who have had a total hysterectomy may choose to stop cervical cancer screening.
Colorectal	Men and woman, age 50+	Fecal occult blood test (FOBT) with at least 50% test sensitivity for cancer, or fecal immunochemical test (FIT) with at least 50% test sensitivity for cancer, **or**	Annual, starting at age 50. Testing at home with adherence to manufacturer's recommendation for collection techniques and number of samples is recommended. FOBT with the single stool sample collected on the clinician's fingertip during a digital rectal examination in the health care setting is not recommended. Guaiac-based toilet bowl FOBT tests also are not recommended. In comparison with guaiac-based tests for the detection of occult blood, immunochemical tests are more patient-friendly, and are likely to be equal or better in sensitivity and specificity. There is no justification for repeating FOBT in response to an initial positive finding.
		Stool DNA test, **or**	Interval uncertain, starting at age 50.

TABLE 7.1		Cancer Screening Guidelines *(Continued)*	

Cancer Site	Population	Test or Procedure	Frequency
		Flexible sigmoidoscopy (FSIG), **or**	Every 5 years, starting at age 50. FSIG can be performed alone, or consideration can be given to combining FSIG performed every 5 years with a highly sensitive FOBT or FIT performed annually.
		Double contrast barium enema (DCBE), **or**	Every 5 years, starting at age 50.
		Colonoscopy	Every 10 years, starting at age 50.
		CT colonography	Every 5 years, starting at age 50.
Endometrial	Women, at menopause	At the time of menopause, woman at average risk should be informed about risks and symptoms of endometrial cancer and strongly encouraged to report any unexpected bleeding or spotting to their physicians.	
Prostate	Men, ages 50+	Digital rectal examination (DRE) and prostate-specific antigen test (PSA)	Men who have at least a 10-year life expectancy should have an opportunity to make an informed decision with their healthcare provider about whether to be screened for prostate cancer, after receiving information about the potential benefits, risks, and uncertainties associated with prostate cancer screening. Prostate cancer screening should not occur without an informed decision-making process.
Cancer-related checkup	Men and women, age 20+	On the occasion of a periodic health examination, the cancer-related checkup should include examination for cancers of the thyroid, testicles, ovaries, lymph nodes, oral cavity, and skin, as well as health counseling about tobacco, sun exposure, diet and nutrition, risk factors, sexual practices, and environmental and occupational exposures.	

Note: Screening recommendations for lung cancer will be released in 2012; please refer to cancer.org for the most current information.

* Beginning at age 40, annual clinical breast examination should be performed prior to mammography.

† New recommendations will be released in early 2012; please refer to cancer.org for the most current guidelines.

Reproduced from: American Cancer Society. *Cancer Facts and Figures 2012.* Atlanta, GA: American Cancer Society, 2012.

testicles. When the healthcare provider holds a flashlight up to the scrotum, the light does not pass through the lump. Other tests include abdominal and pelvic computed tomography (CT) scan, blood tests for tumor markers, and ultrasound of the scrotum.

Treatment

Treatment depends on the type of testicular tumor and the stage of the tumor. Once cancer is found, the first step is to determine the type by examining the cancer cells under a microscope. The next step is to determine how far the cancer has spread to other parts of the body. Stage 1 cancer has not spread beyond the testicle. Stage 2 cancer has spread to lymph nodes in the abdomen. Stage 3 cancer has spread beyond the lymph nodes (it could be as far as the liver, lungs, or brain).

Testicular cancer is one of the most treatable and curable cancers. The survival rate for men in stage 1 is greater than 95%. The disease-free survival rate for stage 2 and 3 cancers is slightly lower, depending on the size of the tumor and when treatment is begun. Three types of treatment exist: surgery to remove the testicle, radiation

Myths and Facts

About Coronary Heart Disease and Cancer

MYTH	FACT
If coronary heart disease runs in your family, you cannot do much to prevent getting it.	Coronary heart disease is related to a number of factors, of which heredity is but one. Other risk factors include smoking, lack of exercise, fatty diets, obesity, and high blood pressure. You can do much to eliminate or diminish the effects of these risk factors.
All cholesterol is bad.	The cholesterol that accumulates on the walls of the arteries, LDL, is bad for you. HDL cholesterol, however, helps to carry blood fats out of the body and therefore is helpful.
You can recognize whether your blood pressure is high, but you can do little to lower it.	High blood pressure occurs without any noticeable symptoms, but with a healthier diet and regular physical activity, you can lower blood pressure, even without medication.
You cannot possibly prevent cancer when it has so many causes.	Although cancer has many causes (e.g., various naturally occurring and artificial chemicals, carcinogens in cigarette smoke, and certain viruses), your exposure to most of these can be minimized through your lifestyle choices.
Cancer affects all groups of people to the same extent.	African-American men and women have a higher cancer death rate than that of white men and women. White men and women contract skin cancer to a much greater extent than do African-American men and women.

therapy using high-dose x-rays or other high-energy rays to prevent the tumor from returning, and/or chemotherapy to kill cancer cells (PubMed Health, 2010).

Diabetes

Diabetes is a disease that has a strong genetic component; that is, it runs in families. I know this only too well. My father had it, my brother has it, my daughter developed it when she became pregnant, and my sister-in-law needed organ transplants as a result of it. And yet, although a tendency to develop diabetes exists in certain families and people, lifestyle behaviors exert a tremendous influence over whether it will occur and, if it does, how severe it will be. The Diabetes Prevention Program, a large prevention study of people at high risk for diabetes, showed that lifestyle changes—losing weight and increasing physical activity—reduced the development of type 2 diabetes by 58% during a 3-year period.

Diabetes is a group of diseases marked by high levels of blood glucose resulting from defects in insulin production, insulin action, or both. **Insulin** is a hormone that is needed to convert sugar, starches, and other food into energy needed for daily life (American Diabetes Association, 2011).

Symptoms

Diabetes is diagnosed by the A1C test, which measures average blood glucose over a 2- to 3-month period of time. Symptoms include excessive thirst, increased urination, fatigue, weight loss, blurred vision, slow-healing sores, tingling in the hands or feet, and red, swollen, tender gums (Mayo Clinic, 2010).

Types of Diabetes

Among the different types of diabetes are the following:

- *Type 1 diabetes.* Previously called juvenile-onset diabetes, type 1 usually strikes children and young adults.

- *Type 2 diabetes.* Previously called adult-onset diabetes, type 2 accounts for 90–95% of all diagnosed cases of diabetes. It usually begins as insulin resistance, a disorder in which the cells do not use insulin properly. As the need for insulin rises, the pancreas gradually loses its ability to produce it.

- *Gestational diabetes.* This form of glucose intolerance is diagnosed during pregnancy. Gestational diabetes requires treatment during pregnancy to optimize maternal blood glucose levels to lessen the risk of complications in the infant. After pregnancy, blood glucose levels may revert to normal levels. However, many women with gestational diabetes develop diabetes within 5–10 years after delivery.

Prevalence of Diabetes

In the United States, 25.8 million children and adults—8.3% of the population—have diabetes. In 2010 alone, 1.9 million new cases of diabetes were diagnosed in people aged 20 and older. Men are slightly more prone to develop diabetes than are women. Of those aged 20 or older, 11.8% of men and 10.8% of women have diabetes. Prevalence rates also differ by race and ethnicity: 7.1% for whites, 8.4% for Asian Americans, 11.8% for Hispanics, and 12.6% for African Americans (Centers for Disease Control and Prevention, 2011).

Complications

Diabetes is associated with a number of important health consequences. Among these are the following (Centers for Disease Control and Prevention, 2011):

- *Heart disease and stroke.* Adults with diabetes have heart disease death rates approximately two to four times higher than those of adults without diabetes, and the risk for stroke is two to four times higher among people with diabetes.

Diabetes: a group of diseases marked by high levels of blood glucose resulting from defects in insulin production, insulin action, or both.

Insulin: a hormone that is needed to convert sugar, starches, and other food into energy needed for daily life.

- *High blood pressure.* From 2005 to 2008, of adults age 20 years or older with diabetes, 67% had blood pressure greater than or equal to 140/90 mmHg or used prescription medications for hypertension (high blood pressure).

- *Blindness.* Diabetes is the leading cause of new cases of blindness among adults 20–74 years of age.

- *Kidney disease.* Diabetes is the leading cause of kidney failure, accounting for 44% of new cases in 2008.

- *Nervous system disease (neuropathy).* About 60–70% of people with diabetes have mild to severe forms of nerve damage.

- *Amputation.* More than 60% of lower-limb amputations not resulting from accidents occur in people with diabetes.

- *Periodontal disease.* Periodontal (gum) disease is more common in people with diabetes. Among young adults, those with diabetes have approximately twice the risk of development of periodontal disease as those without diabetes.

- *Depression.* People with diabetes are twice as likely to have depression.

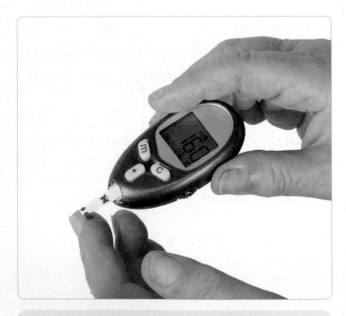

People with diabetes need to check their blood glucose levels regularly to determine if they need more medication or insulin.

Treatment of Diabetes

Diabetes can be treated or managed by diet, insulin, and oral medication to lower blood glucose levels. Type 1 diabetics must have insulin delivered by injection or an insulin pump. The pump monitors blood glucose levels and automatically dispenses insulin as needed. Type 2 diabetics can control their blood glucose by following a healthy diet and exercise program, losing excess weight, and taking oral medication. Some type 2 diabetics may also need insulin to control their blood glucose level.

To determine if you are at risk for diabetes, complete Health Check Up 7.3 (see Health Check Up 7.3 on the companion website). Once completed, place Health Check Up 7.3 in your Health Decision Portfolio.

What You Can Do to Prevent Lifestyle Diseases

Although the following scenario is not physiologically accurate, suspend your disbelief for few moments:

Imagine that various pimples are roaming about in your body. As one tries to emerge on your nose, you press down on it to prevent it from surfacing. Then, another pimple tries to emerge on your forehead. Once again, you press down at that spot to prevent it from surfacing. Other pimples try to emerge elsewhere. After a short while, you run out of arms and fingers to press down on all of the spots at which pimples might surface.

Lifestyle diseases are like pimples. There are too many diseases (*pimples*) to prevent (*press down*) each one separately. Fortunately, lifestyle diseases have common risk factors and therefore common prevention strategies. If you respond to this array of risk factors by using the following strategies, you can prevent many lifestyle diseases all at once:

- Eat a healthful diet consisting of diverse fruits and vegetables; whole grains; lean meats, poultry, or fish; fat-free or low-fat milk and milk products; beans, eggs, and nuts; limited saturated fat and no trans fat; limited salt; and controlled portion sizes.

- Maintain a desirable weight for your height and body structure.

- Engage in regular physical activity.

- Manage stress.

- Refrain from the use of all tobacco products, including cigarettes, cigars, pipes, and chewing tobacco. If you now use tobacco products, know that once ceasing such use, your risk for contracting lifestyle diseases decreases significantly.

- Furthermore, many of the ways recommended to reduce the risk of development of lifestyle diseases are interrelated. For example, consider how these prevention strategies reinforce one another:

  - Engaging in regular physical activity helps control weight and blood pressure and manages stress.

- Eating nutritionally helps prevent overweight and obesity, provides energy for physical activity, and is an important variable in maintaining a healthy blood chemistry (low total cholesterol and lipid levels).

- Avoiding or giving up tobacco products improves endurance during physical activity and helps control blood pressure.

Remember, too, that regular visits to your doctor or your campus health center can help keep you aware of and up-to-date with vaccinations and screenings that can help prevent multiple lifestyle diseases or catch them at an early, treatable stage. Continuing to read and learn about the latest prevention recommendations will also serve you well throughout your life.

SUMMARY

The goal of this chapter is to provide you with the tools you need to prevent lifestyle diseases. To help you do that, a summary of important information included in this chapter is provided.

- Lifestyle diseases are those diseases that result from health behaviors people adopt or do not adopt. Examples of prevalent lifestyle diseases are heart disease, stroke, cancer, diabetes, and sexually transmitted diseases.

- The circulatory system is composed of arteries, capillaries, and veins. Arteries are large blood vessels that leave the heart to supply oxygen and nutrients to organs and tissues of the body. Capillaries are smaller blood vessels that transport oxygen and nutrients from the arteries to all cells of the body and from body cells to veins. Veins are blood vessels that return blood to the heart after oxygen and nutrients are exchanged for carbon dioxide and waste products.

- Some risk factors for lifestyle diseases cannot be modified, such as age and family history. Other risk factors can be modified, such as diet, physical activity level, use of tobacco, and management of stress.

- Cholesterol is a waxy, fat-like substance found in the membranes of cells in all parts of the body. The body uses cholesterol to make hormones, bile acids, vitamin D, and other substances. Cholesterol circulates in the bloodstream in packages called lipoproteins. Two main kinds of lipoproteins carry cholesterol in the blood: LDL and HDL. A low level of HDL increases the risk for heart disease, and a high level of HDL decreases the risk for heart disease.

- Stroke is a circulatory disorder that occurs when a portion of the brain is deprived of the flow of oxygenated blood. The brain can be deprived of blood because of a blockage of the blood vessels supplying the brain (ischemic stroke) or a rupture of those blood vessels (hemorrhagic stroke).

- Risk factors for stroke include high blood pressure, smoking, diabetes, heart diseases, brain aneurysms, age and gender, race and ethnicity, and a personal or family history of stroke.

- Cancer is the uncontrolled growth of abnormal cells in the body (called malignant cells). The three most common cancers in men in the United States are prostate cancer, lung cancer, and colon cancer, and the three most common cancers in women in the United States are breast cancer, colon cancer, and lung cancer.

- Diabetes is a group of diseases marked by high levels of blood glucose resulting from defects in insulin production, insulin action, or both. Insulin is a hormone that is needed to convert sugar, starches, and other food into energy needed for daily life. Symptoms include excessive thirst, increased urination, fatigue, weight loss, blurred vision, slow-healing sores, tingling in the hands or feet, and red, swollen, tender gums.

- To prevent lifestyle diseases or postpone them until old age, eat nutritiously, participate in regular physical activity, maintain a healthy weight, control high blood pressure, refrain from the use of tobacco products, manage stress, and obtain recommended medical screenings.

REFERENCES

American Academy of Dermatology. *Skin Cancer.* 2011. Available at: http://www.aad.org/media-resources/stats-and-facts/conditions/skin-cancer.

American Cancer Society. *Cancer Facts and Figures, 2010.* Atlanta, GA: American Cancer Society, 2010.

American Cancer Society. Breast cancer survival rates by stage. *Learn About Cancer.* 2011a. Available at: http://www.cancer.org/cancer/breastcancer/detailedguide/breast-cancer-survival-by-stage.

American Cancer Society. Colon cancer. *Learn About Cancer.* 2011b. Available at: http://www.cancer.org/Cancer/ColonandRectumCancer/DetailedGuide/colorectal-cancer-survival-rates.

American Cancer Society. *Learn About Cancer: Skin Cancer Facts.* 2011c. Available at: http://www.cancer.org/Cancer/CancerCauses/SunandUVExposure/skin-cancer-facts.

American Dental Hygienists' Association. *Tobacco Use and Heart Disease Fact Sheet.* 2010. Available at: http://www.adha.org/media/facts/tobacco-heart.htm.

American Diabetes Association. *Diabetes Statistics.* 2011. Available at: http://www.diabetes.org/diabetes-basics/diabetes-statistics/.

Andriole, G. L., Crawford, E. D., Grubb, III, R. L., Buys, S. S., Chia, D., Church, T. R., et al. Mortality results from a randomized prostate-cancer screening trial. *New England Journal of Medicine* 360 (2009): 1310–1319.

Cagan, R. L. A Drosophila model of diabetes-related heart disease. *News and Research, American Diabetes Association.* 2010. Available at: http://www.diabetes.org/news-research/research/research-database/a-drosophila-model-of.html.

Centers for Disease Control and Prevention. *National Diabetes Fact Sheet: National Estimates and General Information on Diabetes and Prediabetes in the United States.* Atlanta, GA: U.S. Department of Health and Human Services, Centers for Disease Control and Prevention, 2011.

Diseases and Conditions Index. Stroke. National Heart, Lung, and Blood Institute. 2011. Available at: http://www.nhlbi.nih.gov/health/dci/Diseases/stroke/stroke_what.html.

Increased stroke risk from birth control pills, review finds. *Science News.* October 26, 2009. Available at: http://www.sciencedaily.com/releases/2009/10/091026152820.htm.

Mayo Clinic. Diabetes symptoms: When diabetes symptoms are a concern. *Diabetes.* 2010. Available at: http://www.mayoclinic.com/health/diabetes-symptoms/DA00125.

National Center for Biotechnology Information. *Colon Cancer.* PubMed Health. 2010. Available at: http://www.ncbi.nlm.nih.gov/pubmedhealth/PMH0001308/.

National Heart, Lung, and Blood Institute. *Your Guide to Lowering Your Cholesterol With TLC: Therapeutic Lifestyle Changes.* Washington, DC: National Heart, Lung, and Blood Institute, 2005.

PubMed Health. *Testicular Cancer.* 2010. Available at: http://www.ncbi.nlm.nih.gov/pubmedhealth/PMH0002266/.

Schroder, F. H., Hugosson, J., Roobol, M. J., Tammela, T. L. J., Ciatto, S., Nelen, V., et al. Screening and prostate-cancer mortality in a randomized European study. *New England Journal of Medicine* 360 (2009): 1320–1328.

INTERNET RESOURCES

American Diabetes Association
http://www.diabetes.org/

American Heart Association
http://www.aha.org/

American Cancer Society
http://www.cancer.org

National Stroke Association
http://www.stroke.org/site/PageNavigator/HOME

American Social Health Association
http://www.ashastd.org/

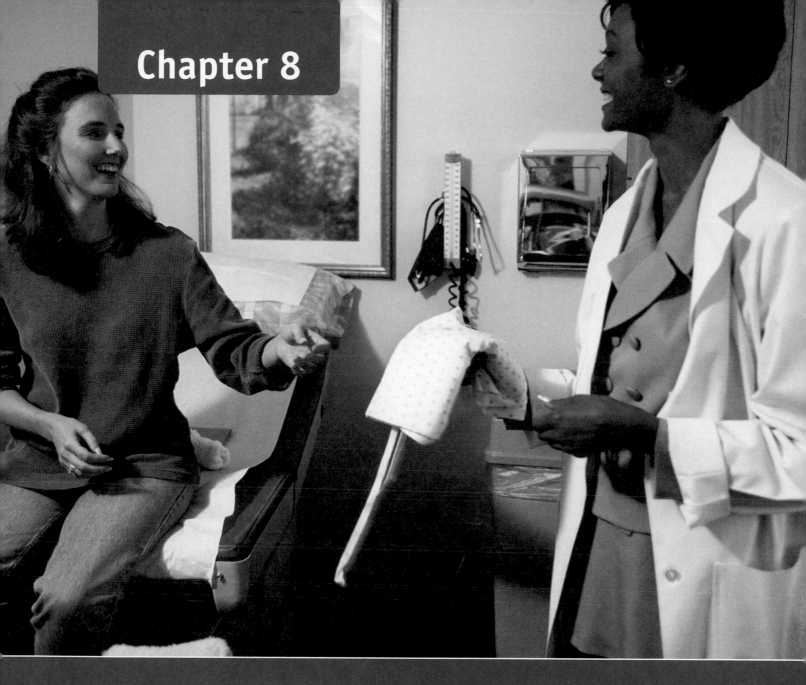

Chapter 8

Being an Informed Health Consumer

 Access Health Check Ups and Health Behavior Change activities on the Companion Website:
go.jblearning.com/Empowering.

Learning Objectives

- Describe how to choose a healthcare provider.
- Discuss how to evaluate healthcare providers and hospitals.
- Define complementary alternative therapies and discuss their pros and cons.
- Describe self-care skills one should acquire and the self-care supplies and medications that should be on hand.
- Explain how to choose health and dental insurance coverage.

Imagine you walk into a grocery store intending to shop for the items on your shopping list. To your surprise, however, at the entrance of the store you are given a large shopping bag and instructed to proceed directly to the cash register. There, the cashier puts a lot of different foods, pharmacy items, and paper goods in your bag and charges you accordingly. At that point, what would you do? Pay for the items and leave the store? Probably not. Refuse to pay, stating you do not want those items and, in fact, came into the store with a list of items you did want? That is more probable.

This scenario may sound farfetched, but something akin to it occurs every day in the United States. Patients visit their healthcare providers with one intention (perhaps a physical exam) and are told they need to have other screenings, tests, or procedures—and often, they unquestioningly agree to these. This does not mean patients should not agree to such procedures, only that patients should not do so without understanding the reasons for the procedures, what they entail, how accurate they are, and how invasive they will be. In other words, we should be informed consumers when we go grocery shopping *and* when we seek healthcare. This chapter is designed to help you take a more active role in your healthcare.

Choosing a Healthcare Provider

One of the most important decisions you make regarding your healthcare is choosing a primary healthcare provider. This may be an internist, family practitioner, or some other medical provider. One of the best pieces of advice with respect to choosing a healthcare provider is to do it *before* you need care. In that way, you will have the time to make an informed decision rather than being rushed to receive treatment when you are ill. In addition, if you are already a patient, you will be more likely to receive care promptly.

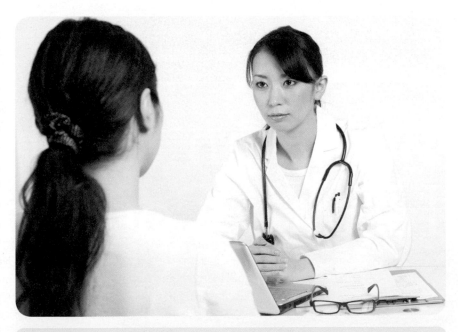

Choosing a doctor should be done systematically.

What I Need to Know

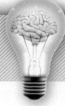

How to Check Up on a Doctor

You can check on a doctor you are considering to use as your physician by using the following resources. Note that some of these are free, whereas others charge a fee.

Free:

■ *Administrators in Medicine* (www.docfinder .org). Information on licensing and disciplinary actions taken against doctors in 18 states; links to state medical boards of remaining states.

■ *American Board of Medical Specialties* (www .abms.org). List of board-certified doctors. Board certification means the doctor has completed an approved residency program and passed a detailed written exam in at least one of 24 specialty areas, such as family practice, internal medicine, or obstetrics and gynecology.

■ *American Medical Association DoctorFinder* (webapps.ama-assn.org/doctorfinder). Comprehensive information, including educational history, board certification, and hospital admitting privileges, for the 40% of

doctors who belong to the American Medical Association.

Requires a Fee:

■ *Consumers' Checkbook Guide to Top Doctors* (www.checkbook.org). Searchable database (with an annual subscription fee) of the top-rated doctors in 30 fields based on a survey of about 260,000 physicians. You can also receive a print copy by mail for the same price.

■ *Federation of State Medical Boards Physician Profiles* (www.docinfo.org). Disciplinary sanctions, education, licensure history, and practice locations for U.S.-licensed physicians and some physician assistants. All information comes from the group's comprehensive, nationally consolidated data bank.

■ *HealthGrades* (www.healthgrades.com). Reports on doctors, including education and training, board certification, professional misconduct or disciplinary actions, and satisfaction scores from patients.

Choosing a Doctor

You have probably heard of the patient who tells the doctor, "It hurts when I do this," and the doctor replies, "Well, then don't do that." This is not a doctor you want. You want someone with medical knowledge and skills, but you also want a doctor who is more sympathetic than one who tells you, "Then don't do that." You want to be comfortable with his or her *bedside manner*, the way the doctor listens, communicates, and responds to your needs.

There are criteria you can use to make sure you select a doctor with solid appropriate expertise *and* good bedside manner. Health Check Up 8.1 will help you generate a list of doctors to consider for service as your primary care physician. Once that list is generated, Health Check Up 8.2 will help you select the doctor that best meets your needs (see Health Check Ups 8.1 and 8.2 on the companion website). Once completed, place Health Check Ups 8.1 and 8.2 in your Health Decision Portfolio.

You may be thinking that choosing a doctor is as simple as going with one recommended by a family member or friend. Your medical status, however, is not like anyone else's. The fact that a doctor is good for a family member or friend does not mean that doctor will be good for you. So, be careful with something as important as your health. Even if you are seriously considering a recommended doctor for your healthcare, take the time to use Health Check Ups 8.1 and 8.2 before finalizing that choice. Next, check out any doctor being considered. The accompanying What I Need to Know box shows how to conduct that evaluation.

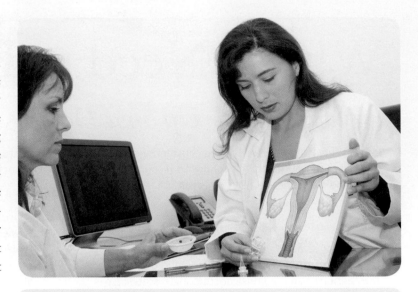

Gynecologists sometimes serve as primary care physicians for women.

The Primary Care Physician: The Gatekeeper

Primary care doctors are trained to serve as your main doctor over the long term. They provide medical care when needed, encourage health-related behaviors and discourage risky behaviors to help you remain healthy, and oversee and coordinate your health and medical care. Primary care doctors can also refer you to other medical specialists when necessary. The primary care doctor is your first point of contact, a sort of "gatekeeper" for your medical and health needs.

Medical doctors (MDs) make up the majority of primary care providers: MDs have received training in 4-year medical schools and performed residencies after medical school in which they learned a specialty branch of medicine in a hospital setting. Internists and family practice physicians are the two largest groups of primary care physicians (Agency for Healthcare Research and Quality, 2001). Some women choose obstetrician/gynecologists as their primary care doctor, and many parents choose pediatricians to serve as the primary care doctor for their children. In addition, physician assistants, nurse practitioners, and certified nurse midwives deliver primary care. Physician assistants must practice in partnership with physicians, although nurse practitioners and certified nurse midwives can work independently. **Doctors of osteopathy (DOs)** are another type of primary care giver. A DO is different from an MD in that he or she has received training in hands-on manual medicine and the body's musculoskeletal system and specializes in a hands-on approach to make sure that the body is moving freely.

Regardless of which kind of primary care provider you choose, one skill you should develop is how to talk to your doctor to get the most out of the care provided. The accompanying What I Need to Know box advises you how to speak with your doctor during office visits.

Primary care doctors: provide medical care when needed, encourage health-related behavior and discourage risky behaviors to help patients remain healthy, and oversee and coordinate patients' health and medical care; the first point of contact, a sort of gatekeeper for the medical and health needs of patients.

Medical doctors (MDs): physicians who have received training in 4-year medical schools and performed residencies in which they learned a specialty branch of medicine.

Doctors of osteopathy (DOs): physicians who have received training in hands-on manual medicine and the body's musculoskeletal system.

What I Need to Know

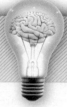

How to Communicate with Doctors

The single most important way you can stay healthy is to be an active member of your own healthcare team. One way to get high-quality healthcare is to find and use information and take an active role in all the decisions made about your care.

This information can help you communicate effectively with your doctor.

Give Information. Don't Wait to Be Asked!

- You know important things about your symptoms and your health history. Tell your doctor what you think he or she needs to know. It is important to tell your doctor personal information—even if it makes you feel embarrassed or uncomfortable.

- Bring a *health history* list with you, and keep it up to date.

- Always bring any medicines you are taking or a list of those medicines (include what strength and when and how often you take them; for example, 100 mg sertraline, once a day, at 8 a.m.). Talk about any allergies or reactions you have had to your medicines.

- Bring other medical information, such as x-ray films, test results, and medical records.

Get Information

- Ask questions. If you don't, your doctor may think you understand everything that was said.

- Write down your questions before your visit. List the most important ones first to make sure they get asked and answered.

- You might want to bring a family member or friend along to help you ask questions. This person can also help you understand and/or remember the answers.

- Take notes.

- Let your doctor know if you need more time. If there is not time that day, perhaps you can speak to a nurse or physician assistant on staff. Or, ask if you can call later to speak with someone.

Take Information Home

- Ask for written instructions.

- Take any brochures that might help you. If not, ask how you can get such materials or ask for website links that would be helpful.

Once You Leave the Doctor's Office, Follow Up

- If you have questions, call.

- If your symptoms get worse or if you have problems with your medicine, call.

- If you had tests and do not hear from your doctor, call for your test results.

- If your doctor said you need to have certain tests, make appointments at the lab or other offices to get them done.

- If your doctor said you should see a specialist, make an appointment.

- Get copies of all test results for your records. Also request that x-ray films be given to you. These may be available on disk, but the actual films are more reliable. Keep your records organized at home. Years from now, you may need to compare new tests with ones you had in college. It may be difficult to access the original results unless you keep them yourself.

For more on healthcare quality and materials to help you make healthcare decisions, go to the website of the Agency for Healthcare Research and Quality (www.ahrq.gov).

REPRODUCED FROM: *Quick Tips—When Talking with Your Doctor*. AHRQ Publication No. 01-0040a. Rockville, MD: Agency for Healthcare Research and Quality, May 2002. Available at: http://www.ahrq.gov/consumer/quicktips/doctalk.htm.

Choosing a Dentist

There are several factors to consider when choosing a dentist. Among these are location and hours, cost, personal comfort, professional qualifications, and availability of emergency care (WebMD, 2009; Colgate World of Care, 2011).

■ *Location.* Choose a dentist close to home or work. This will make it easier to schedule visits and to arrive on time.

■ *Hours.* What are the office hours? Are they convenient for your schedule?

■ *Cost.* Does the dentist accept your insurance? Does the dentist offer multiple payment options (credit cards, personal checks, payment plans)? If your insurance plan requires referrals to specialists, can this dentist provide them? What is the dentist's office policy on missed appointments? Also, be aware that costs vary by practice. If you can, get estimates of what your dentist might charge for common procedures such as fillings, crowns, or root canal therapy. Even if you have dental insurance, you may be paying part of the costs yourself.

■ *Personal comfort.* One of the most important things to consider when you choose a dentist is whether you feel comfortable with that person. Are you able to explain symptoms and ask questions? Do you feel like the dentist hears and understands your concerns? Would you feel comfortable asking for pain medicine, expressing your fear or anxiety, or asking questions about a procedure? What type of anesthesia is the dentist certified to administer to help you relax and feel more comfortable during any necessary dental treatment?

■ *Professional qualifications.* The dentist's office staff should be able to tell you about the dentist's training, and the practice should have policies on infection control. If the staff seems uncomfortable answering your questions or you are uncomfortable with their answers, consider finding another dentist. You can also obtain information about a dentist's qualifications from the local dental society or your insurance carrier. Most organizations of specialty dentists also list the qualifications of their members.

■ *Emergency care.* Find out what happens if you have an emergency either during normal office hours or at night or on a weekend. A dentist should not refer you to a hospital emergency room. You should be able to contact your dentist (or a suitable substitute) at any time by calling an answering service, cell phone, or pager.

Friends or family can also be good sources to aid you in choosing a dentist. Ask them the following questions:

■ How well does the dentist explain treatment options?

■ Do you feel comfortable asking questions?

■ How does the office handle emergencies?

■ How long do you have to wait for an appointment?

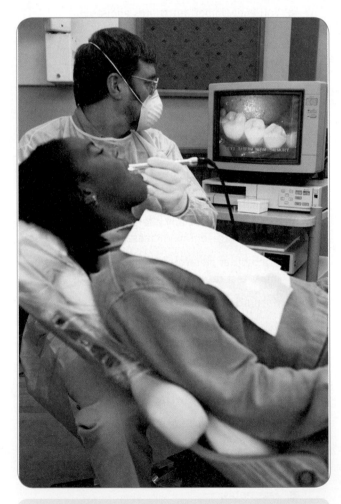

One of the most important considerations when you choose a dentist is whether you feel comfortable with that person.

- How long do you have to sit in the waiting room?

- How are bills handled?

Evaluating Healthcare Providers

Just because you choose a particular healthcare provider does not mean you are stuck with that person. You should periodically evaluate the care you receive; if it does not meet your standards, choose another provider.

Evaluating Your Doctor

One means of evaluation is to determine whether your doctor is providing the basic preventive healthcare and screenings recommended by national and professional guidelines. Table 8.1 shows these guidelines.

In addition, decide if you are satisfied with the access you have to your doctor. Is the office reachable by telephone or email? Can you make appointments easily and be seen in a reasonable period of time? Are any laboratory results communicated to you in a timely fashion? Has the doctor been able to diagnose your illnesses accurately, and has treatment been effective? Is the doctor easy to talk to and responsive to your questions and concerns?

Recall the scenario at the beginning of this chapter, which described having no choice at a supermarket but having to pay for grocery items anyway. This kind of scenario need not apply to your initial choice of a doctor or to your continued choice to stay with him or her. You are the one in charge of getting your money's worth for your healthcare.

Evaluating Your Dentist

There are several factors you should consider when evaluating your dentist. One is whether you are you satisfied with the charges you pay for dental services. Dental fees vary widely. One investigation involved two patients with completely healthy mouths and teeth who were seen by six dentists. One patient was given estimates for dental work by the six dentists that ranged from $645 to $2,563, and the other patient's estimated costs ranged from $2,135 and $7,960 (Dodes, 1997). Other investigations have disclosed similar variation in prices quoted by dentists. If

the charges for your dental services seem excessively high or you suspect unnecessary procedures are being recommended, consider choosing another dentist.

Next, evaluate your satisfaction with any dental work you have had done (How to Choose a Dentist, 1997):

- How does your bite feel?

- Is any of the dental work irritating your gums?

- Does the treated tooth look like a tooth?

- Does dental floss or your tongue catch on the tooth?

- Did the dentist take time to polish your fillings?

- Do you feel pain when drinking hot or cold liquids?

- Was any debris left in your mouth after treatment?

If you are not satisfied with the dental care you receive, go through the process detailed earlier to choose another dentist that better meets your needs.

Choosing and Evaluating Hospitals

If you need hospitalization, you will most likely choose a hospital recommended by your physician or, in the case of an emergency, you will simply go to the hospital to which the ambulance transports you. However, for elective surgeries (such as arthroscopic surgery on your knee) or for procedures for which you have sufficient advance notice (such as birth delivery), you have a choice as to which hospital you use. In these instances, it is important to consider quality, because research shows that some hospitals simply do a better job than others. For example, studies comparing hospitals that offer the same kind of surgery have found that *more-experienced* hospitals (those that perform the surgery more often) have better outcomes for their patients.

One criterion to consider is whether the hospital is accredited. Hospitals can, but are not required to, seek accreditation from The Joint Commission, an independent, nonprofit organization. The Joint Commission uses 28 areas of performance that include infection control, patients' rights, social services, and surgical procedures. Six different accreditation levels may be awarded:

TABLE 8.1 Basic Preventive Healthcare and Screenings Recommended by National and Professional Guidelines

Test or Procedure	To Detect or Prevent	How Often
Physical exam		
Abdomen	Enlarged liver or spleen, aortic aneurysm	Every few years, especially in men after age 50
Breasts	Breast cancer	Every 1–2 years starting at age 40
Heart	Murmur, irregular heartbeat	Every visit
Height and weight	Overweight; also osteoporosis in postmenopausal women	Every visit
Neck	Thyroid nodules and narrowed carotid arteries	Every few years, especially after age 60
Pelvic	Cancer and other problems in bladder, ovaries, rectum, uterus, vagina	Annually until age 30, then every 2 to 3 years
Rectal	Colorectal and prostate cancer	Every 1–2 years starting at age 40
Testicles and groin	Inguinal hernia and cancer	Every few years, especially between age 20 and 35
Immunizations		
Hepatitis B	Hepatitis B, a liver disease	Once by age 20
Influenza	Flu	Annually
Pneumococcal	Pneumonia	Once at age 65
Tetanus booster	Tetanus	Every 10 years
Varicella	Chicken pox	Given to anyone who has not had chicken pox
Screening tests: definitely or probably needed		
Blood pressure	Hypertension	Every visit
Bone densitometry	Osteoporosis	Every 2–3 years after menopause in women; at least once after age 65 in men
Colonoscopy or sigmoidoscopy plus fecal occult blood test (FOBT)	Colon and rectal cancer	Starting at age 50, colonoscopy every 10 years or sigmoidoscopy every 5 years, plus FOBT annually
Complete lipid profile	High LDL-cholesterol or tri-glyceride levels or low HDL level	Every 5 years starting at age 20
Eye exam	Glaucoma, macular degeneration, and other vision problems	Every 3–5 years before age 45 and every 1–3 years after that
Fasting plasma glucose (FPG)	Diabetes and metabolic syndrome	Every 3 years starting at age 45
Mammography	Breast cancer	Every 1–2 years starting at age 40
Pap smear and human papillomavirus (HPV) testing	Cervical cancer (Pap smear) and virus that causes it (HPV test)	Annual Pap smear through age 30, then Pap smear alone or combined with HPV test every 2–3 years; can usually stop testing after hysterectomy or age 65
Thyroid-stimulating hormone (TSH)	Thyroid disease	Every 5 years starting at age 35

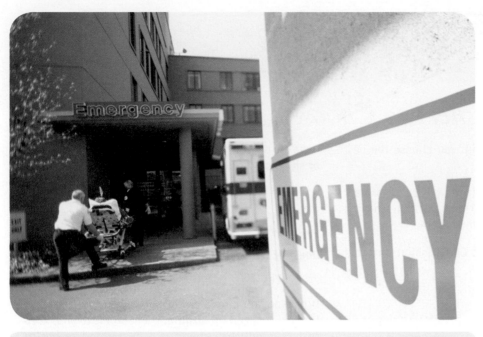

Sometimes patients must use the hospital with which their doctor is affiliated. Other times, however, patients have a choice about which hospital they will use.

■ *Provisional Accreditation.* This only applies to new hospitals that have passed an initial assessment. They will be assessed twice more in the next 6 months, at which time their status will change depending on the results.

The federal government has made available an on-line source to compare hospitals. All you need do is go to http://www.hospitalcompare.hhs.gov and type in your area code. You then have the opportunity to compare up to three hospitals at a time against each other based on the following criteria:

■ *Accreditation with Recommendations for Improvement.* The hospital meets most standards, but regarding at least one critical area it does not. The hospital is given a time frame in which to meet this standard; if it fails to do so, accreditation is withdrawn. About 90% of hospitals that apply are given this status.

■ *Full Accreditation.* The hospital meets all standards in every area of performance. This accreditation is earned by about 4% of hospitals that apply.

■ *Accreditation with Commendation.* In these cases, the hospital not only meets all standards but also proves to be outstanding overall. This accreditation is also earned by about 4% of hospitals that apply.

■ *Conditional Accreditation.* The hospital's performance is considered marginal at best. The hospital is given a time frame in which to improve certain areas or risk losing Conditional Accreditation. This accreditation is earned by about 1% of hospitals that apply.

■ *Denied Accreditation.* The hospital fails to meet Joint Commission standards. Less than 1% of hospitals that apply are denied accreditation.

■ Patients who reported that their nurses *always* communicated well.

■ Patients who reported that their doctors *always* communicated well.

■ Patients who reported that they *always* received help as soon as they wanted.

■ Patients who reported that their pain was *always* well controlled.

■ Patients who reported that staff *always* explained medicines before administering them.

■ Patients who reported that their room and bathroom were *always* clean.

■ Patients who reported that the area around their room was *always* quiet at night.

■ Patients at each hospital who reported that *yes*, they were given information about what to do during their recovery at home.

What I Need to Know

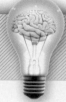

Using a Worksheet to Choose a Hospital

The following questions can help you choose the best hospital for your needs.

You may not have a choice right now because of your health plan or doctor, but keep these questions in mind for when you might make a change.

Does the hospital meet Joint Commission national quality standards?

___ Yes   ___ No

You can order The Joint Commission's performance reports free of charge by calling 630-792-5800. Or, check its website at www.jointcommission.org for a hospital's performance report or for its accreditation status.

How does the hospital compare with others in my area?

_____

_____

_____

_____

One effective way to learn about hospital quality is to look at hospital report cards developed by state governments and consumer groups. Some states—for example, Pennsylvania, California, and Ohio—have laws that require hospitals to report data on the quality of their care. The information is then given to the public so consumers can compare hospitals. Some groups gather information on how well hospitals perform and how satisfied their patients are. An example is the Cleveland Health Quality Choice Program, which is made up of businesses, doctors, and hospitals. Consumer groups also publish guides to hospitals and other healthcare facilities in various cities. You can find out what kind of information is available where you live by calling your state department of health, healthcare council, or hospital association. Also, ask your doctor what he or she thinks about the hospital.

Does my doctor have privileges at the hospital (is he or she permitted to admit patients)?

___ Yes   ___ No

If not, you would need to be under the care of another doctor while at the hospital.

Does my health plan cover care at the hospital?

___ Yes   ___ No

If not, do you have another way to pay for your care? If going to a certain hospital is important to you, keep that in mind when choosing a doctor and/or health plan. In general, you will need to go to a hospital where your doctor has *privileges*.

Does the hospital have experience with my condition?

___ Yes   ___ No

For example, *general* hospitals treat a wide range of routine conditions, such as hernias and pneumonia, whereas *specialty* hospitals have a lot of experience with certain conditions (such as cancer) or certain groups (such as children). You may be able to choose one hospital for gallbladder surgery and another hospital if you need care for a heart condition.

Has the hospital had success with my condition?

___ Yes   ___ No

Research shows that hospitals that do many of the same types of procedures tend to have better success with them. In other words, *practice makes perfect*. Ask your doctor or the hospital if there is information on how often the procedure is done there, how often the doctor does the procedure, and how well the patients do (patient outcomes). Note that some health departments and other organizations publish reports on outcomes for certain procedures.

- Patients who gave their hospital a rating of 9 or 10 on a scale from 0 (lowest) to 10 (highest).

- Patients who reported *yes*, they would definitely recommend the hospital.

A worksheet for choosing a hospital is presented in the accompanying What I Need to Know box.

Deciding Whether to Use Complementary or Alternative Medicine

Some people believe that conventional medical procedures are not enough to keep them healthy or to treat effectively the conditions they develop. Many of these people turn to complementary or alternative medicine. In fact, the 2007 National Health Interview Survey conducted by the federal government found that 38% of American adults use complementary or alternative medicine (Centers for Disease Control and Prevention, 2004).

What Is Complementary or Alternative Medicine?

Complementary or alternative medicine (CAM) comprises diverse medical and health care systems, practices, therapies, and products that are not currently considered to be part of conventional medicine (Table 8.2). **Conventional medicine** (also called Western or allopathic medicine) is medicine as practiced by holders of MD or DO degrees and by allied health professionals, such as physical therapists, psychologists, and registered nurses. *Complementary medicine* refers to the use of CAM together with

conventional medicine, such as use of relaxation techniques together with prescribed medications to lessen pain. *Alternative medicine* refers to the use of CAM in place of conventional medicine, such as spinal manipulation by a chiropractor rather than back surgery (National Center for Complementary and Alternative Medicine, 2010).

TABLE 8.2	Common Complementary or Alternative Therapies

Natural Products
Dietary supplements: such as multivitamins
Probiotics: live microorganisms (usually bacteria) that are similar to microorganisms found in the digestive tract
Botanical medicines: such as herbal medicine
Mind and Body Medicine
Meditation
Yoga
Acupuncture
Deep-breathing exercises
Guided imagery
Hypnotherapy
Progressive relaxation
Qi gong
Tai chi
Manipulative and Body-Based Practices
Spinal manipulation
Massage therapy
Other CAM Practices
Movement therapies: such as pilates and rolfing
Manipulation of energy fields: such as magnet therapy, light therapy, qi gong, Reiki, and healing touch
Whole Medical Systems
Ayurvedic medicine
Traditional Chinese medicine
Homeopathy
Naturopathy

REPRODUCED FROM: National Center for Complementary and Alternative Medicine. *What Is Complementary and Alternative Medicine?* 2011. Available at: http://nccam.nih.gov/health/whatiscam/#types.

Complementary or alternative medicine (CAM): diverse medical and healthcare systems, practices, therapies, and products that are not currently considered to be part of conventional medicine.

Conventional medicine: medicine as practiced by holders of MD or DO degrees and by allied health professionals, such as physical therapists, psychologists, and registered nurses.

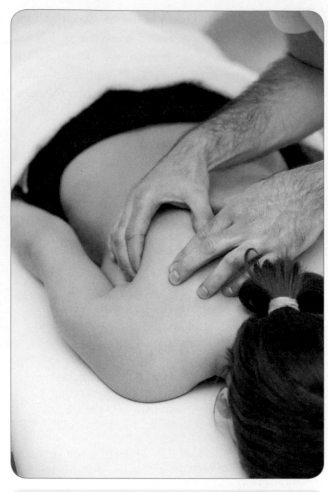

A person considering use of complementary or alternative medicine therapies should read the research on the safety and effectiveness of those therapies before pursuing them.

What Does the Research Show?

If you are considering use of a CAM therapy, consult with the *National Center for Complementary and Alternative Medicine* to determine what research has been conducted regarding that therapy and what the results showed. The center's research can be accessed at its website: http://nccam.nih.gov/research.

Self-Care

Medical self-care is defined as the things that individuals do to deal with minor illness and injuries at home.

This includes preventing, detecting, and treating illness and disease. It is estimated that 80% of health problems can be treated at home (Carlson, 2009). Furthermore, it is estimated that 70% of visits to physicians are for conditions that could be treated at home. When you take an over-the-counter drug for a headache, this is an example of medical self-care. Other examples of health issues that can be treated at home are acne, many allergies, bruises and minor burns, colds, and most cases of back pain, influenza, headache, vomiting and diarrhea, and sore throat (Tajeu, 2005).

Self-Care Skills

To perform self-care, you need to develop certain skills. Generally, you need to know how to prevent common illnesses, be able to recognize signs and symptoms of illness, know how to treat these illnesses, and recognize when it is necessary to seek care from a healthcare provider. Among the specific skills and knowledge you should acquire are the following:

1. Which immunizations to receive and when.

2. How to eat nutritionally and maintain a healthy weight.

3. How to exercise at the recommended frequency, intensity, and duration and the proper amount of sleep to get each night.

4. How to use drugs appropriately: refrain from use of alcohol or use it in moderation, refrain from use of tobacco, and use over-the-counter medications as recommended.

5. Which health screenings to obtain and when (see Table 8.1).

6. How to control stress through the use of stress-management techniques.

> **Medical self-care:** those things individuals do to deal with minor illness and injuries at home; this includes preventing, detecting, and treating illness and disease.

Myths *and* Facts

About Complementary and Alternative Medicine

MYTH	FACT
There are rigorous, well-designed clinical trials for most complementary and alternative therapies.	Well-designed clinical trials for many complementary and alternative therapies are lacking; therefore, the safety and effectiveness of many CAM therapies are uncertain. The National Center for Complementary and Alternative Medicine is sponsoring research designed to fill this knowledge gap by building a scientific evidence base about CAM therapies—whether they are safe and whether they work for the conditions for which people use them and, if so, how they work.
Although CAM therapies may not be effective, they are not harmful.	CAM therapies can potentially be unsafe. For example, manipulation of the spine can result in injury. Furthermore, if CAM therapies are substituted for traditional medical practices rather than used as supplements to those practices, effective treatment is withheld and illnesses and disease may be exacerbated.
Dietary supplements are among the safest CAM therapies and can be used by almost everyone.	Dietary supplements may interact with medications or other supplements, may have side effects of their own, or may contain potentially harmful ingredients not listed on the label. In addition, most supplements have not been tested in pregnant women, nursing mothers, or children.
Costs of CAM therapies are not of concern because health insurance companies will reimburse patients for these services.	Most CAM therapies are expensive, long term, and costs are not reimbursable from health insurance providers.

7. How to behave safely: drive and bike safely, practice safer sex, follow firearm safety rules, and keep poisonous products out of the reach of children.

8. How to take a temperature, count pulse rates, and take blood pressure.

9. First aid skills such as CPR, the Heimlich maneuver, wrapping a sprain, and applying compression bandages (to stop bleeding) and butterfly bandages (to keep deep cuts closed).

10. How to acquire and maintain your medical records and personal health history. Health Check Up 8.3 guides you through this process (see Health Check Up 8.3 on the companion website).

Once completed, place Health Check Up 8.3 in your Health Decision Portfolio.

11. How to evaluate health-related websites (see the HONcode box later in the "Using the Internet" section).

Self-Care Supplies and Medications

There are specific supplies and medications you should have at home in order to perform basic self-care procedures:

1. Adhesive bandages
2. Support bandages for wrapping sprains
3. Sterile gauze
4. Antiseptic ointments or wipes
5. Cotton balls
6. Petroleum jelly
7. Thermometer
8. Tweezers
9. Cold packs
10. Heating pad
11. Medicine spoon
12. Sunscreen

Among the medications you should have are the following:

1. Acetaminophen (Tylenol)
2. Aspirin
3. Ibuprofen (e.g., Advil or Motrin)
4. Antacids (e.g., Rolaids or Tums)
5. An antidiarrhea medication (e.g., Kaopectate or Imodium-AD)
6. Cough suppressant (e.g., Robitussin-DM)
7. Decongestant (e.g., Sudafed)
8. Laxative (e.g., Metamucil or Correctol)
9. Throat anesthetic (e.g., Sucrets)

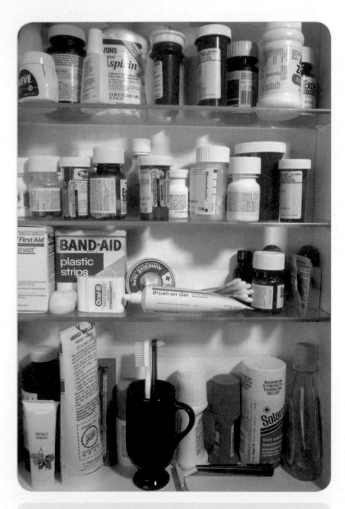

To administer medical self-care requires preparation in terms of maintaining necessary supplies and medications.

10. Toothache anesthetic (e.g., Anbesol)

11. Ointments or creams to relieve rashes and itching

12. Antibiotic ointments

13. Syrup of ipecac to induce vomiting (when poisoning is suspected)

Complete Health Check Up 8.4 to identify those self-care supplies and medications you already have on hand and those you need to acquire (see Health Check Up 8.4 on the companion website). Once completed, place Health Check Up 8.4 in your Health Decision Portfolio.

Self-Care Resources

There are many resources that can help you provide medical self-care. Several of these are listed here:

American College of Emergency Physicians. *American College of Emergency Physicians First Aid Manual, Second Edition*. London, England: DK Adult, 2004.

Fries, J. F. and Vickery, D. M. *Take Care of Yourself, 9th Edition: The Complete Illustrated Guide to Medical Self-Care*. Cambridge, MA: Da Capo Lifelong Books, 2009.

Mayo Clinic Health Solutions. *Embody Health: Guide to Self-Care*. Rochester, MN: Mayo Clinic Health Solutions, 2009.

Porter, R. *The Merck Manual Home Health Handbook: Third Home Edition*. Whitehouse Station, NJ: Merck, 2009.

Powell, D. *Healthier at Home*. Farmington Hills, MI: American Institute for Preventive Medicine Press, 2005.

Using the Internet

One of the most commonly used tools for medical self-care skills is the internet. Fifty-nine percent of the U.S. adult population access health information online. In fact, online searches for health information are the third most popular online pursuit, after email and use of a search engine for general information. A study conducted by the Pew Internet Project found (Fox, 2011):

■ Sixty-six percent of internet users look online for information about a specific disease or medical problem.

■ Fifty-six percent of internet users look online for information about a certain medical treatment or procedure.

■ Forty-four percent of internet users look online for information about doctors or other health professionals.

■ Thirty-six percent of internet users look online for information about hospitals or other medical facilities.

■ Thirty-three percent of internet users look online for information related to health insurance, including private insurance, Medicare, or Medicaid.

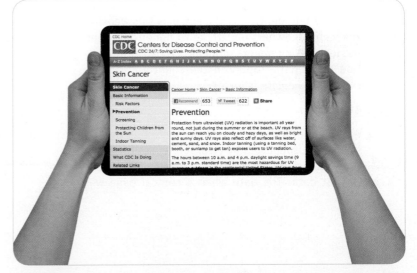

When obtaining health-related information on the internet, make sure you know who runs the site, who pays for the site, what the source of information is, and if that information is reliably documented and up-to-date.

What I Need to Know

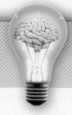

HONcode Principles

The Health on the Net Foundation evaluates health websites to determine if they can be trusted. If a website meets these standards, it can display an HON symbol. To be sure the health information you obtain via the internet is valid, look for the HON symbol on a website. The **HONcode** principles that are used to certify a health-related website appear below.

1. **Authoritative**

   All medical or health advice provided and hosted on this site is only given by medically trained and qualified professionals unless a clear statement is made that a piece of advice offered is from a non-medically qualified individual or organization.

2. **Complementarity**

   The information provided on this site is designed to support, not replace, the relationship that exists between a patient/site visitor and his/her existing physician.

3. **Privacy**

   Confidentiality of data relating to individual patients and visitors to a medical/health website, including their identity, is respected by this website. The website owners undertake to honor or exceed the legal requirements of medical/health information privacy that apply in the country and state where the website is located.

4. **Attribution**

   Where appropriate, information contained on this site will be supported by clear references to source data and, where possible, have specific HTML links to that data. The date when a clinical page was last modified will be clearly displayed (e.g., at the bottom of the page).

5. **Justifiability**

   Any claims relating to the benefits/performance of a specific treatment, commercial product, or service will be supported by appropriate, balanced evidence in the manner outlined above in Principle 4.

6. **Transparency**

   The designers of this website will seek to provide information in the clearest possible manner and provide contact addresses for visitors who seek further information or support. The webmaster will display his/her email address clearly throughout the website.

7. **Financial disclosure**

   Support for this website will be clearly identified, including the identities of commercial and non-commercial organizations that have contributed funding, services, or material for the site.

8. **Advertising policy**

   If advertising is a source of funding, it will be clearly stated. A brief description of the advertising policy adopted by the website owners will be displayed on the site. Advertising and other promotional material will be presented to viewers in a manner and context that facilitates differentiation between it and the original material created by the institution operating the site.

REPRODUCED FROM: Health on the Net Foundation. *HONcode Principles.* 1997. Available at: http://www.hon.ch/HONcode/Patients/Conduct .html.

■ Twenty-two percent of internet users look online for information about environmental health hazards.

Given the likelihood that you, too, will use this self-care skill to learn more about a health-related issue, it is

HONcode: a symbol that health-related websites can display if certified valid by the Health on the Net Foundation.

essential that you know how to evaluate critically the information you obtain. Review skills you learned earlier in this text about assessing the validity of health information you find on the internet.

When to Consult with a Healthcare Provider

It is important to know when self-care is inappropriate and a healthcare professional should be consulted. If any of the following emergency conditions occur, a call to a physician, hospital, or 9-1-1 should be made immediately (Tajeu, 2005):

■ Heavy bleeding or if bleeding does not stop after 15 minutes of pressure is applied.

■ Unconsciousness.

■ A stupor or dazed condition occurs.

■ Cold sweats with chest pain, abdominal pain, or lightheadedness.

■ Difficulty breathing.

■ Seizure.

■ Spinal or neck injury.

■ Head injury followed by confusion, deep sleepiness, vomiting, or inability to move arms or legs.

■ Choking.

■ Chemical or acid burns or serious burns from fire and/or smoke inhalation.

■ Headache accompanied by stiff neck, drowsiness, confusion, paralysis, numbness, slurred speech, or visual disturbance.

Choosing Health Insurance

In 2014, the major provisions of the health reform law passed in 2010 will start. Health insurers will be required to offer comprehensive plans and accept all customers regardless of any preexisting conditions. By 2014, all Americans will be required to have health coverage except in cases of severe financial hardship. The government will subsidize health insurance costs for low-income households.

Below are some ways to evaluate a health insurance plan in which you are considering to enroll (Consumer Reports Health, 2010):

Make sure everything is covered. Insurance should cover hospitalization, doctor visits, emergency services, diagnostic tests, and prescription drugs. Verify that there are no major exclusions listed.

Choice of doctors. Consider whether you can choose your own doctors or must use a doctor in the plan. If you can go out of the plan, how much does it cost you out-of-pocket? Are the doctors in the plan of sufficient quality that you would not object to using them?

Ask your employer. Your human resources department may be able to help you choose an appropriate plan. Many large employers offer online tools to compare plans.

Consult HealthCare.gov. Some 5,500 products from about 1,000 insurers are listed by state. Also included are cost information and tools to compare plans.

Review the rankings of health plans. Check out the rating of insurance plans you are considering. Rankings of private health insurance plans are available at http://www.consumerreports.org/health/insurance/best-health-insurance-1.htm.

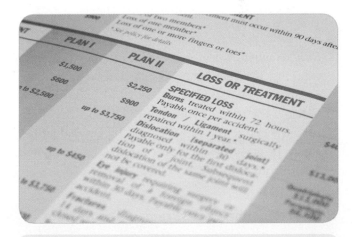

Health insurance companies may differ on which medical conditions they cover, the amount of copayments and deductibles, premium costs, and other variables. Gather as much information as you can before choosing a company for your health insurance.

What I Need to Know

Questions to Ask When Prescribed Medications

One of the medical self-care skills that you should acquire is adherence to medication regimens prescribed by your physician. If your doctor prescribes a medication for you, you should understand how to take the medication. Here are some questions to ask your doctor regarding prescribed medications:

- How do you spell the name of the medication?

- Can I take a generic version of this medicine (to save money)?

- What is the medicine for?

- How am I supposed to take it?

- When should I take my medicine?

- How much medicine should I take?

- How long do I need to take the medicine?

- When will the medicine start working?

- Can I stop taking my medicine if I feel better?

- Can I get a refill?

- Are there any side effects?

- When should I tell someone about a side effect?

- Do I need to avoid any food, drinks, or activities?

- Does this new prescription mean I should stop taking any other medicines I'm taking now?

- Can I take vitamins with my prescription?

- What should I do if I forget to take my medicine?

- What should I do if I accidentally take more than the recommended dose?

- Is there any written information about this medication I can take home with me?

- Are there any tests I need to take while I'm on this medicine?

REPRODUCED FROM: *Build Your Question List*. Rockville, MD: Agency for Healthcare Research and Quality, 2009. Available at: http://www .ahrq.gov/questionsaretheanswer/questionBuilder.aspx.

Run the numbers. Employee share of group insurance continues to rise. That means it is important to select a plan that balances cost, coverage, and quality of care. What is the monthly premium you must pay? One basic tradeoff to consider is this: A higher **deductible**, **copay**, or **out-of-pocket limit** can lower your overall monthly premium.

The Various Health Insurance Plan Options

Managed healthcare plans are types of health insurance policies that help employers offer their employees discounted medical insurance services by negotiating reduced charges with hospitals and physicians. This group of healthcare providers is called a *network*. There are three basic types of managed healthcare plans: health maintenance organizations, preferred provider organizations, and point of service.

Deductible: the amount of the covered expenses a patient must pay each year before the plan starts to reimburse the patient.

Copay: fees needing to be paid when visiting a doctor, hospital, or emergency room.

Out-of-pocket limit: the maximum amount of money per year a patient would have to pay for healthcare.

Health Maintenance Organization

A **health maintenance organization (HMO)** is a health insurance plan that negotiates payments with specific doctors, hospitals, and clinics that are part of a network. Patients must receive all of their medical care from network providers, except in emergencies, for the reduced fees to be provided. Premiums are usually lower in HMOs than in preferred provider organization and point of service plans.

Preferred Provider Organizations

A **preferred provider organization (PPO)** is similar to an HMO, but the insured person can choose the physician he or she wants to see instead of being solely restricted to the PPO providers. An insured person can choose between a member or nonmember provider. The member provider would be the least expensive choice for the insured. Using a nonmember provider requires additional costs.

Point of Service

In **point of service (POS)** health insurance plans, insured patients can choose their own physician as long as that physician has previously agreed to provide services at a discounted fee. In a POS plan, the insured would have to use the chosen physician as a gateway first before moving on to a specialist. In other words, whenever there is a medical issue, the POS physician must always be contacted first and, if deemed appropriate, that physician will refer the patient to a specialist (Sage, 2011a, b).

Indemnity Plans

In addition to managed care plans, there are indemnity health insurance plans. **Indemnity plans** offer more flexibility in choice of doctors and hospitals because there are no networks involved. Usually, you can choose any doctor you wish, you can change doctors at any time, and you usually will not need a referral to see a specialist or to go for x-ray procedures or tests. Indemnity insurance pays a portion of the bill—usually 80%—after the deductible has been met, although this may vary. You pay the remainder. Indemnity policies typically have an out-of-pocket limit. This means that once your expenses reach a certain amount in a given calendar year, the fee for

covered benefits typically will be paid in full by your insurance plan.

The Various Dental Insurance Options

Many people choose not to pay for dental insurance. Instead, they decide to pay for each service rendered according to the fees established by the dentist. This is called *fee-for-service*. If you are lucky (and diligent about brushing and flossing) and your teeth and gums remain healthy, you can save money by not paying dental insurance premiums. However, if you have a dental problem such as need for a root canal or a dental crown, the costs can be prohibitive. If you decide not to gamble on your dental health, you might consider enrolling in a dental insurance plan. In that case, you have several options as described in the sections that follow.

Direct Reimbursement

Direct reimbursement dental plans allow patients to go to the dentist of their choice. Depending on the plan, the

---

Health maintenance organization (HMO): a health insurance plan that negotiates payments with specific doctors, hospitals, and clinics that are part of a network; members must receive all of their medical care from network providers, except in emergencies, for the reduced fees to be provided.

Preferred provider organization (PPO): a health insurance plan that negotiates payments with specific doctors, hospitals, and clinics that are part of a network, but members can choose the physician they want to see instead of being solely restricted to the network providers.

Point of service (POS): a health insurance plan in which members can choose their own physician as long as that physician has previously agreed to provide services at a discounted fee.

Indemnity plans: managed care plans in which there are no networks involved so patients can change doctors at any time and usually do not need a referral to see a specialist or to go for x-ray procedures or tests.

patient pays the dentist directly and then submits a paid receipt as proof of treatment. The plan then reimburses the member a percentage of the dental care costs.

Indemnity Plans

In an indemnity dental plan, the insurance company pays claims based on the procedures performed, usually as a percentage of the charges. Generally, an indemnity plan allows patients to choose their own dentists. Most plans have a maximum allowance for each procedure, which does not usually cover the total cost of the dental care.

Preferred Provider Organization

A PPO dental plan is an indemnity plan combined with a network of dentists under contract to the insurance company to deliver specified services for set fees. Contracted dentists must usually accept the fee schedule as dictated by the plan. Patients who see a dentist who is not part of the plan incur a greater out-of-pocket expense.

Dental Health Maintenance Organization

Under a dental health maintenance organization (DHMO) plan, patients must receive treatment at a contracted office in order to receive a benefit. If considering a DHMO, ask the following questions:

- What is the average waiting period for an initial appointment?
- What is the average period between appointments?
- What is the dentist/patient ratio for the program?
- Does the plan have adequate specialist participation?
- How does the program provide for emergency treatment?
- What provisions are in the program for emergency care away from home?

Issues to Consider When Choosing Dental Insurance

Because the benefits and limitations vary significantly between types of dental plans, there are several issues you should consider when making your selection:

- What dentists are in the plan (*in-network*), and can patients choose their *in-network* dentists? If an *out-of-network* dentist is chosen, what services are covered?
- Does the patient have input into the type of dental service provided?
- Does the plan cover diagnosis to identify dental problems, preventive services such as cleanings, and services in case of emergency? Are full-mouth x-ray procedures covered?
- Does the plan cover specialized services such as crowns and root canals?
- Are major dental procedures covered such as dental implants?
- If away from home and dental services are needed, are these services covered by the plan?

SUMMARY

The goal of this chapter is to provide you with the tools you need to be an informed consumer. To help you do that, a summary of important information included in this chapter is provided.

- When choosing a healthcare provider, make that choice *before* you need care. In this way, you will have the time to make an informed decision rather than being rushed to receive treatment when you are ill.

- There are several websites that can provide you with useful information about a doctor you are considering for your healthcare. Some of these websites are free, whereas others charge a fee.

- Primary care doctors are trained to serve as your main doctor over the long term and are your first point of contact for your medical needs. They provide medical care when needed, encourage health-related behavior and discourage risky behaviors to help you remain healthy, and oversee and coordinate your health and medical care. Primary care doctors can also refer you to other medical specialists when necessary.

- There are several factors to consider when choosing a dentist. Among these are location, hours, cost, personal comfort, professional qualifications, and availability of emergency care.

- Once a doctor or dentist is selected to provide you with healthcare, continue to evaluate that care over time. If dissatisfied, choose a different doctor or dentist.

- Hospitals can be evaluated in several ways. One way is to determine if the hospital is accredited by The Joint Commission. The federal government has a website you can access to compare hospitals on a number of criteria.

- Many people decide to use CAM. CAM therapies are diverse medical and healthcare systems, practices, and products that are not currently considered to be part of conventional medicine. Complementary medicine refers to the use of CAM together with conventional medicine, whereas alternative medicine refers to the use of CAM in place of conventional medicine.

- Medical self-care is defined as those things that individuals do to deal with minor illness and injuries at home. This includes preventing, detecting, and treating illness and disease. It is estimated that 80% of health problems can be treated at home, and 70% of visits to physicians are for conditions that could be treated at home. To perform medical self-care, you need certain skills and should keep medical supplies and medications on hand.

- One of the most used medical self-care skills is the use of the internet. Fifty-nine percent of the U.S. adult population access health information online. Online searches for health information are the third most popular online pursuit, after email and use of a search engine. The Health on the Net Foundation evaluates health websites to determine if they can be trusted and permits approved websites to display a symbol attesting to the validity of the information provided there.

- It is important to know when self-care is not sufficient and a health professional should be consulted. Among conditions requiring a health professional are heavy bleeding, unconsciousness, difficulty breathing, and choking.

- Health insurance can take different forms. There are three basic types of managed healthcare plans: HMOs, PPOs, and POS. An HMO is a health insurance plan that negotiates payments with specific doctors, hospitals, and clinics that are part of a network. Patients must receive all of their medical care from network providers. A PPO is similar to an HMO, but the insured can choose the physician he or she wants to see instead of being solely restricted to the PPO providers. In POS health insurance plans, insured patients can choose their own physician as long as that physician has previously agreed to provide services at a discounted fee.

- Indemnity insurance plans are different from managed healthcare insurance plans. Indemnity plans offer more flexibility in choice of doctors and hospitals because there are no networks involved. Usually, you can choose any doctor you wish, with insurance paying a portion of the bill—usually 80%. You pay the remainder, usually 20% of the total bill.

■ Dental insurance plans come in different varieties. There are direct reimbursement plans, indemnity plans, PPO plans, and DHMO plans.

■ When selecting a dental insurance plan, consider whether the plan allows you to choose your own dentist, the dental services covered, if the plan allows for referrals to specialists, and the emergency care available.

REFERENCES

Agency for Healthcare Research and Quality. *Your Guide to Choosing Quality Health Care*. Washington, DC: U.S. Department of Health and Human Services, 2001.

Carlson, G. *Medical Self–Care: What Is It?* 2009. Missouri Families.com. Available at: http://missourifamilies.org/features/healtharticles/health32.htm.

Centers for Disease Control and Prevention. More than one-third of U.S. adults use complementary and alternative medicine, according to new government survey. *NCHS Press Room*. May 27, 2004. Available at: http://www.cdc.gov/nchs/pressroom/04news/adultsmedicine.htm.

Colgate World of Care. *Oral & Dental Health Basics: Choosing a Dentist*. 2011. Available at: http://www.colgate.com/app/Colgate/US/OC/Information/OralHealthBasics/CheckupsDentProc/TheDentalVisit/ChoosingADentist.cvsp.

Consumer Reports Health.org. *How to Choose a Good Health-Care Plan*. 2010. Available at: http://www.consumerreports.org/health/insurance/health-insurance/how-to-pick-health-insurance/compare-health-plans.htm?loginMethod=auto.

Dodes, J. Coverage questioned (letter to the editor). *ADA News*, September 15, 1997.

Fox, S. Food safety, drug safety, and pregnancy information are among eight new topics included in our survey. *Pew Internet Project*. 2011. Available at: http://pewinternet.org/Reports/2011/HealthTopics/Summary-of-Findings/Food-safety.aspx.

How to Choose a Dentist. *Consumers Research*, March 1997: 2024.

National Center for Complementary and Alternative Medicine. *What Is Complementary and Alternative Medicine?* 2010. Available at: http://nccam.nih.gov/health/whatiscam/.

Sage, B. 10 key considerations when comparing health care plans. *About.com Guide*. 2011a. Available at: http://personalinsure.about.com/cs/healthinsurance1/a/aa070703a.htm.

Sage, B. What is the difference between HMO, PPO, and POS? *About Com Personal Insurance*. 2011b. Available at: http://personalinsure.about.com/cs/healthinsurance1/a/aa011704a.htm.

Tajeu, K. S. Self-care for you and your family. *Alabama Cooperative Extension System (Alabama A&M University and Auburn University)*. 2005. Available at: http://www.aces.edu/pubs/docs/C/CRD-0064/. (All rights to the original material are reserved by the Alabama Cooperative Extension System.)

WebMD. *Oral Health Guide: Finding a Dentist*. 2009. Available at: http://www.webmd.com/oral-health/guide/finding-dentist.

INTERNET RESOURCES

Agency for Health Research and Quality
  http://www.ahrq.gov

Consumers Reports Health
  http://www.consumerreports.org/health

Legacy Health
  http://www.legacyhealth.org

Joint Commission Center for Transforming Healthcare
  http://www.centerfortransforminghealthcare.org/

Consumer Health Foundation
  http://www.consumerhealthfdn.org

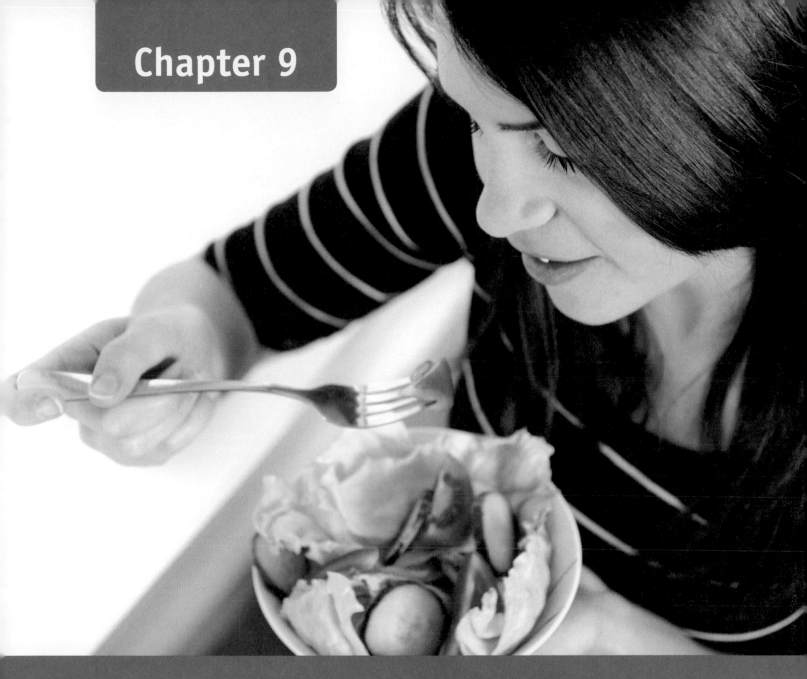

Chapter 9

Taking Charge of Your Diet and Weight

 Access Health Check Ups and Health Behavior Change activities on the Companion Website:
go.jblearning.com/Empowering.

Learning Objectives

■ Discuss how body image is influenced by media and societal trends.

■ Explain the relationship between nutrition and health, both good health and ill health.

■ Describe the role of dietary fiber and list foods that are high in fiber.

■ Cite how body mass index is used to determine whether a person is underweight, overweight, or obese and discuss the causes of overweight and obesity.

■ Explain what factors contribute to effective weight-loss programs.

■ Describe the components of SuperTracker and how it can be used as a guide to more nutritional eating.

■ Discuss several different eating disorders and the most effective treatments.

As I age, I notice more and more imperfections in the way I look. I have developed tires around my waist—I guess as a precaution against drowning. My hair is thinning, the good news being it takes less time to shampoo and dry. And, my facial skin seems to hang a little lower than it did when I was younger. This is not to say that I hadn't noticed imperfections prior to these, only that these latest ones seem particularly insulting because they appear to be ganging up on me rather than attacking me one-by-one as they used to. Perhaps you, too, have noticed some imperfections that concern you. In fact, if you have not, you haven't been looking. Most of us are unhappy about some aspects of our bodies. This chapter seeks to view these concerns with proper perspective and considers three important related variables: diet, nutrition, and weight.

Body Image

Body image refers to the mental image we have of our physical appearance. Many factors influence body image, including how much we weigh, how our weight is distributed, our values about physical appearance, our concepts of good physical appearance, our ethnic and cultural background, what we see in people around us, what we hear through the media, and what we hear from others.

Those of us with a better body image tend to have higher self-esteem.

Body image in our society is often problematic. Many people are dissatisfied with their bodies and experience the associated negative consequences. Generally, women want to lose weight and men want to gain muscle. Women report concern about their body size, buttocks, breasts, thighs, facial features, and body hair (Hunt, Thienhaus, and Ellwood, 2008).

In one study, girls in grades 5 through 12 said they wanted to lose weight because of the pictures in magazines (Field et al., 1999). Notably, only 29% of the 548 girls interviewed were overweight. Even more alarming, one-third of these girls were fifth and sixth graders. Fifty percent of these fifth and sixth grade girls reported that they read fashion magazines at least two to five times per month. Those who read these magazines were three times as likely to have unrealistic body expectations.

In contrast, males tend to be more concerned about increased muscle definition and their body shape as opposed

Body image: the mental image we have of our physical appearance.

to weight (University of Iowa, 2002). As with women, however, studies have shown that the viewing and purchasing of muscle and fitness magazines is associated with body dissatisfaction in males (Duggan and McCreary, 2004).

Complete Health Check Up 9.1 to determine how healthy your body image is (see Health Check Up 9.1 on the companion website). Once completed, place Health Check Up 9.1 in your Health Decision Portfolio.

The Elusive Perfect Body

What does the perfect body look like? The answer to that question depends on the purposes we have in mind

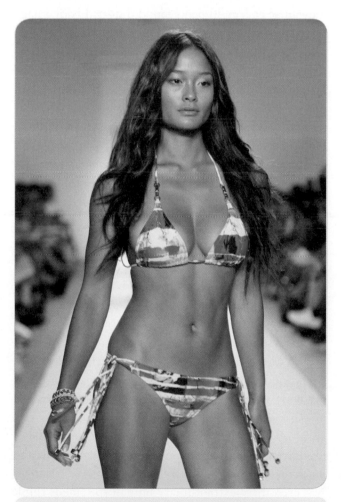

Although models in magazines, television, and film appear perfect, the images are usually computer enhanced to cover up their imperfections—which everyone has.

for the body. For example, the perfect body for a swimmer is typically tall and lean, whereas for a female gymnast, the perfect body is usually small and fit. The point is that a body that works for one purpose may not work for another.

So, there is no perfect body. You are (probably) not a competitive swimmer or gymnast. What is your "perfect" body? Perhaps it is one that allows you to do things you enjoy, live life to the fullest, and feel positive about how you look. These are, in fact, achievable goals. This chapter will show you how.

Why Models Look So Perfect

The covers of major fashion and sports magazines, and the ads inside, usually depict men and women with seemingly perfect bodies. The same can often be said about actors in movies. Their bodies seem almost too perfect to believe. Can these people really look like this all the time? The answer, of course, is no. Models prepare meticulously for that millisecond when the camera's shutter captures their pose. (And there are dozens, if not hundreds, of "takes.") Movie stars may spend months before shooting begins working with a personal trainer and controlling their diets to sculpt their bodies. Clothes, makeup, and lighting are carefully chosen to create the desired image. Hair styling and face and body makeup further enhance the image. As if that were not enough, after the photo or film is taken, editing refines the image to make it perfect. For example, magazines may edit photos to slim female models' waists and thighs and augment their breast size before publication of the photos. Magazines make similar adjustments to photos of male athletes and male models.

The lesson to learn here is not to believe everything you see. Even the most beautiful and handsome models do not have perfect bodies. Consequently, it is unrealistic for us to expect to have perfect bodies. If we believe that a perfect body is possible and we cannot acquire one, we subject ourselves to a lifetime of dissatisfaction about an important part of who we are.

Cultural Influences

Consider that the average American woman is 5 feet 4 inches tall and weighs 163 pounds, whereas the average female model is 5 feet 9 inches tall and weighs 109 pounds. The average male is 5 feet 10 inches tall and weighs 190 pounds (Ogden, Fryar, Carroll, and Flegal, 2004), whereas the average male model is more than 6 feet tall and is thin. Girls grow up influenced by Barbie dolls with unrealistic body size and appearance. In fact, if Barbie were a real person, she would be 6 feet tall, weigh 100 pounds, and wear a size 4. Her measurements would be 39/21/33 (Answers.com, 2011). Add beauty pageants to the mix, and the situation becomes even more problematic. A study of the winners of the Miss America Pageant from 1922 to 1999 found that an increasing number of winners were in the range of *undernutrition*, as measured by body mass index (Rubinstein and Caballero, 2000). Although pageant winners' heights increased by about 2% over the years, their weights decreased by 12%. And, boys are not immune to similar influences. They are subjected to muscular and defined bodies of action figures and video game avatars when young and to models with six-pack abs and sculptured bodies when older—boys often see those as the body images to strive to achieve.

The result of these influences is widespread dissatisfaction with body appearance. Eighty-five percent of first-year male and female college students desire to change their body weight (Williams, 1996). In a study of normal-weight college students, almost 90% yearned to be thinner (*Science News*, 2007). And, half of underweight women wanted to lose even more weight or stay just where they were (instead of gaining to reach a healthy weight). In contrast, most overweight women did not want to work on their health behaviors to achieve a healthy weight. Seventy-eight percent of overweight college males also wanted to weigh less. However, 59% of this group had an inaccurate notion of how much they needed to lose no longer to be classified as overweight (in other words, they underestimated). The researchers suggest "that the idealized body weight and shape, especially among underweight females and overweight individuals of both genders, are not in accordance with population-based standards defining healthy body weight."

Cultural and ethnic background also influences average body weight and concepts of body image. The Health and Nutrition Examination Study, conducted by the National Center for Health Statistics, reports that 50% of African-American women and 43% of Hispanic women are overweight or obese, as are 45% of Mexican-American women. This is in contrast to 33% of white women being overweight or obese (Flegal, Carroll, Odgen, and Curtin, 2010). Men tend to have more similar rates with 37.3% of African-American men, 35.9% of Mexican men, 34.3% of Hispanic men, and 31.9% of white men being overweight or obese. Another study found that a much higher percentage of Caucasians reported body image concerns than did Latino or African Americans; the latter two groups did not differ significantly from each other (Barry and Grilo, 2002).

The typically Western pattern of body dissatisfaction has influenced the traditional notions of female beauty among women in other parts of the world as well. Studies of Taiwanese college students found distorted body image and related risk factors leading to eating disorders to be common. Studies of Chinese undergraduates in Hong Kong and undergraduates in Iran found body shape dissatisfaction among female college students, even when they were not overweight or obese. A global study of adolescents concluded that body weight dissatisfaction was highly prevalent and more common among girls than boys, among overweight than non-overweight individuals, and among older adolescents than younger adolescents (Sabbah et al., 2009).

Body Esteem

What do you think about your body and how it functions? This is called *body esteem* or *body cathexis*. To find out, complete Health Check Up 9.2 (see Health Check Up 9.2 on the companion website). Once completed, place Health Check Up 9.2 in your Health Decision Portfolio. Every individual thinks well about some parts of his or her body and not so well about other parts. When the most gorgeous, seemingly perfect models and movie stars are asked about their physiques, it is not unusual for them to complain that their noses are too big, or they have too much flab on their thighs, or their breasts could be larger. Not even these extraordinary human specimens think their bodies are ideal. Health Check Up 9.2 allows you to identify any body parts that you think need to improve; you will then strategize ways to either improve them or

Myths *and* Facts

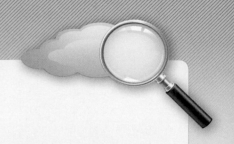

What Americans Think About Body Image and Weight

MYTH	FACT
Most Americans are satisfied with their bodies.	Various studies have found Americans to be highly dissatisfied with their bodies. Women are typically more dissatisfied than men, but both sexes want a better body. Women tend to want to improve their weight, whereas men tend to want to improve their abdomens and have "washboard abs."
If you are unlucky enough to be born with a body type that you believe is unattractive, you can't really do anything to improve your body image.	You may not be able to do anything to improve certain parts of your body, but you can do things to be more accepting of your body. For example, you can use selective awareness to identify parts of your body that you value, so you appreciate them more. You can perceive your body more positively (i.e., improve your body image) if you realize that parts of it are worthy of your admiration.
The perfect body is one that is thin and tall, with muscle tone and low body fat.	One size doesn't fit all. Different body types are best for different purposes. Body fat may be desirable for a football player, short stature may be best for a jockey, and a thin, tall physique may be best for a ballerina. All three of these athletic body types can be healthy, as can numerous other body shapes and sizes.
Exercise burns calories and can be good for losing weight, but it increases your appetite. Therefore, the best way to lose weight is by dieting, not exercise.	Studies have shown that the best way to lose weight is through a combination of diet and exercise. Exercise alone is a more effective weight-loss method than is dieting alone. One reason for this is that exercise actually decreases one's appetite.
Eating disorders result from a loss of control over one's eating patterns.	Eating disorders often result from an obsession with control (by people who believe they have little control over most aspects of their lives besides their food intake).

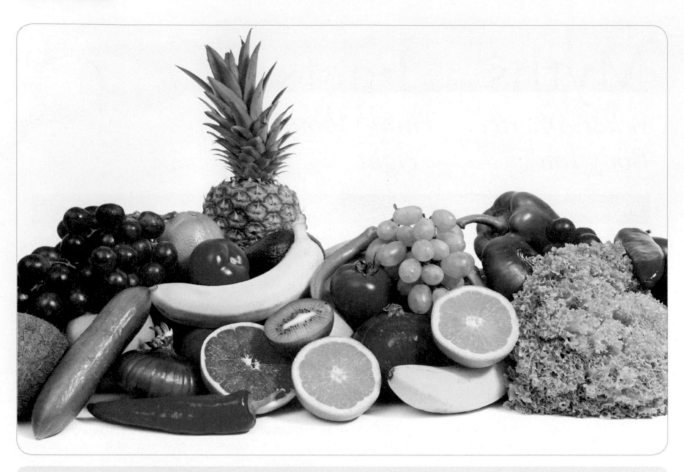

To be healthy requires eating foods that supply the right nutrients and avoiding foods that do not.

perceive them as less bothersome. In this way, you can improve your body esteem.

Nutrients and Good Health

To maintain good health, you need to eat foods that provide certain nutrients. Table 9.1 lists the nutrients you need, their function, and the foods that contain them. In the discussion of overweight and obesity later in this chapter, components of a healthy diet are further described.

How healthy is your dietary behavior? Complete Health Check Up 9.3 to find out (see Health Check Up 9.3 on the companion website). Once completed, place Health Check Up 9.3 in your Health Decision Portfolio. Once you determine how healthy your dietary behavior is, complete Health Check Up 9.4 to identify barriers to your eating

more healthfully (see Health Check Up 9.4 on the companion website). Once completed, place Health Check Up 9.4 in your Health Decision Portfolio.

Overweight and Obesity

Body mass index (BMI) is a measure of body fat based on height and weight that is often used to define underweight, overweight, and obesity. For adults, BMI values are categorized as:

> **Body mass index (BMI):** a measure of body fat based on height and weight that is often used to define underweight, overweight, and obesity.

TABLE 9.1	The Six Classes of Nutrients

Nutrient Class	Major Roles in the Body	Rich Food Sources
Carbohydrates	Provide energy	Grain products, beans, vegetables, fruits, honey, sugar-sweetened soft drinks, candy
Lipids	Triglycerides: provide energy Cholesterol: component of most steroid hormones, needed for bile production, skin maintenance, vitamin D synthesis, and nerve function	Vegetable oils, nuts, margarines, fatty meats, cheeses, cream, butter, fried foods
Proteins	Growth, repair, and maintenance of all cells; production of enzymes, antibodies, and certain hormones	Dried beans, peas, nuts, soy products, meats, shellfish, fish, poultry, eggs, and dairy products (except cream and butter)
Vitamins	Metabolism, reproduction, development, and growth	Widespread in foods: nuts, beans, peas, fruits and vegetables, whole grains, meats, enriched breads and cereals, fortified milk
Minerals	Metabolism, development, and growth	Widespread in foods: nuts, whole grains, meats, fish, poultry, dairy products, vegetables, fruits, enriched breads and cereals
Water	Essential for life: many chemical reactions require water; it helps maintain normal body temperature (nearly every food contributes to body temperature) and transports nutrients	Water, nonalcoholic and caffeine-free beverages, fruits, vegetables, milk

REPRODUCED FROM: Alters, S. and Schiff, W. *Essential Concepts for Healthy Living*, Sixth Edition. Burlington, MA: Jones & Bartlett Learning, 2012, p. 273.

- Underweight: BMI under 19

- Normal weight: BMI between 19 and 24.9

- Overweight: BMI between 25 and 29.9

- Obese: BMI of 30 or higher

Complete Health Check Up 9.5 to compute your BMI and find out your weight category (see Health Check Up 9.5 on the companion website). Once completed, place Health Check Up 9.5 in your Health Decision Portfolio.

As depicted in Tables 9.2 and 9.3, overweight and obesity are public health issues in the United States. Recent studies find that 34% of Americans are obese (BMI of 30 or higher): 32% of men and 36% of women. Furthermore, another 34% are overweight (BMI between 25 and 29.9), for a total of 68% of Americans who are overweight or obese (Flegal et al., 2010; Freedman, 2011). This is a noticeable increase from the year 2000, when 28% of American men were obese, and 33% of women were obese.

What Causes Overweight and Obesity?

To put it simply, overweight and obesity are the result of an imbalance between calories ingested versus the number of calories expended. You can determine the number of calories you expend each day by completing Health Check Up 9.6 (see Health Check Up 9.6 on the companion website). Once completed, place Health Check Up 9.6 in your Health Decision Portfolio. Of course, weight management is much more complex. Several factors cause people to be overweight or obese, as described in the following sections.

What I Need to Know

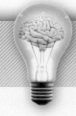

The Role of Dietary Fiber

Dietary fiber, also known as roughage or bulk, includes all parts of plant foods that your body cannot digest or absorb. Unlike other food components such as fats, proteins, or carbohydrates—which your body breaks down and absorbs—fiber isn't digested. Therefore, it passes relatively intact through your stomach, small intestine, and colon and out of your body. Eating fiber decreases the risk of some types of cancer, obesity, cardiovascular disease (by lowering blood pressure and cholesterol levels), and the risk of diabetes (by lowering glucose levels) (U.S. Department of Agriculture, 2007). In addition, fiber normalizes bowel movements by increasing the weight and size of the stool and by softening it.

Foods high in fiber also help with weight loss because they require more chewing time. Time allows your body to recognize when you are no longer hungry. In this way, you are less likely to overeat. A high-fiber diet also tends to make meals feel more filling. An added benefit is that high-fiber diets also tend to be less *energy dense*, which means they have fewer calories for the same volume of food.

An adequate intake of fiber for adult men is at least 30 grams, and for adult women it is at least 20 grams. Yet, the average American consumes only 15 grams of fiber a day (U.S. Department of Agriculture, 2007; Harvard School of Public Health, 2011b). Sources of fiber include grain products (white flour, cereals, whole-wheat flours, and rice), vegetables (white potatoes, tomatoes, deep-yellow vegetables, dark-green vegetables),

legumes, nuts and soy products, and fruits (fresh bananas, citrus fruits, fresh apples).

Strategies for consuming an adequate amount of fiber include (Mayo Clinic, 2009; Harvard School of Public Health, 2011a):

- Ingest whole fruit rather than juice. Whole fruit contains more fiber and fewer calories than liquid fruit.

- Choose a breakfast cereal containing 5 grams or more of fiber per serving. Choose cereals with "bran" or "fiber" in the name. (Then check the fiber content in the nutritional information on the side of the box.)

- Add fruit to breakfast cereals and eat fruit at every meal. Apples, bananas, oranges, pears, and berries are good sources of fiber.

- Choose whole grains. For example, look for breads that list whole wheat, whole-wheat flour, or another whole grain as the first ingredient on the label, and look for a brand with at least 2 grams of dietary fiber per serving.

- Eat more beans—they are an inexpensive source of fiber.

- Make snacks count by snacking on fresh fruit, raw vegetables, low-fat popcorn, and whole-grain crackers. A handful of nuts is also a good high-fiber snack.

Lack of Energy Balance

If more calories are ingested than expended through daily activity, weight gain results. One pound is gained for every surplus of 3,500 calories. Even though there may only be a small difference in the energy balance each day, over time this small difference will result in a large weight gain. For example, if you ingested only 100 calories a day more than you expended, over a month you would ingest 3,000

more calories than you use up. Over a year, you would take in 36,000 more calories than you use up. Whoops! Now you weigh 10 pounds more than you did last year.

Dietary fiber: known as roughage or bulk, it includes all parts of plant foods that your body cannot digest or absorb.

TABLE 9.2	Prevalence of Obesity and Overweight in the United States

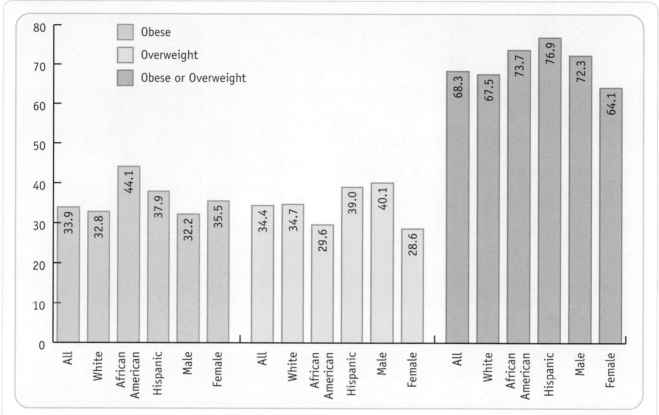

Obese
Overweight
Obese or Overweight

All — 33.9 | White — 32.8 | African American — 44.1 | Hispanic — 37.9 | Male — 32.2 | Female — 35.5

All — 34.4 | White — 34.7 | African American — 29.6 | Hispanic — 39.0 | Male — 40.1 | Female — 28.6

All — 68.3 | White — 67.5 | African American — 73.7 | Hispanic — 76.9 | Male — 72.3 | Female — 64.1

DATA FROM: Flegal, K. M., Carroll, M. D., Odgen, C. L., and Curtin, L. R. Prevalence and trends in obesity among US adults, 1999–2008. *Journal of the American Medical Association* 303 (2010): 235–241.

To correct this energy imbalance requires either taking in fewer calories or increasing the level of physical activity. Often, both are required (**FIG. 9.1 ▶**).

Environment

Often the environment discourages healthy habits, leading to overweight and obesity. Examples of how this occurs include (National Heart, Lung, and Blood Institute, 2011a):

- *School and work schedules.* People often say that they do not have time to be physically active because of hours required to spend on school or work. When they finally have the time, they are too tired to engage in physical activity.

- *Oversized food portions.* Americans are surrounded by huge food portions in restaurants, fast food places, gas stations, movie theaters, supermarkets, and even home. Some of these meals and snacks can feed two or more people. Eating of large portions means too many calories are ingested. Over time, this will cause weight gain if it is not balanced with physical activity.

- *Food advertising.* Americans are surrounded by advertisements from food companies. Children are often the targets of ads for high-calorie, high-fat snacks and sugary drinks. They then develop a habit of eating these foods as they get older. The goal of these ads is to sway people to buy these high-calorie foods, and often they succeed.

- *Lack of neighborhood sidewalks and safe places for recreation.* Not having area parks, trails, sidewalks, and affordable gyms makes it hard for people to be physically active.

TABLE 9.3 — Changes in Obesity from 2000 to 2008

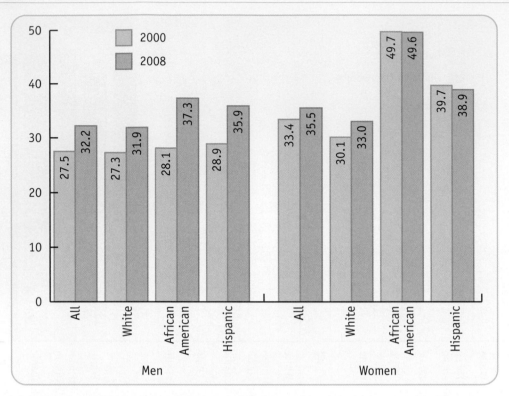

DATA FROM: Flegal, K. M., Carroll, M. D., Odgen, C. L., and Curtin, L. R. Prevalence and trends in obesity among US adults, 1999–2008. *Journal of the American Medical Association* 303 (2010): 235–241.

■ *Lack of access to healthy foods.* Some people do not live in neighborhoods that have supermarkets that sell healthy foods, such as fresh fruits and vegetables. Furthermore, for some people these healthy foods are too costly or travel to supermarkets out of the neighborhood that have these healthy foods is too inconvenient or expensive.

Do any of these conditions affect you? If so, try to strategize to minimize their effect on your diet and weight.

Genes and Family History

Studies of identical twins raised apart show that genes have an influence on a person's weight. Overweight and obesity tend to run in families. Your chances of being overweight are greater if one or both of your parents are overweight or obese.

Although genes play a role, other family factors are also involved. For example, families share food and physical activity habits. This is why a child who has overweight parents who eat high-calorie foods and are inactive will likely be overweight, too. In contrast, if the family adopts healthy food and physical activity habits, the child's chance of being overweight or obese is reduced.

Health Conditions

Some people may become overweight or obese because of hormonal conditions such as underactive thyroid (hypothyroidism), Cushing's syndrome, and polycystic ovarian syndrome.

Emotional Factors

Emotional factors may also influence weight gain. Some people eat more than usual when they are bored, angry,

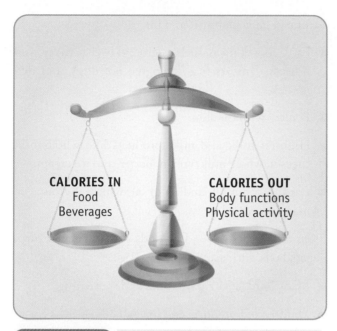

CALORIES IN
Food
Beverages

CALORIES OUT
Body functions
Physical activity

FIGURE 9.1 A calorie balance scale. Reproduced from: Centers for Disease Control and Prevention. *Healthy Weight—It's Not a Diet, It's a Lifestyle!* 2011. Available at: http://www.cdc.gov/healthyweight/calories/index.html.

or stressed. Over time, overeating will lead to weight gain and may cause overweight or obesity.

Notably, the federal government recently passed regulations that require labeling of calories in foods served in chain restaurants. The hope is that consumers seeing the caloric count of high-calorie foods will choose more healthy options. And yet, this does not seem to be the case in localities that have previously passed such regulations. People still choose the high-calorie foods. Certainly, emotional factors are part of the explanation for this finding. What do you think are other plausible explanations?

Age

As people age, their basal metabolism—the amount of energy needed to stay alive such as for breathing and heat regulation—slows down, and they require less energy (calories). In addition, as people age they lose muscle, especially if they are less active. A lower basal metabolism along with muscle loss can slow down the rate at which the body burns calories. Therefore, if people do not reduce their calorie intake as they get older, they may gain weight.

Lack of Sleep

Studies find that the less people sleep, the more likely they are to be overweight or obese. People who report that they sleep 5 hours a night, for example, are more likely to become obese compared with people who sleep 7–8 hours a night. Hormones that are released during sleep control appetite and the body's use of energy. For example, insulin controls the rise and fall of blood sugar levels during sleep. People with severe sleep disturbances have insulin and blood sugar levels that are similar to those in people who have diabetes. In addition, people with severe sleep disturbances have high levels of the hormone *ghrelin* (which causes hunger) and low levels of the hormone *leptin* (which normally helps curb hunger).

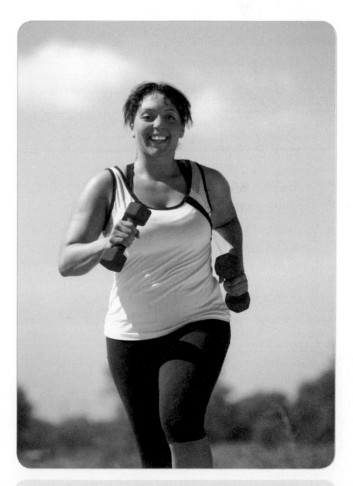

Anyone can benefit from regular physical activity.

Preventing Overweight and Obesity

Overweight and obesity can be prevented by making healthy decisions such as following a healthy eating plan, watching food portion sizes, being active, reducing sedentary "screen time" (time spent using television, computers, DVDs, smart phones, and video games), and regularly keeping track of your weight.

A Healthy Eating Plan

A healthy eating plan gives your body the nutrients it needs every day. It has enough calories for good health, but not so many that you gain weight. Healthy foods are low in saturated fat, *trans* fat, cholesterol, sodium (salt), and added sugar.

Healthy Foods

Healthy foods include (National Heart, Lung, and Blood Institute, 2011b):

- Fat-free and low-fat milk and milk products (such as low-fat yogurt and cheese).

- Lean meat, fish, poultry, cooked beans, and peas.

- Whole-grain foods, such as oatmeal, brown rice, and couscous, and whole-grain versions of pasta, cereal, bagels, bread, tortillas, and crackers.

- Fruits, which can be fresh, canned (in fruit juice or water, but not corn syrup!), frozen, or dried.

- Vegetables, which can be fresh, canned (without salt), frozen, or dried.

- Canola and olive oils and soft (tub) margarines made from these oils, which are heart healthy. Consume these in small amounts because they are high in calories.

- Unsalted nuts, like walnuts and almonds, in limited amounts (nuts contain beneficial nutrients but are high in calories).

Foods to Limit

Foods that are high in saturated fat, *trans* fat, and cholesterol raise blood cholesterol levels and also may be high in calories. These fats raise the risk of heart disease and stroke, so they should be limited.

Saturated fat is mainly found in:

- Fatty cuts of meat, such as ground beef, sausage, and processed meats (e.g., bologna, hot dogs, and deli meats).

- Poultry with the skin.

- High-fat milk and milk products like whole-milk cheeses, whole milk, cream, butter, and ice cream.

- Lard, coconut oil, and palm oil, which are found in many processed foods.

Trans fat is mainly found in foods with partially hydrogenated oils, such as:

- Many hard (stick) margarines and shortening.

- Many baked products and snack foods, such as crackers, cookies, and doughnuts.

- Foods fried in hydrogenated shortening, such as fast food french fries and chicken.

Finally, it is important to limit foods and drinks with added sugars, like high-fructose corn syrup. Added sugars supply extra calories without providing healthful nutrients like vitamins and minerals. Added sugars are found in many desserts, canned fruit packed in syrup, fruit drinks, and non-diet drinks.

Weight-Loss Strategies

If you are trying to manage your weight or lose weight, researchers have identified several strategies you might want to use.

The Food Weight Strategy

Studies have shown that people tend to eat a constant *weight* of food. Ounce for ounce, our food intake is fairly consistent. Knowing this, you can control your weight by eating foods that are lower in calories and fat for a given amount of food. For example, replacing a full-fat food product that weighs 2 ounces with a low-fat product that weighs the same helps you cut back on calories. Another helpful practice is to eat foods that contain a lot of water, such as vegetables, fruits, and soups.

Behavioral Strategies

Changing your behaviors or habits related to food and physical activity is important for losing weight. The first step is to understand which habits lead you to overeat or have an inactive lifestyle. The next step is to change these habits. Below are some simple tips to help you adopt healthier habits.

- *Change your surroundings.* You may be more likely to overeat when watching television, when treats are available in the dorm or at work, or when you are with a certain friend. Change these situations to your advantage: for example, take a different route so you can avoid walking by the candy jar in your dorm or the vending machine at work.

- *Reinforce healthful alternatives.* You also may find it hard to motivate yourself to engage in physical activity regularly; just sitting on the couch seems easier. However, you can change your habits by making the alternative fun. For example, instead of watching television, dance to your favorite music. You might even reward yourself by downloading a new song after several successful days of dancing instead of watching television.

- *Use chaining.* To perform a behavior requires a number of steps. For example, eating healthfully when you are cooking for yourself requires planning of a shopping list and menus, getting to the store, and setting aside time to cook. Imagine these steps to be links in a chain. The more links a behavior requires, the more likely it is that the behavior will not be performed. The fewer the number of links, the more likely the behavior will occur. There are various ways to reduce the links in the chain leading to healthy eating. For example, if you decide what healthy foods you will eat in the cafeteria or at home beforehand, that decision is eliminated for later on. If you are cooking a healthy dinner, you can lay out as many of the ingredients as possible in the morning to eliminate the step of having to do that later on. As a result, it will be more likely that you will actually prepare and eat that healthy meal.

- *Keep a record.* Keeping a daily record of your food intake, amount of physical activity, and your weight will also help you manage your weight and behaviors related to your weight. A record is an easy way to track how you are doing and, when necessary, to identify when to make changes.

- *Seek support.* Ask for help or encouragement from your friends and family. You can get support in person, through email, or by talking on the phone. You can also join a weight-loss support group on your campus or in the community.

- *Reward success.* Reward your success for meeting your weight-loss goals or other achievements with something you would like to do, not with food. Choose rewards that you will enjoy, such as a movie, music CD, a massage, or personal time.

Weight-Loss Medications

When other methods fail, some doctors may recommend medications to patients needing to lose weight for health reasons. To be safe, these medications should only be used under doctor's orders. Orlistat (Xenical) is the only Food and Drug Administration (FDA)-approved weight-loss medicine. This prescription medication generally results in a weight loss between 5 and 10 pounds. Most of the weight loss occurs within the first 6 months of taking the medicine. Orlistat reduces the absorption of fats, fat calories, and vitamins A, D, E, and K by the body. Potential side effects are mild, such as oily and loose stools. The FDA has also approved Alli, an over-the-counter weight-loss aid for adults. Alli is the lower-dose form of orlistat. Alli is meant to be used along with a reduced-calorie, low-fat diet and physical activity. Most people taking Alli lose 5 to 10 pounds over 6 months. Like orlistat, Alli reduces the absorption of fats, fat calories, and vitamins A, D, E, and K to promote weight loss, and it has the same potential side effects (National Heart, Lung, and Blood Institute, 2011c).

Popular Weight-Loss Diets and Programs

Obviously, many people want to lose weight, and they are willing to pay a lot of money to do so. It is estimated that in 2008, in the United States alone, approximately

What I Need to Know

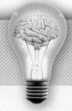

Watching Television Is Bad for Your Health

The more time you spend in front of the television, the more likely it is you will die at an earlier age. This is what recent research studies have concluded. For more than 6 years, Dunstan and colleagues followed 8,800 adults with no prior history of heart disease. These researchers found that those who watched 4 hours of television a day were 80% more likely to die of heart disease and 46% more likely to die from any cause than those who watched 2 hours of television a day. Furthermore, each 1-hour increase in television viewing was associated with an 18% increase in death from heart disease and an 11% increase in death from all causes. These trends occurred even when the researchers controlled for diet and exercise.

Another study by Grøntved and Hu also found time spent viewing television to be associated with the development of heart disease, diabetes, and death from all causes. For every 2-hour increase of daily television viewing, 176 more cases of type 2 diabetes per 100,000 individuals per year occurred, 38 more cases of heart disease per 100,000 individuals per year occurred, and 104 more deaths from all causes per 100,000 individuals per year occurred.

Putting this into sobering perspective, Americans watch an average of 8 hours of television daily! The potential for Americans to improve their health by turning off the television is huge.

ADAPTED FROM: Dunstan, D. W., Barr, E. L. M., Healy, G. N., Salmon, J., Shaw, J. E., Balkau, B. D., Magliano, J., Cameron, A. J., Zimmet, P. Z., and Owen, N. Television viewing time and mortality: The Australian Diabetes, Obesity and Lifestyle Study (AusDiab). *Circulation* 121 (2010): 384–391; Grøntved, A. and Hu, F. B. Television viewing and risk of type 2 diabetes, cardiovascular disease, and all-cause mortality: A meta-analysis. *Journal of the American Medical Association* 305 (2011): 2448–2455.

$61 billion a year was spent on weight-loss products and programs (Worldometer, undated).

The Key to Successful Weight-Loss Diets

There are many different weight-loss programs and many different weight-loss approaches. Still, the effective programs have several common features. In a statistical analysis of key behaviors correlating most strongly with having a healthy BMI, six factors were identified (Consumer Reports Health.org, 2009):

- *Watching portions.* Carefully control portion size (this was the most highly correlated with having a lower BMI).

- *Limiting fat.* Restrict fat to less than one-third of daily caloric intake.

- *Eating fruits and vegetables.* Eat five or more servings daily.

- *Consuming whole grains.* Choose whole-wheat breads and cereals over refined (white) grains.

- *Eating at home.* Eat at home rather than at restaurants or ordering take-out food.

- *Exercising.* Participate in vigorous aerobic exercise (which increases breathing and heart rates) for at least 30 minutes at least 3 days a week, and weight train at least once a week.

Notably, in this study several common diet practices were found *not* to be related to a healthy BMI. These included eating many small meals and never eating between meals.

Weight-Loss Programs

There are several diet plans that work. These include Jenny Craig, Slim-Fast, Weight Watchers, the Ornish plan, the Atkins diet, and the Zone. Each of these takes a somewhat different approach. For example, Jenny Craig provides meals so as to control food choices (1,315 calories per day), Ornish is a very-low-fat diet (1,525 calories per day) that includes behavioral components as well (such as meditation), Atkins is a high-fat diet (1,915 calories per day), and Weight Watchers uses a point scale to provide guidance on food choices and offers social support (1,865 calories per day).

After evaluating various diet plans, *U.S. News & World Report* and Consumers Union rated diets somewhat differently. *U.S. News & World Report* used a panel of health experts to evaluate diets based on the following criteria: easy to follow, nutritious, safe, and effective for weight loss and against diabetes and heart disease. The government-endorsed Dietary Approaches to Stop Hypertension (DASH) came out number one (*U.S. News & World Report*, 2012).

The DASH diet is rich in fruits, vegetables, fat-free or low-fat milk and milk products, whole grains, fish, poultry, beans, seeds, and nuts. Compared with the typical American diet, it also contains less salt and sodium, less sweets, added sugars, and sugar-containing beverages, less fats, and less red meats. This heart healthy way of eating is also lower in saturated fat, *trans* fat, and cholesterol and rich in nutrients that are associated with lowering of blood pressure—mainly potassium, magnesium, calcium, protein, and fiber. DASH has been shown to lower blood pressure, reduce cholesterol, improve insulin sensitivity, and to be effective for weight loss (National Heart, Lung, and Blood Institute, 2006).

Consumers Union, in contrast, rated Jenny Craig as the most effective weight-loss diet (Consumer Reports Health.org, 2011). The Consumers Union rating is consistent with research showing that prepackaged meals are a key component to the success of diet programs (Wing, 2010). Furthermore, a recent study found that 92% of dieters stick with a Jenny Craig–type of program (Rock et al., 2010). Other researchers have found that addition of exercise to a diet plan enhances weight loss (Goodpaster et al., 2010), as does participation in a support group (Diet and Nutrition, 2011).

Guidelines to Healthful Eating

The U.S. government periodically brings experts together to review the current state of nutrition knowledge and to make recommendations consistent with that knowledge. As such, the organization and presentation of nutritional guidelines have evolved over the years from the *Five Food Groups*, to the *SuperTracker*, to *ChooseMyPlate*.

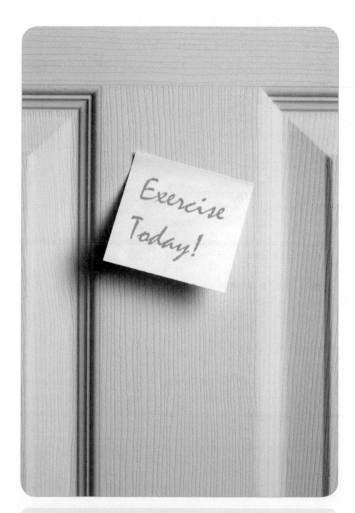

When discussing the health belief model earlier in this text, the importance of *cues to action* was cited. Reminders in the form of notes placed on bathroom doors are excellent cues to exercise.

Still, the basis for healthful eating, as presented earlier in this chapter, has for the most part remained the same. This includes foods to eat and foods to avoid, as well as the quantity recommended to eat.

ChooseMyPlate.gov

The latest nutrition tool developed by the U.S. Department of Agriculture is a website entitled *ChooseMyPlate .gov*, which can be accessed at http://www.choosemyplate .gov. ChooseMyPlate.gov helps people learn more about what types of foods they should eat and in what amounts, and which foods they should avoid. On that website is an illustration of a plate (**FIG. 9.2**). Clicking on a part of the plate brings up information about that part of the diet.

The recommendations on the ChooseMyPlate.gov website are based on the U.S. Department of Agriculture's *Dietary Guidelines for Americans, 2010,* and recommends:

- *Balancing calories*
  - Enjoy your food, but eat less.
  - Avoid oversized portions.
- *Foods to increase*
  - Make half your plate fruits and vegetables.
  - Make at least half of your grains whole grains.
  - Switch to fat-free or low-fat (1%) milk.
- *Foods to reduce*
  - Compare sodium in foods like soup, bread, and frozen meals—and choose the foods with lower numbers.
  - Drink water instead of sugary drinks.

SuperTracker

SuperTracker is another online dietary and physical activity assessment tool developed by the U.S. Department of Agriculture (**FIG. 9.3**). It can be accessed online at https://www.supertracker.usda.gov. SuperTracker

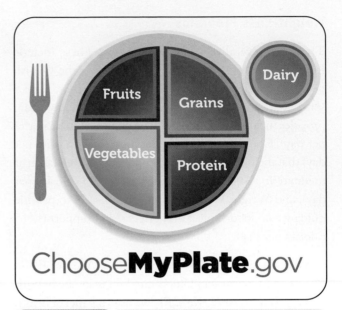

FIGURE 9.2   ChooseMyPlate. Reproduced from: U.S. Department of Agriculture. *ChooseMyPlate.* Available at: http://www.choosemy plate.gov.

officially replaced the MyPyramid Tracker in June 2012, and integrates the latest information from MyPlate and the 2010 Dietary Guidelines for Americans. Super-Tracker provides information on your diet quality and physical activity status, provides weight management guidance, and helps you set goals to achieve long-lasting health and wellness. The Food-A-Pedia feature enables you to access dietary and nutrition information for over 8,000 foods. Using this feature, you are able to compare two foods side-by-side for a closer analysis of calories, fats, sugars, and food groups.

SuperTracker: an online dietary and physical activity assessment tool that provides information on diet quality and physical activity status, provides weight management guidance, and helps you set goals to achieve long-lasting health and wellness.

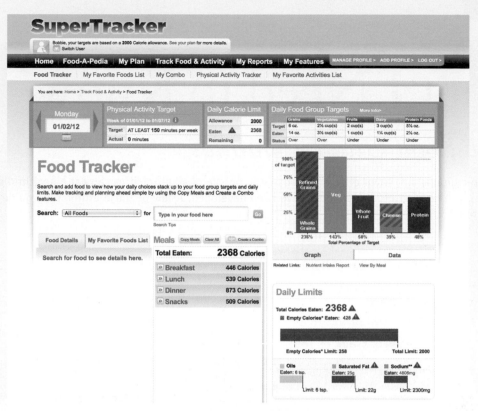

Bobbie's Food Groups and Calories Report

Your plan is based on a **2000 Calorie** allowance.

Food Groups	Target	Average Eaten	Status
⊞ Grains	6 ounce(s)	14 ounce(s)	Over
⊞ Whole Grains	≥ 3 ounce(s)	1 ounce(s)	Under
⊞ Refined Grains	≤ 3 ounce(s)	13 ounce(s)	Over
⊞ Vegetables	2½ cup(s)	3½ cup(s)	Over
⊞ Dark Green	1½ cup(s)/week	0 cup(s)	Under
⊞ Red & Orange	5½ cup(s)/week	1¾ cup(s)	Under
⊞ Beans & Peas	1½ cup(s)/week	¼ cup(s)	Under
⊞ Starchy	5 cup(s)/week	0 cup(s)	Under
⊞ Other	4 cup(s)/week	1¾ cup(s)	Under
⊞ Fruits	2 cup(s)	1 cup(s)	Under
⊞ Whole Fruit	No Specific Target	1 cup(s)	No Specific Target
⊞ Fruit Juice	No Specific Target	0 cup(s)	No Specific Target
⊞ Dairy	3 cup(s)	1¼ cup(s)	Under
⊞ Milk & Yogurt	No Specific Target	¼ cup(s)	No Specific Target
⊞ Cheese	No Specific Target	1 cup(s)	No Specific Target
⊞ Protein Foods	5½ ounce(s)	2½ ounce(s)	Under
⊞ Seafood	8 ounce(s)/week	0 ounce(s)	Under
⊞ Meat, Poultry & Eggs	No Specific Target	2½ ounce(s)	No Specific Target
⊞ Nuts, Seeds & Soy	No Specific Target	0 ounce(s)	No Specific Target
⊞ Oils	6 teaspoon	6 teaspoon	OK

Limits	Allowance	Average Eaten	Status
⊞ Total Calories	2000 Calories	2368 Calories	Over
⊞ Empty Calories*	≤ 258 Calories	428 Calories	Over
⊞ Solid Fats	*	375 Calories	*
⊞ Added Sugars	*	53 Calories	*

*Calories from food components such as added sugars and solid fats that provide little nutritional value. Empty Calories are part of Total Calories.

Note: If you ate Beans & Peas and chose "Count as Protein Foods instead," they will be included in the Nuts, Seeds & Soy subgroup.

FIGURE 9.3   SuperTracker: A U.S. government food guidance plan. Courtesy of: USDA.

What I Need to Know

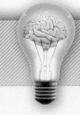

Ethnic Food Guide Pyramids

Different ethnic groups may favor different foods. Still, people of all ethnicities can eat a healthful diet. To assist with this goal, ethnic food guide pyramids have been developed. A few of these ethnic food guide pyramids are presented here for illustration.

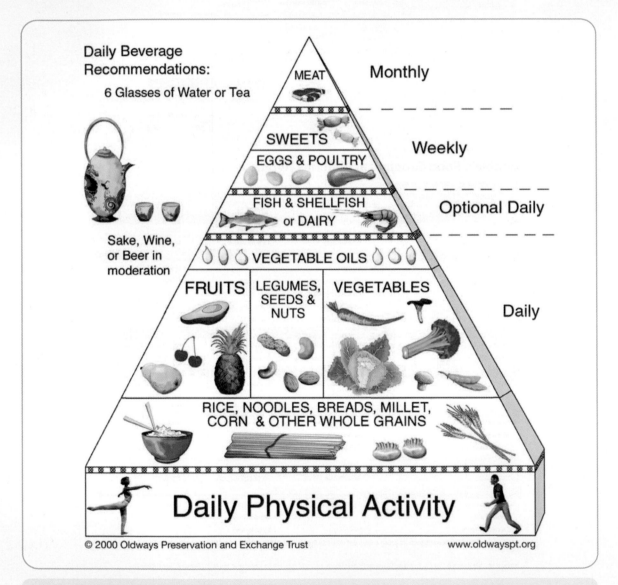

Asian diet pyramid. *Source:* © 2000 Oldways Preservation & Trust.

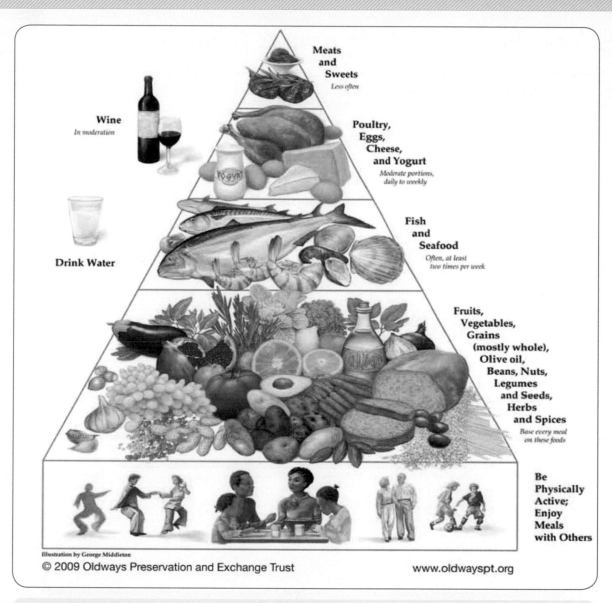

Mediterranean diet food guide pyramid. *Source:* © 2009 Oldways Preservation & Exchange Trust, www.oldwayspt.org.

(Continues)

What I Need to Know

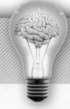

Ethnic Food Guide Pyramids (Cont.)

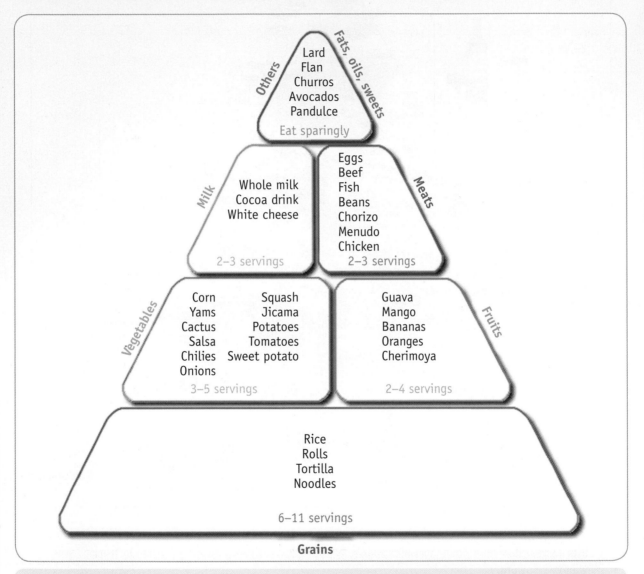

Others — **Fats, oils, sweets**
Lard
Flan
Churros
Avocados
Pandulce
Eat sparingly

Milk
Whole milk
Cocoa drink
White cheese
2–3 servings

Meats
Eggs
Beef
Fish
Beans
Chorizo
Menudo
Chicken
2–3 servings

Vegetables
Corn   Squash
Yams   Jicama
Cactus Potatoes
Salsa   Tomatoes
Chilies Sweet potato
Onions
3–5 servings

Fruits
Guava
Mango
Bananas
Oranges
Cherimoya
2–4 servings

Rice
Rolls
Tortilla
Noodles
6–11 servings

Grains

Mexican food guide pyramid. Reproduced from: Southeastern Michigan Dietetics Association. *Mexican Food Guide Pyramid*. Available at: http://www.semda.org/info/pyramid.asp?ID=27. This pyramid is being used as is and SEMA offers no guarantees for its use and cannot be held liable for any damages incurred by its use.

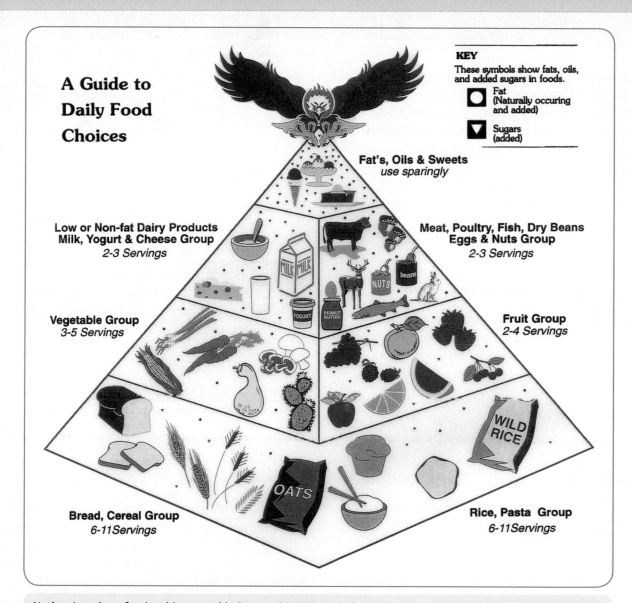

A Guide to Daily Food Choices

KEY
These symbols show fats, oils, and added sugars in foods.

◯ Fat (Naturally occuring and added)

▽ Sugars (added)

Fat's, Oils & Sweets
use sparingly

Low or Non-fat Dairy Products Milk, Yogurt & Cheese Group
2-3 Servings

Meat, Poultry, Fish, Dry Beans Eggs & Nuts Group
2-3 Servings

Vegetable Group
3-5 Servings

Fruit Group
2-4 Servings

Bread, Cereal Group
6-11Servings

Rice, Pasta Group
6-11Servings

Native American food guide pyramid. *Source:* CANFIT, Berkeley, CA. For more information, call 510-644-1533 or info@canfit.org. Used with permission.

- *Assess your food intake.* After you enter a day's worth of dietary information, the Food Tracker dietary assessment gives you an overall evaluation by comparing the amounts of food you ate to current food group targets. The Food Tracker also gauges your daily limits for oils, saturated fat, and sodium.

- *Assess your physical activity.* After you enter a week's worth of physical activity information, the Physical Activity Tracker calculates your total Moderate Intensity Equivalent (MIE) Minutes based on the types of activities you perform and the duration for which each is performed. When you're finished, you can populate a Physical Activity Report, which compares your results to the Physical Activity Guidelines for Americans.

The Vegetarian Food Guide Pyramid

Vegetarianism encourages the inclusion of plants and plant-based products in the diet and discourages the consumption of animal products. However, the degree to which vegetarians adhere to this concept defines the type of vegetarian they are. The vegetarian spectrum includes (Manohar, 2011):

- *Vegans:* Strict vegetarians who do not eat meat of any kind, eggs, dairy products, or any processed foods containing any animal-derived ingredients such as gelatin.

- *Fruitarians:* Vegetarians who only eat fresh fruits.

- *Lacto-ovo-vegetarians:* Vegetarians who do not eat pork, beef, poultry, fish, or animal flesh of any kind, but do consume eggs and dairy products.

- *Lacto vegetarians:* Vegetarians who do not eat any type of animal meat or even poultry and eggs, but consume milk.

- *Ovo vegetarians:* Vegetarians who do not eat any kind of animal flesh or meat and do not even consume milk, but eat eggs.

- *Pescetarian:* Vegetarians who refrain from eating all types of meat with the exception of fish.

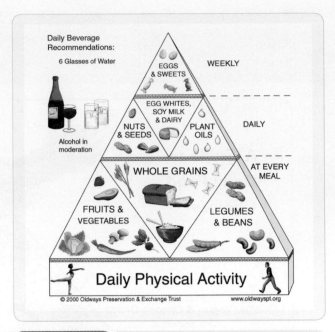

FIGURE 9.4   The vegetarian food guide pyramid. *Source:* © 2000 Oldways Preservation & Exchange Trust, www.oldwayspt.org.

- *Flexitarians:* Vegetarians who mostly stick to a vegetarian diet but occasionally eat meat.

- *Pollo-vegetarians:* People who eat poultry—such as chicken, turkey, and duck—but no other type of animal flesh and meat.

Vegetarian diets can meet all of the recommendations for nutrients and, therefore, compose a healthful diet (**FIG. 9.4** ▲). The key is to consume a variety of foods and the right amount of foods to meet your calorie needs. Follow the food group recommendations for your age, sex, and activity level to get the right amount of food and the variety of foods needed for nutrient adequacy. Nutrients that vegetarians may need to focus on in particular include protein, iron, calcium, zinc, and vitamin B_{12}.

Reading Food Labels

One of the most important skills to have in the management of your diet is the ability to understand the **Nutrition Facts label** that appears on the packaging of most foods

What I Need to Know

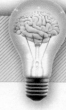

Tips for Creating Vegetarian Meals

Below are some tips to ensure a nutritionally sound vegetarian diet. (Note that nonvegetarians can also use these tips to create healthy meals and diets.)

- Build meals around protein sources that are naturally low in fat, such as beans, lentils, and rice. Don't overload meals with high-fat cheeses to replace the meat.

- Calcium-fortified soy-based beverages can provide calcium in amounts similar to that of milk. They are usually low in fat and do not contain cholesterol.

- Many foods that typically contain meat or poultry can be made vegetarian. This can increase vegetable intake and cut saturated fat and cholesterol intake; for example, vegetable pizza, vegetable lasagna, tofu-vegetable stir fry, and bean burritos or tacos.

- A variety of vegetarian products look (and may even taste) like their nonvegetarian

counterparts but are usually lower in saturated fat and contain no cholesterol. A variety of kinds are available, made with soy beans, vegetables, and/or rice. For example, rather than hamburgers, try veggie burgers. Add vegetarian meat substitutes to soups and stews to boost protein without adding saturated fat or cholesterol.

- Most restaurants can accommodate vegetarian modifications to menu items by substituting meatless sauces, omitting meat from stir-fries, and adding vegetables or pasta in place of meat. These substitutions are more likely to be available at restaurants that make food to order.

- Many Asian and Indian restaurants offer a varied selection of vegetarian dishes.

REPRODUCED FROM: United States Department of Agriculture. *Tips and Resources: Vegetarian Diets*. Undated. Available at: http://www. mypyramid.gov/tips_resources/vegetarian_diets_print.html.

(Food and Drug Administration, 2011). **FIG. 9.5 ▶** presents a sample Nutrition Facts label. Product-specific information (serving size, calories, and nutrients) is provided in the main or top section (see numbers 1–4 and number 6 in Figure 9.5). The bottom part (number 5) contains a footnote with Daily Values (DVs) for 2,000- and 2,500-calorie diets. This footnote provides recommended dietary information for important nutrients, including fats, sodium, and fiber.

The first thing to check on a Nutrition Facts label is the serving size and the number of servings in the package. Serving sizes are standardized to make it easier to compare similar foods. Serving sizes are provided in familiar units, such as cups or pieces, followed by the metric amount (the number of grams). The size of the serving on the food package influences the number of calories

and all the nutrient amounts listed on the top part of the label. In Figure 9.5, one serving of macaroni and cheese equals one cup. If you ate the whole package, you would eat *two* cups. That doubles the calories and other nutrient numbers, including the Percent Daily Values as shown in the sample label.

Nutrition Facts label: appearing on the packaging of most foods, it contains product-specific information (serving size, calories, and nutrient information), Daily Values (DVs) for 2,000- and 2,500-calorie diets, and dietary information for important nutrients, including fats, sodium, and fiber.

Sample label for Macaroni & Cheese

Nutrition Facts

1 Start here

Serving Size 1 cup (228g)
Servings Per Container 2

2 Check calories

Amount Per Serving

Calories 250   Calories from Fat

	% Daily Value*
Total Fat 12g	**18%**
Saturated Fat 3g	**15%**
Trans Fat 3g	
Cholesterol 30mg	**10%**
Sodium 470mg	**20%**
Total Carbohydrate 31g	**10%**
Dietary Fiber 0g	**0%**
Sugars 5g	
Protein 5g	
Vitamin A	**4%**
Vitamin C	**2%**
Calcium	**20%**
Iron	**4%**

3 Limit these nutrients

6 Quick guide to % DV
• 5% or less is low
• 20% or more is high

4 Get enough of these nutrients

* Percent Daily Values are based on a 2,000 calorie diet.
Your Daily Values may be higher or lower depending on
your calorie needs.

5 Footnote

	Calories:	2,000	2,500
Total Fat	Less than	65g	80g
Sat Fat	Less than	20g	25g
Cholesterol	Less than	300mg	300mg
Sodium	Less than	2,400mg	2,400mg
Total Carbohydrate		300g	375g
Dietary Fiber		25g	30g

FIGURE 9.5   Deciphering the Nutrition Facts label. Reproduced from: Food and Drug Administration. *How to Understand and Use the Nutrition Facts Label*. 2011. Available at: http://www.fda.gov/Food/ResourcesForYou/Consumers/NFLPM/ucm274593.htm.

The Role of Exercise in Weight Management

Regardless of claims by developers of weight-management programs, whether you gain or lose weight is ultimately dependent on the amount of calories taken in and the amount of calories expended. Because 3,500 calories equals 1 pound, if you were to ingest 500 more calories each day than you use up, you would be 1 pound heavier at the end of that week. So it stands to reason that to lose weight—that is, to use up more calories than ingested—you can decrease the number of calories taken in by controlling your diet or increase the number of calories used up by increasing your physical activity. The most effective approach is to do both.

Eating Disorders

If you were told you could be attractive and feel better about your body but would develop intestinal problems, decayed teeth, malnutrition, dehydration, stomach ruptures, esophagus tears, serious heart, kidney, and liver damage, and death, would you agree to that Faustian bargain? Well, that is exactly what some people do. They adopt an eating disorder that subjects them to serious health consequences, such as those above, in order to perceive that their bodies look better (Hughes, 2005). Ironically, they usually wind up looking worse—gaunt, hollow faced, thin legged—and appearing fatigued. Among the more common eating disorders are anorexia nervosa, bulimia, and muscle dysmorphia.

Anorexia Nervosa

Anorexia nervosa (often called just *anorexia*) is an eating disorder characterized by emaciation, a relentless pursuit of thinness and unwillingness to maintain a normal or healthy weight, a distortion of body image and intense fear of gaining weight, a lack of menstruation among girls and women, and extremely disturbed eating behavior. Some people with anorexia lose weight by dieting and exercising excessively; others lose weight by self-induced vomiting or by misusing laxatives, diuretics, or enemas.

Many people with anorexia see themselves as overweight, even when they are starved or are clearly malnourished. Control over food and weight becomes an obsession. People with anorexia typically weigh themselves repeatedly, portion foods carefully, and eat only very small quantities of only certain foods. Some who have anorexia recover with treatment after only one episode. Others get well but have relapses. Still others have a more chronic form of anorexia, in which their health deteriorates over many years as they battle the illness.

People with anorexia are up to 10 times more likely to die as a result of their illness compared to those without the disorder. The most common complications that lead to death are cardiac arrest and electrolyte and fluid imbalances. Suicide is another cause of death.

Many people with anorexia also have coexisting psychiatric and physical illnesses, including depression, anxiety, obsessive behavior, substance abuse, cardiovascular and neurologic complications, and impaired physical development. Other symptoms may develop over time, including thinning of the bones (osteoporosis), brittle hair and nails, dry and yellowish skin, growth of fine hair over the body, mild anemia and muscle weakness, severe constipation, low blood pressure, and lethargy (National Institute of Mental Health, 2010a).

Treatment for anorexia involves four components: restoring the person to a healthy weight, treating the psychological issues related to the eating disorder, reducing or eliminating behaviors or thoughts that lead to disordered eating, and preventing relapse. Different forms of psychotherapy, including individual, group based, and family based, can help address the psychological reasons for the illness. Some studies suggest that family-based therapies in which parents assume responsibility for feeding their afflicted adolescent are the most effective in helping a person with anorexia gain weight and improve eating habits and mood (National Institute of Mental Health, 2010a).

> **Anorexia nervosa:** an eating disorder characterized by emaciation, a relentless pursuit of thinness, a distortion of body image, and intense fear of gaining weight.

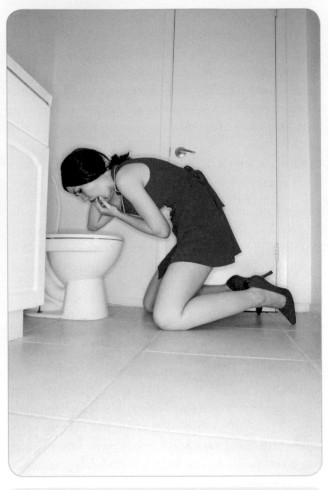

People with eating disorders place their health in great jeopardy. Even though many of them realize the danger to their health, their obsession to take control of their bodies overwhelms rational decision making. Medical and psychological intervention is necessary.

Bulimia

Bulimia nervosa (*bulimia*) is another eating disorder. It is characterized by recurrent and frequent episodes of eating unusually large amounts of food (binge eating) and feeling a lack of control over the eating. This binge eating is followed by a type of behavior that compensates for the binge, such as purging (e.g., vomiting and/or excessive use of laxatives or diuretics), fasting, and/or excessive exercise.

Unlike people with anorexia, people with bulimia can fall within the normal weight range for their age and height. However, like people with anorexia, they often fear gaining of weight, want desperately to lose weight, and are

intensely unhappy with the appearance of their bodies. Typically, bulimic behavior is done secretly because it is often accompanied by feelings of disgust or shame. The binging and purging cycle usually repeats several times a week. Similar to anorexia, people with bulimia often have coexisting psychological illnesses, such as depression, anxiety, and/or substance abuse problems. Many physical conditions result from the purging aspect of the illness, including electrolyte imbalances, gastrointestinal problems, and oral and tooth-related problems. Other symptoms include chronically inflamed and sore throat, swollen glands in the neck and below the jaw, worn tooth enamel and increasingly sensitive and decaying teeth, gastroesophageal reflux disorder, intestinal distress and irritation from laxative abuse, kidney problems from diuretic abuse, and severe dehydration from purging of fluids (National Institute of Mental Health, 2010b).

As with treatment for anorexia, treatment for bulimia often involves a combination of approaches and depends on the needs of the individual. To reduce or eliminate binging and purging behaviors, a patient may undergo nutritional counseling and psychotherapy, especially cognitive behavior therapy (CBT), or be prescribed medication. Some antidepressants—such as fluoxetine (Prozac), which is the only medication approved by the FDA to treat bulimia—may help patients who also have depression and/or anxiety. Prozac also appears to help reduce binge-eating and purging behavior, reduces the chance of relapse, and improves eating attitudes (National Institute of Mental Health, 2010b).

Muscle Dysmorphia

Being preoccupied with muscle development may involve a disturbance in behaviors similar to those seen in cases

Bulimia nervosa: an eating disorder characterized by recurrent and frequent episodes of eating unusually large amounts of food (binge eating), followed by behavior that compensates for the binge, such as purging.

Muscle dysmorphia: sometimes referred to as bigorexia or reverse anorexia, it is a preoccupation with muscle development.

of anorexia nervosa. **Muscle dysmorphia**, sometimes referred to as *bigorexia* or *reverse anorexia*, affects hundreds of thousands of men and many women. Even though these men and women have well-developed physiques, they perceive themselves as being muscularly underdeveloped to the point that they will shy away from situations that expose their bodies. They are so preoccupied with developing their bodies that they miss important events, continue training through injury, or even lose their jobs.

Although the causes of muscle dysmorphia are unknown, it is suspected that two forces are at work. First, it is hypothesized that muscle dysmorphia is a form of obsessive-compulsive behavior directed at control of the body. Second, depictions of "perfect" bodies, as portrayed in the media, pressure people to conform to an unrealistic ideal shape. Notably, in a study in which American and European college men were asked to pick a body type they thought women would find attractive, on average they chose pictures of men with 20–30 more pounds of muscle than that of a normal man. In contrast, when women were asked which man they found most attractive, they chose the normal-sized man most of the time (Pope, 2000).

One of the health issues associated with muscle dysmorphia is the use of anabolic steroids. In pursuit of a more muscular body, it is common for bigorexics to use steroids despite experiencing side effects such as increased aggression, acne, breast enlargement, baldness, impotence, and testicular shrinkage. The mindset is such that the risk of these side effects is worth the increased muscle mass (Kennard, 2010).

Treatment for muscle dysmorphia consists of a combination of educational and psychotherapeutic techniques. Counseling is directed at having patients develop more realistic and achievable goals regarding their bodies. To determine if you have muscle dysmorphia, complete Health Check Up 9.7 (see Health Check Up 9.7 on the companion website). Once completed, place Health Check Up 9.7 in your Health Decision Portfolio.

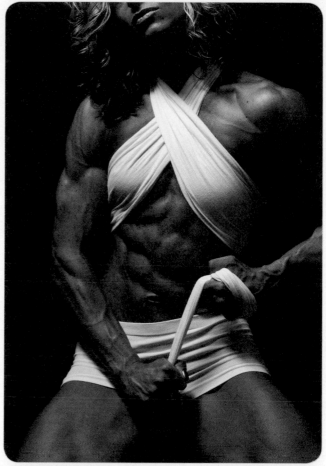

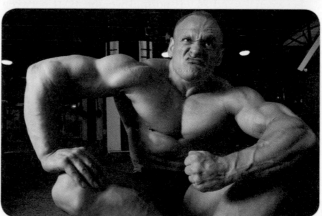

The desire to develop a muscular physique is normal. When it becomes an obsession, however, it can interfere with other parts of a healthy lifestyle.

SUMMARY

The goal of this chapter is to provide you with the tools you need to take charge of your diet and weight. To help you do that, a summary of important information included in this chapter is provided.

- Body image refers to the mental image we have of our physical appearance. Many factors influence body image, including how much we weigh, how our weight is distributed, our values about physical appearance, our concepts of good physical appearance, our ethnic and cultural background, what we see in people around us, what we hear through the media, and what we hear from others.

- Body esteem, or body cathexis, is what you think about your body, body parts, and body functions. Every individual thinks well about some parts of his or her body and not so well about other parts.

- BMI is a measure of body fat based on height and weight that is often used to define underweight, overweight, and obesity. For adults, BMI values are categorized as follows: BMI under 19 is underweight, BMI between 19 and 24.9 is normal weight, BMI between 25 and 29.9 is overweight, and BMI of 30 or higher is obese.

- Overweight and obesity are the result of an imbalance between calories ingested versus the amount of calories expended; that is, calories in and calories out. Overweight and obesity are influenced by the environment, genes and family history, health conditions, emotional factors, age, and lack of sleep.

- Overweight and obesity can be prevented by making healthy decisions such as following a healthy eating plan, watching food portion sizes, being active, reducing screen time (television, computers, DVDs, smart phones, and video games), and regularly keeping track of your weight.

- Effective weight-loss programs have several common features: watching portions, limiting fat, eating fruits and vegetables, consuming whole grains, eating at home, and exercising.

- SuperTracker and ChooseMyPlate are online dietary and physical activity assessment tools developed by the U.S. Department of Agriculture. They provide information on diet quality and physical activity status, offer related nutrition messages, and list links to nutrient and physical activity information.

- One of the most important skills to develop to manage diet is the ability to use the Nutrition Facts label that appears on the packaging of most foods. The Nutrition Facts label contains product-specific information (serving size, calories, and nutrient information), DVs for 2,000- and 2,500-calorie diets, and dietary information for important nutrients, including fats, sodium, and fiber.

- Among the more common eating disorders are anorexia nervosa, bulimia, and muscle dysmorphia. Anorexia nervosa is an eating disorder characterized by emaciation, a relentless pursuit of thinness, a distortion of body image, and an intense fear of gaining weight. Bulimia nervosa is characterized by recurrent and frequent episodes of eating unusually large amounts of food (binge eating) followed by purging (e.g., vomiting, excessive use of laxatives or diuretics). Muscle dysmorphia, sometimes referred to as bigorexia or reverse anorexia, is a preoccupation with muscle development.

REFERENCES

Answers.com. *If Barbie Were Life Size What Would Her Measurements Be?* 2011. Available at: http://wiki.answers.com/Q/If_Barbie_were_life_size_what_would_her_measurements_be#ixzz1fhZFNQfo.

Barry, D. T. and Grillo, C. M. Eating and body image disturbances in adolescent psychiatric inpatients: Gender and ethnicity patterns. *International Journal of Eating Disorders* 32 (2002): 335–343.

Consumer Reports Health.org. 6 secrets of the slim for your diet plan. 2009. Available at: http://www.consumerreports.org/health/healthy-living/diet-nutrition/diets-dieting/dieting-on-a-budget/six-secrets-of-the-slim/dieting-on-a-budget-slimming-secrets.htm. © 2010 by Consumers Union of U.S. Inc., Yonkers, NY 10703-1057, a nonprofit organization. Reprinted with permission from ConsumerReports.org. for educational purposes only. No commercial use or reproduction permitted.

Consumer Reports Health.org. CRH: Jenny Craig rated best diet; Weight Watchers scores a distant third. 2011. Available at: http://pressroom.consumerreports.org/pressroom/2011/05/crh-jenny-craig-rated-best-diet-weight-watchers-scores-a-distant-third-.html.

Diet and Nutrition. *Consumer Reports Health.org.* 2011. Available at: http://www.consumerreports.org/health/healthy-living/diet-nutrition/diets-dieting/diet-reviews/overview/index.htm.

Duggan, S. J. and McCreary, D. R. Body image, eating disorders, and drive for muscularity in gay and heterosexual men: The influence of media images. In Morrison, T. G., ed. *Eclectic Views on Gay Male Pornography: Pornucopia.* Binghamton, NY: Haworth Press, 2004, 45–58.

Field, A. E., Cheung, L., Wolf, A. M., Herzog, D. B., Gortmaker, S. L., and Colditz, G. A. Exposure to the mass media and weight concerns among girls. *Pediatrics* 103 (1999): 36.

Flegal, K. M., Carroll, M. D., Odgen, C. L., and Curtin, L. R. Prevalence and trends in obesity among US adults, 1999–2008. *Journal of the American Medical Association* 303 (2010): 235–241.

Food and Drug Administration. *How to Understand and Use the Nutrition Facts Label.* 2011. Available at: http://www.fda.gov/food/labelingnutrition/consumerinformation/ucm078889.htm#twoparts.

Freedman, D. S. Obesity—United States, 1988–2008. *Morbidity and Mortality Weekly Report* 60 Supplement (2011): 73–77.

Goodpaster, B. H., DeLany, J. P., Otto, A. D., Kuller, L., Vockley, J., South-Paul, J. E., Thomas, S. B., Brown, J., McTigue, K., Hames, K. C., et al. Effects of diet and physical activity interventions on weight loss and cardiometabolic risk factors in severely obese adults: A randomized trial. *Journal of the American Medical Association* 304 (2010): 1795–1802.

Harvard School of Public Health. *The Nutrition Source: Fiber.* 2011a. Available at: http://www.hsph.harvard.edu/nutritionsource/what-should-you-eat/fiber/.

Harvard School of Public Health. *The Nutrition Source: Fiber; Start Roughing It!* 2011b. Available at: http://www.hsph.harvard.edu/nutritionsource/what-should-you-eat/fiber-full-story/index.html.

Hughes, R. A. Mind, mood, and message: Pathways in community behavioral health. *St. Luke's Health Initiatives: Arizona Health Futures Issue Brief.* 2005. Available at: http://www.slhi.org/publications/issue_briefs/pdfs/ib-2005-January.pdf

Hunt, T. J., Thienhaus, M. D., and Ellwood, A. The mirror lies: Body dysmorphic disorder. *American Family Physician* 78 (2008): 217–222.

Kennard, J. Bigorexia: Reverse anorexia. *About.com. Men's Health.* 2010. Available at: http://menshealth.about.com/cs/menonly/a/bigorexia.htm.

Manohar, U. Different types of vegetarians. *Buzzle.com.* 2011. Available at: http://www.buzzle.com/articles/different-types-of-vegetarians.html.

Mayo Clinic. *Dietary Fiber: Essential for a Healthy Diet.* 2009. Available at: http://www.mayoclinic.com/health/fiber/NU00033.

National Heart, Lung, and Blood Institute. *In Brief: Your Guide To Lowering Your Blood Pressure With DASH.* Washington, DC: National Heart, Lung, and Blood Institute, 2006.

National Heart, Lung, and Blood Institute. Overweight and obesity: What causes overweight and obesity? *Diseases and Conditions Index.* 2011a. Available at: http://www.nhlbi.nih.gov/health/dci/Diseases/obe/obe_causes.html.

National Heart, Lung, and Blood Institute. How can overweight and obesity be prevented? *Diseases and Conditions Index.* 2011b. Available at: http://www.nhlbi

.nih.gov/health/dci/Diseases/obe/obe_prevention .html.

National Heart, Lung, and Blood Institute. How are overweight and obesity treated? *Diseases and Conditions Index*. 2011c. Available at: http://www.nhlbi.nih .gov/health/dci/Diseases/obe/obe_treatments.html.

National Institute of Mental Health. *Anorexia Nervosa*. 2010a. Available at: http://www.nimh.nih.gov/health /publications/eating-disorders/anorexia-nervosa.shtml.

National Institute of Mental Health. *Bulimia*. 2010b. Available at: http://www.nimh.nih.gov/health /publications/eating-disorders/bulimia-nervosa.shtml.

Ogden, C. L., Fryar, C. D., Carroll, M. D., and Flegal, K. M. Mean body weight, height, and body mass index, United States, 1960–2002. *Advance Data from Vital and Health Statistics* 347 (October 27, 2004).

Pope, H. G., Gruber, A. J., Mangweth, B., Bureau, B., deCol, C., Jouvent, R., and Hudson, J. I. Body image perception among men in three countries. *American Journal of Psychiatry* 157 (2000): 1297–1301.

Rock, C. L., Flatt, S. W., Sherwood, N. E., Karanja, N., Bilge Pakiz, B., and Thomson, C. A. Effect of a free prepared meal and incentivized weight loss program on weight loss and weight loss maintenance in obese and overweight women: A randomized controlled trial. *Journal of the American Medical Association* 304 (2010): 1803–1810.

Rubinstein, S. and Caballero, B. Is Miss America an undernourished role model? *Journal of the American Medical Association* 238 (2000): 1569.

Sabbah, H. A., Vereecken, C. A., Elgar, F. J., Tonja Nansel, T., Aasvee, K., Abdeen, Z., Ojala, K., Ahluwalia, N., and Maes. L. Body weight dissatisfaction and communication with parents among adolescents in 24 countries: International cross-sectional survey. *BMC Public Health* 9 (2009): 52.

University of Iowa. Eating disorders and body dissatisfaction have historically been tagged as women's problems. *Health Reports*. December 30, 2002. Available at: http://www.uihealthcare.com/reports /internalmedicine/021230whome.html.

U.S. Department of Agriculture. *SuperTracker*. Undated. Available at: https://www.supertracker.usda.gov.

U.S. Department of Agriculture. Center for Nutrition Policy and Promotion. The food supply and dietary fiber: Its availability and effect on health. *Nutrition Insight 36*, November 2007.

U.S. News & World Report. Health: Best Diets Overall. 2012. Available at: http://health.usnews.com/best-diet /best-overall-diets.

Williams, S. J. Medical sociology, chronic illness and the body: A rejoinder to Michael Kelly and David Field. *Sociology of Health and Illness* 18 (1996): 699–709.

Wing, R. R. Treatment options for obesity: Do commercial weight loss programs have a role? *Journal of the American Medical Association* 304 (2010): 1837–1838.

Worldometer. World Statistics Updated in Real Time. Undated. Available at: http://www.worldometers.info /weight-loss/.

INTERNET RESOURCES

National Institute of Child Health and Human Development
http://www.nichd.nih.gov/health/topics/diet_and_nutrition.cfm

American Heart Association: Nutrition Center
http://www.heart.org/HEARTORG/
GettingHealthy/NutritionCenter/Nutrition-Center_UCM_001188_SubHomePage.jsp

Nutrition.gov
http://www.nutrition.gov/nal_display/index.php?info_center=11&tax_level=1

Self Nutrition Data: Know What You Eat
http://nutritiondata.self.com/

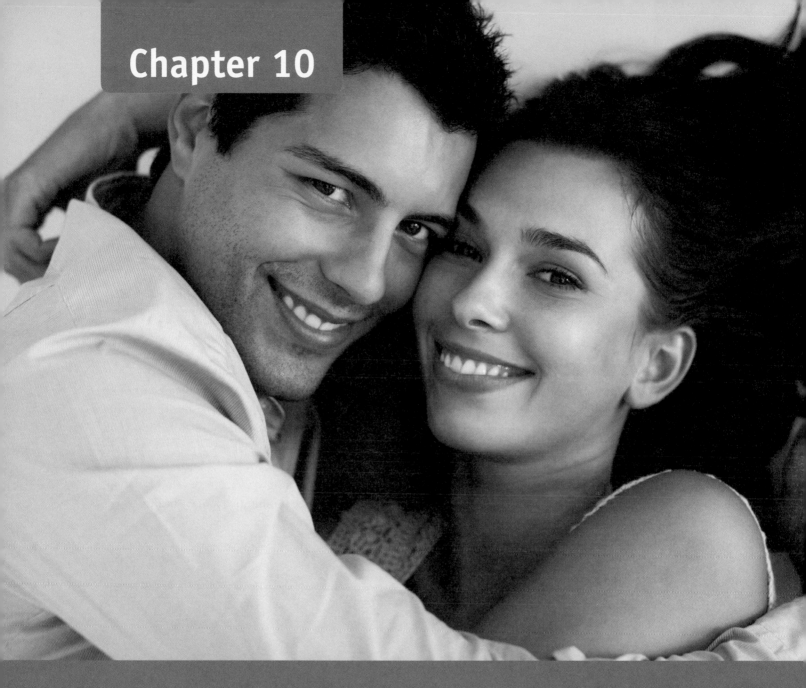

Chapter 10

Developing Healthy and Satisfying Relationships

 Access Health Check Ups and Health Behavior Change activities on the Companion Website:
go.jblearning.com/Empowering.

Learning Objectives

■ Discuss strategies to develop friendships.

■ Define different types of love, and describe how they interact with one another.

■ Identify symptoms of unhealthy relationships.

■ Describe the health effects of marriage and how to select a life partner.

■ Discuss the challenges facing single-parent families and strategies to respond to these challenges.

D o you want to be healthy and live longer? Of course you do. Did you know that your relationships affect your longevity? It's true, and to a greater degree than you might think. Researchers conducted a systematic review of the literature on the extent to which social relationships influence mortality risk and which aspects of social relationships are most predictive of mortality (Holt-Lunstad, Smith, and Layton, 2010). They found that people with stronger social relationships had a 50% increased likelihood of survival than those with weaker social relationships. The researchers concluded that the influence of social relationships on the risk of death are comparable with the influence of well-established risk factors such as smoking and alcohol consumption and actually exceed the influence of other risk factors such as physical inactivity and obesity.

Other studies provide consistent and compelling evidence linking a low quantity or quality of social relationships with a host of conditions, including development and progression of cardiovascular disease, recurrent heart attacks, atherosclerosis, high blood pressure, cancer and delayed cancer recovery, and slower wound healing (Robles and Kiecolt-Glaser, 2003; Everson-Rose and Lewis, 2005; Uchino, 2004; Ertel, Glymour, and

Berkman, 2009). Poor quality and low quantity of social ties have also been associated with impaired immune function, factors associated with adverse health outcomes, and mortality (Kiecolt-Glaser, McGuire, Robles, and Glaser, 2002; Robles and Kiecolt-Glaser, 2003).

This chapter decribes how you can develop satisfying relationships and, as a result, live longer, healthier, and happier.

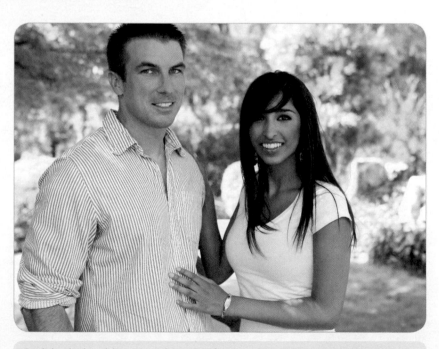

Social relationships can take many forms—friendship, romantic love, or family bonds. Regardless of their form, positive social relationships are an important ingredient in maintenance of health.

Friendship

One type of relationship associated with significant benefits is friendship. In fact, some studies found that friends have a greater effect on health than do family members (Giles, Glonek, Luszcz, and Andrews, 2005). Development of friendships, then, is an important health-enhancing strategy. Although there is no sure way to develop a network of friends, there are some recommendations that can increase the likelihood of friendships occurring:

■ Spend more time with people. In other words, hang out in places in which other people hang out. Staying at home watching television, playing computer games, or listening to music is not a good way to meet people and make friends.

■ Identify an interest of yours and locate organizations, on or off campus, that cater to that interest. For example, if you play a musical instrument, find a band or orchestra to join. If you enjoy reading, join a book club. Interaction with people with whom you share a common interest is a good way to make friends.

■ Join an intramural sports team on campus or play pickup games in the campus gym or recreation center. You do not have to be exceptionally talented to participate in sports. You will find people of various skill levels who enjoy playing games.

There are many ways to make friends, including engaging in volunteer activities or community service.

■ Volunteer on campus or in the community. Participation in volunteer activities usually involves groups of people getting together to plan and conduct a service of some sort. These occasions are good times to meet people with whom you share a common passion.

Making new friends is only half the battle. Maintenance of friendships is just as important. Of course, being trustworthy (not revealing secrets told to you by friends), being honest, being reliable (being there when a friend is in need), and being a good listener are all necessary to maintain friendships. However, one of the most overlooked ingredients to maintain friendships is a shared intimacy: sharing feelings, joys and sorrows, accomplishments and failures, and life goals bring people closer. Do you have shared intimacy with your close friends? To determine how intimate your friendships are, complete Health Check Up 10.1 (see Health Check Up 10.1 on the companion website). Once completed, place Health Check Up 10.1 in your Health Decision Portfolio. You may want your friends to complete Health Check Up 10.1 as well.

Romantic Relationships

If you've ever been in love, you know how good it can feel. With old friends and family back home, many college students find a need to fill the void with new love relationships. Development of these relationships, however, requires a lot of work. Any new relationship requires adaptation to a new set of rules and standards. How often do we see each other? How often do we call? Where should we go out? Who should pay? With whose friends should we hang out? The answers to these questions often depend on the type of love relationship.

Types of Love

There are different types of love and different types of lovers. **Erotic love (eros)** is a passionate, all-enveloping love. When erotic lovers meet, the heart races and a fluttering in the stomach and a shortness of breath occur. **Ludic love (ludus)** is a playful, flirtatious love. It involves no long-term commitment and is basically for amusement. Ludic love is usually played with several partners at once. **Storgic love (storge)** is a calm, companionate love. Storgic lovers are quietly affectionate and have long-term goals for the relationship, such as marriage and children. **Manic love (mania)** is a combination of erotic and ludic love. A manic lover's needs for affection are insatiable. He or she is often racked with highs of irrational joy, lows of anxiety and depression, and bouts of extreme jealousy. Manic attachments seldom develop into lasting love.

Some love relationships involve two people who are different in many respects, including the types of lovers they are. Imagine that a ludic lover is in a love relationship with a storgic lover. One is playing games with no intention of a lasting or exclusive relationship, and the other is thinking of a long-term relationship that may include marriage and children. When love relationships are frustrating or unfulfilling, it may be because of misunderstandings regarding the types of love involved.

What are your expectations for a romantic relationship? If you are currently in a love relationship, is the type of love you express compatible with what you receive? Recognizing that your goals for romance may change during different stages of your life, do you think you will someday pursue a different type of love from the one you want now? Do you look forward to this transition? Why or why not?

> **Erotic love (eros):** a passionate, all-enveloping love. When erotic lovers meet, the heart races and a fluttering in the stomach and a shortness of breath occur.
>
> **Ludic love (ludus):** a playful, flirtatious love. It involves no long-term commitment and is basically for amusement. Ludic love is usually played with several partners at once.
>
> **Storgic love:** a calm, companionate love. Storgic lovers are quietly affectionate and have goals of marriage and children for the relationship.
>
> **Manic love (mania):** a combination of erotic and ludic love. A manic lover's needs for affection are insatiable. He or she is often racked with highs of irrational joy, lows of anxiety and depression, and bouts of extreme jealousy.

As with other decisions in your life, you can control the types of relationships that you enter; by understanding what you want, you can increase your odds of finding a compatible lover.

To determine what type of lover you are, complete Health Check Up 10.2 (see Health Check Up 10.2 on the companion website). Once completed, place Health Check Up 10.2 in your Health Decision Portfolio. If you are now involved in a love relationship, perhaps you'll want your lover to complete Health Check Up 10.2 as well.

There are online *love tests* that match people on a variety of characteristics and personality traits. Some of the variables they measure are adventurousness, communication style, relationship role, temperament, romanticism, importance of wealth, and need for independence. Each month, approximately 20 million people use online matching services such as Match.com, Americansingles.com, and Date.com (*Online Dating Magazine*, 2007). Online personal ads generated more than $400 million in 2003, up from $72 million in 2001. It seems that a lot of people are looking for love and are willing to pay to find it.

Breakups

Whereas being in love can be very satisfying, breakups can be very hard. Sometimes relationships break up because the partners are too dissimilar (one may be interested in going to sporting events and the other in staying home to study) or because they have different expectations of the relationship (one may be a ludic lover and the other a storgic lover). College students are at a stage of life in which they are experimenting with different kinds of relationships, so it is not surprising that many of these do not develop into long-term relationships. In fact, college students usually experience several breakups during their college years. People tend to maintain romantic relationships when their partners meet their fundamental psychological needs and break up when they do not (Patrick, Knee, Canevello, and Lonsbary, 2007).

One of the needs found to be very important in maintaining of relationships is called **attachment anxiety**, which describes a strong dependence on a partner to affirm one's worthiness of having his or her needs met (Mikulincer and Shaver, 2007). People with high attachment anxiety

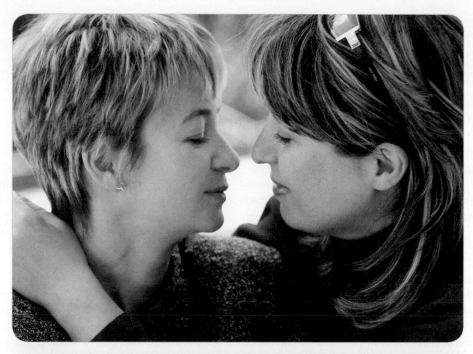

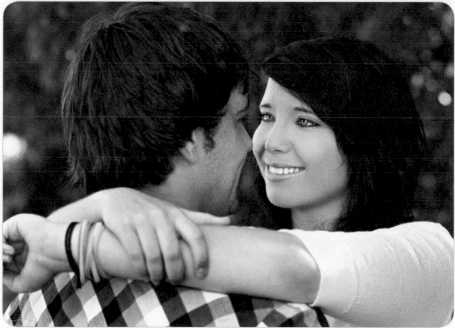

Love develops and changes over time. An erotic lover may become a storgic lover with a greater commitment to maintaining a long-term love relationship.

seem to be less psychologically willing or able to break up a relationship even when their partners fail to meet their psychological needs. For these people, being in any relationship may be preferable to being alone (Slotter and Finkel, 2009).

Attachment anxiety: being dependent on one's partner to affirm one's worthiness of having his or her needs met. People with high attachment anxiety seem to be less psychologically willing or able to break up a relationship.

What I Need to Know

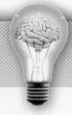

Hormones Influence Love and Affection

How often do you hug? Do you like to sit close and hold each other's hands? Recent research shows such physical contact is good for your health. Not only between loving partners but also between parents and children, and even between close friends, physical affection can help the brain, the heart, and other body systems you might never have imagined.

Recently, scientists supported by National Institutes of Health have begun to understand the chemistry and biology of love. At the center of how our bodies respond to love and affection is a hormone called **oxytocin**. Most of our oxytocin is made in the area of the brain called the hypothalamus. Oxytocin makes us feel good when we're close to family and other loved ones, including pets. It does this by acting through what scientists call the dopamine reward system. **Dopamine** is a brain chemical that plays a crucial part in how we perceive pleasure. Problems with the dopamine reward system can lead to clinical depression and other mental illness.

Oxytocin does more than make us feel good. It lowers the levels of stress hormones in the body, thereby reducing blood pressure, improving mood, increasing tolerance for pain, and perhaps even increasing the speed at which wounds heal. Oxytocin also seems to play an important role in strengthening our relationships. It has been linked, for example, to how much we trust others.

Researchers have found that people who have a more positive relationship with their partner have higher levels of oxytocin. In addition, it is clear from these research studies that physical contact affects oxytocin levels. People who get lots of hugs and other warm contact tend to have the highest levels of oxytocin. Frequent warm contact may somehow prime the oxytocin system and make it quicker to activate whenever there is warm contact.

Animal studies have found oxytocin is especially important for females to form bonds with their mates. In males, a related hormone called vasopressin also plays a role. Oxytocin and vasopressin are not miracle compounds, however. Giving these hormones to animals does not suddenly cause them to form loving bonds. Animals must have a certain genetic makeup that responds to these hormones in the first place. For humans, the full picture is even more complex. Although humans are genetically programmed to form social bonds, doing so is influenced by early experiences. In the end, an intricate interaction of genes and experience makes some people form social bonds more easily than others.

We may not yet fully understand how love and affection develop between people—or how love affects our health—but research is giving us some guidance. Give those you love all the affection you can. It can't hurt, and it may bring a bounty of health benefits.

ADAPTED FROM: The power of love: Hugs and cuddles have long-term effects. *NIH News in Health*. 2007. Available at: http://newsinhealth.nih.gov/2007/February/docs/01features_01.htm.

Oxytocin: a hormone produced by the hypothalamus that makes people feel good, lowers the levels of stress hormones in the body, reduces blood pressure, improves mood, and increases tolerance for pain. Physical contact increases oxytocin levels.

Dopamine: a brain chemical that plays a crucial part in how we perceive pleasure. Many drugs of abuse act through the dopamine reward system. Problems with the dopamine reward system can lead to clinical depression and other mental illness.

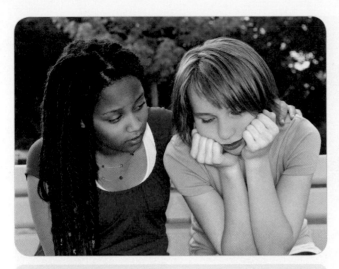

One strategy to overcome the heartbreak over a failed relationship is to share feelings and thoughts and obtain the support of family and friends.

When a breakup does occur, students experiencing the most distress are those who are highly invested in the relationship in terms of time and commitment, whose partners break up with them (being left by the other), whose partners have an interest in other relationships and have more alternatives to pursue that interest, and those who are fearful of abandonment in the first place (Sprecher, Felmlee, Metts, Fehr, and Vanni, 1998). Because most relationship breakups are not by mutual agreement (Sprecher, 1994), usually the partner who did not initiate the breakup experiences significant distress.

What strategies can you use to recover from your next breakup better? First, realize that as with any loss, a grieving process—including symptoms such as shock, anger, and intense sadness—is to be expected. This process takes time, but, eventually, healing does occur. Two strategies are especially important in working through a breakup:

- *Share feelings and thoughts with friends and family.* The social support and perspective they offer may help you understand that although the loss of this relationship is painful, it may be for the best in the long run. Friends and family also help you maintain your sense of self-worth by letting you know you are a person that others love and care about and that you are worthy of being loved.

- "Get back on the horse." That is, make a conscious decision to interact with friends, go out socially, and open yourself up to new relationships. Staying at home and pouting will only exacerbate your sadness.

Unhealthy Relationships

Two issues that are associated with unhealthy relationships need attention: emotionally abusive and controlling relationships; and sexual violence. Both are causes of concern and need remediation. If these issues cannot be eliminated in your relationships, it is reason enough to end those relationships.

Emotionally Abusive and Controlling Relationships

In some relationships, one partner may expect to make all the important decisions, even to what clothes his or her partner wears. This is a form of relationship abuse and a sign of a controlling relationship. Relationship abuse is a pattern of abusive and coercive behaviors used to maintain power and control over a former or current intimate partner. Abuse can be emotional, financial, sexual, or physical and can include threats, isolation, and intimidation, with abuse usually escalating over time (Center for Relationship Abuse Awareness, 2010c). When we think of abuse in an intimate relationship, we tend to think of physical abuse. Verbal abuse, however, is more common and can be quite harmful. Examples of verbal abuse include (Center for Relationship Abuse Awareness, 2010a):

- Degrading a person in front of the person's friends and family

- Telling hurtful "jokes" despite a person's requests to stop

- Taking a person's statements out of context

- Name calling

- Insult

- Humiliation

- Criticism

237

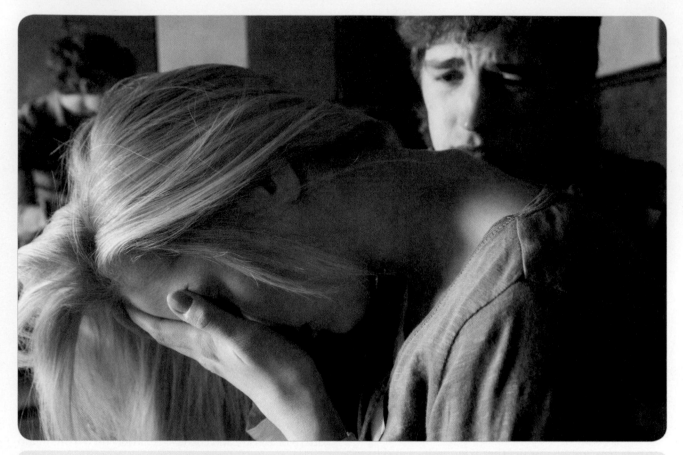

When a breakup is not mutual, the partner "left behind" may go through a grieving process.

- Blame

- Accusation

- Questioning a person's sanity

To determine whether a relationship you are in is an emotionally abusive or controlling one, ask yourself the following questions (Center for Relationship Abuse Awareness, 2010b):

- Do you feel nervous around your partner?

- Do you have to be careful to control your behavior to avoid your partner's anger?

- Do you feel pressured by your partner when it comes to sex?

- Are you afraid of disagreeing with your partner?

- Does your partner criticize you or humiliate you in front of other people?

- Is your partner always checking up on you or questioning you about what you do without your partner?

- Does your partner repeatedly and wrongly accuse you of seeing or flirting with other people?

- Does your partner tell you that if you changed he or she would not abuse you?

- Does your partner's jealousy stop you from seeing friends or family?

- Does your partner make you feel like you are wrong, stupid, crazy, or inadequate?

- Has your partner ever scared you with violence or threatening behavior?

- Does your partner prevent you from going out or doing things you want to do?

- Are you expected to do things to please your partner, rather than to please yourself?

- Do you feel that in the opinion of your partner, nothing you ever do is good enough?

- Does your partner say, "I will kill myself if you break up with me" or "I will hurt/kill you if you break up with me"?

- Does your partner make excuses for the abusive behavior? For example: saying, "It's because of alcohol or drugs," or "I can't control my temper," or "I was just joking"?

If you determine you are in an emotionally abusive or controlling relationship, there are several things you can do. If you decide your partner cannot change, walk away. It is a far better idea to cut your losses by ending the relationship, no matter how emotionally attached you may have become, than trying to change your partner. This kind of controlling behavior is far more likely to escalate and intensify, rather than decline, as the relationship progresses (Baldino, 2011). No one deserves to be abused in this manner. If you choose this option, you need to assess whether your partner might become physically abusive. If you decide this is a possibility, follow the suggestions in the next section to protect yourself. You may also want to contact the police or a local domestic violence center or call the National Domestic Violence Hotline at (800) 799-SAFE.

If you decide the relationship can be salvaged, consider counseling for you and your partner to change the relationship dynamic. Be cautious, however, about rationalizing the abusive and controlling behavior. More often than not, your controlling partner has been this way for a long time, and change will be extremely difficult and unlikely.

Relationship Violence

An American College Health Association study found that 4% of male college students and 9% of female college students report being sexually touched against their will. One percent of male college students and 4% of female college students state that sexual penetration (vaginal, oral, or anal) was attempted against their will, and 1% of males and 2% of females were actually sexually penetrated without their consent (American College Health Association, 2009). The great majority of these sexual assaults are committed by someone known to the victims or by someone they are dating.

The National Crime Prevention Council (2006) cites warning signs that can help you determine if your dating relationship is susceptible to violence or sexual assault. Ask yourself:

- Is your partner jealous or possessive?

- Does your partner dislike your parents or friends?

- Do you get a lot of negative teasing from your partner, even in front of friends?

- Does your partner have a quick temper?

- Does your partner "playfully" slap you and shove you?

- Does your partner's behavior change because he or she drinks or uses drugs?

- Does the burden of making the relationship work fall mainly on you?

- Are you expected to change your behavior to suit your partner?

- Are you afraid of what your partner might do when angry, whether with you or with someone else?

- Are you afraid to express feelings of your own or make decisions about what to wear, where to go, or whom to like?

- Does your partner demand to know where you are at all times?

- Does your partner make you afraid to say no to sex?

- Does your partner respect your wish to practice safe sex?

- Are you afraid to end the relationship?

If you answered yes to any of the above, reconsider maintaining this relationship. You are placing yourself at jeopardy for violence or sexual assault if you do not. Recognize, however, that ending a relationship with a violent partner may provoke that partner to retaliate violently. In some cases, a report to the police and obtaining of a restraining order from the courts is necessary. A restraining order requires your partner to maintain a certain distance from you and prohibits contact (e.g., by phone, email, or messaging). You may also have to change your email address and phone number or, in extreme cases, move your residence. Your campus health center may also be able to assist you with suggestions of whom to consult with and what advice to implement.

Cohabitation

These days, more and more people in romantic relationships are saying, "Hey, why don't we move in together?" As a result, **cohabitation**, which is living with a romantic partner to whom one is not married, is on the rise. Whereas in 1976 the number of people in opposite-sex cohabiting relationships in the United States numbered 1.3 million, by 2006 it was reported there were more than 5 million Americans cohabiting with someone of the opposite sex and more than 700,000 same-sex cohabiting partners (U.S. Census Bureau, 2008). People between the ages of 20 and 24 years are most likely to cohabit, with people ages 25–29 years next most likely.

About a third of all adults, and 40% under the age of 50, have been in a cohabiting relationship (Pew Research Center, 2007). Approximately 25% of unmarried women ages 25–39 are currently living with a partner, and another 25% have lived with a partner sometime in the past (Popenoe and Whitehead, 2006). Cohabitations generally dissolve or become marriages within a year or two (Bumpass and Lu, 2000). Currently, almost half of all first marriages are preceded by cohabitation compared with virtually none 50 years ago (Bumpass and Hsien-Hen, 2000; Teachman, 2003). In one study, when asked why they decided to live together rather than marry, 21% of cohabiting couples stated they wanted to be sure this was the person for them, 15% responded the timing for marriage was not right, 12% reported it was convenient or easier than marriage, and 10% decided to live together for financial reasons (Pew Research Center, 2007). In another study, spending more time together and convenience were the two most common reasons given for cohabiting (Rhoades, Stanley, and Markman, 2009).

If you or a friend is thinking about living with a romantic lover, you should be aware of the **cohabitation effect**. This refers to the consistent finding that couples who live together before marriage are at greater risk for marital distress and divorce (Cohan and Kleinbaum, 2002; Kamp Dush, Cohan, and Amato, 2003; Kline et al., 2004; Stanley, Whitton, and Markman, 2004). Although the reasons for this negative effect on the stability of marriage are unknown, research studies consistently find this effect.

Marriage

As Shakespeare wrote, "To be or not to be. That is the question." So it is with deciding to get married, although, depending in which state they live, gay couples may not have this choice. The percentage of married Americans 18 years of age and older dropped from 57% in 2000 to slightly more than 50% in 2009 (see Table 10.1). This is the lowest percentage recorded since information on marital status was first collected by the U.S. Census Bureau more than 100 years ago. Marriage rates have dropped among all major racial and ethnic groups and for both men and women.

Notably, Americans with less education have experienced a steep decline in marriage in recent years, whereas marriage rates have held fairly steady for those with at least a bachelor's degree. Between 2000 and 2010, the proportion of married young adults dropped 10 percentage points (to 44%) for those with a high school diploma or less. For those with at least a bachelor's degree, the percentage married dropped only four percentage points, to 52%.

Marriage rates have especially dropped among young adults ages 25–34 years. In a dramatic reversal, the proportion of adults ages 25–34 years in the United States

Cohabitation: living with a romantic partner to whom one is not married.

Cohabitation effect: the finding that couples who cohabit premaritally are at greater risk for marital distress and divorce.

| TABLE 10.1 | Marriage Statistics, 2009: Percentage Married by Age, Race, and Ethnicity | | | |

Parameter	Now Married	Divorced or Separated	Never Married	Widowed
Total population	50.3	12.6	30.8	6.3
Males (age)				
20–34 years	32.8	5.2	62.0	0.1
35–44 years	64.0	14.2	21.4	0.4
45–54 years	66.8	18.2	14.0	1.0
55–64 years	72.4	17.2	7.9	2.5
65 years and older	71.4	10.2	4.6	13.8
Females (age)				
20–34 years	39.7	7.9	52.1	0.3
35–44 years	64.3	18.3	16.4	1.1
45–54 years	64.1	22.0	10.8	3.2
55–64 years	62.3	21.6	7.0	9.1
65 years and older	40.3	11.6	4.6	43.4
Race/ethnicity				
White	53.5	12.5	27.3	6.7
African American	30.6	16.1	47.0	6.3
American Indian/Alaska Native	39.1	15.9	39.7	5.3
Asian	59.5	6.2	29.9	4.5
Hispanic	47.1	11.5	38.0	3.5

DATA FROM: U.S. Census Bureau. *United States: Marital Status. American Community Survey.* 2011. Available at: http://factfinder.census.gov/servlet/STTable?_bm=y&-geo_id=01000US&-qr_name=ACS_2009_5YR_G00_S1201&-ds_name=ACS_2009_5YR_G00_.

who have never been married now exceeds those who are married. Whereas in the year 2000, 55% of adults ages 25–34 were married, in 2009, 45% were married. During the same time period, the percentage of those who have never been married increased sharply, from 34% to 46%. Several factors have contributed to the steady decline in marriage: rising divorce rates, an increase in women's educational attainment and labor force participation, and a rise in cohabitation as an alternative or precursor to marriage (Mather and Lavery, 2011).

Although marriage rates have dropped among young adults, most Americans still go on to marry later in life. The probability of adults getting married at some point during their lifetimes is nearly 90%.

Health-Related Effects of Marriage

The trend of declining marriage rates for younger Americans is significant because marriage is associated with many benefits for families and individuals, including higher income, better health, and longer life expectancy. (This does not mean you need to be married to obtain these benefits, rather that they are easier to obtain in a marital relationship than in a nonmarital one.)

Marriage is perhaps the most studied social relationship, with research finding significant effects on the health of both men and women. In a study conducted by the National Center for Health Statistics (Schoenborn, 2004), married respondents ages 18–24 years were the least likely to be in poor or fair health (10.5%) compared with adults of all ages who were widowed (19.6%), divorced or separated (16.7%), living with a partner (14.0%), and those who had never married (12.5%). They were also least likely to have any type of activity limitations: limitations in work activity (e.g., unable to work or limited in kind or amount of work), limitations in activities of daily living (e.g., bathing and dressing), instrumental activities of daily living (e.g., shopping and household chores), and limitations in physical or social functioning (e.g., walking, climbing, and carrying). In addition, marriage relates to a range of health outcomes: It is associated with reduced cardiovascular disease, chronic conditions, mobility limitations, and depressive symptoms and is also associated with greater self-rated health (Zhang and Hayward, 2006; Hughes and Waite, 2009).

One of the reasons for the strong relationship between marriage and health is that marriage encourages healthy behaviors. Studies consistently find that entry into first marriage is associated with a significant decline in both heavy drinking and overall alcohol consumption among young adults. Entry into marriage is also associated with a decline in marijuana use. There have been fewer studies of the effects of divorce on substance abuse by young adults. However, the research that has been done suggests that divorce increases alcohol consumption and marijuana use for both men and women. The magnitude of the increase is similar to the magnitude of the decrease associated with entering marriage.

Marriage is associated less strongly with a few potentially unhealthy outcomes. For example, marriage leads to modest weight increases for both men and women—however, in most cases, the increase is less than 5 pounds, which is not enough to have substantial effects on a person's overall health. Available evidence also suggests that marriage leads to reductions in physical activity—particularly for men (Wood, Goesling, and Avellar, 2007). Perhaps the time devoted to a marriage partner and the responsibilities associated with marriage results in less time for exercise?

The weight of the evidence so far is with the positive effects of marriage on health. Several reasons have been suggested to explain this relationship. As stated earlier, marital partners encouraged each other to behave in

healthier ways. In addition, marriage can provide a sense of meaning and purpose in life, offering psychological and spiritual benefits. Lastly, because married people are more likely to have health insurance and to be financially stable, they are more likely to be healthy.

So, should you get married or engage in a lifelong relationship with a romantic partner? Perhaps. A good marriage or lifelong relationship can be beneficial to your health, but a bad marriage can be detrimental. The trick is to marry someone or select a life partner with whom you will create a good partnership.

How to Select a Life Partner

Deciding whether to marry or have a life partner is a decision with implications for your health. Even more important, however, is choosing the right person for this relationship. Unfortunately, there is no formula for selection of an appropriate life partner. Still, there are several suggestions offered by sociologists and other marriage researchers and counselors.

- *Look past the looks.* Although your ideal life partner may be physically attractive, if the relationship lasts as planned, both partners will experience all the natural physical consequences of aging. Body parts will sag, wrinkles will appear, and senses will dull. What is important over the long term is personality, attitude, character traits, and common interests.

- *Identify traits that are important to you.* Is a sense of humor necessary in your ideal life partner? Is honesty? Fidelity? Education and/or intelligence? Of course you would like to have a life partner with all of these traits, but that may be unrealistic. Which of these traits are *most* important to you—that is, which are "deal breakers" if they are lacking in your partner—and on which can you compromise?

- *Agree on important issues.* Life partnerships entail a myriad of decisions, some important and others not so much. Life partners should agree on the important ones. For example, how will finances be managed and by whom? Do you want children and, if so, how many? How will children be disciplined? Will both partners work outside the home? Are you and your

Myths *and* Facts

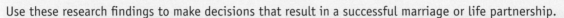

Ten Research Findings on Marriage and Choosing a Marriage Partner

Use these research findings to make decisions that result in a successful marriage or life partnership.

MYTH	FACT
Marrying your high school sweetheart soon after graduation from high school will secure your relationship.	People who marry in their teens are two to three times more likely to divorce than people who marry in their twenties or older.
The most likely way to find a future marriage or life partner is through a lucky blind date.	Despite the romantic notion that people meet and fall in love through chance or fate, almost 60% of married people were introduced by family, friends, coworkers, or other acquaintances.
Opposites attract; the most successful marriages are between people with opposite personalities that are complementary.	Opposites may attract, but they may not live together harmoniously as married couples. People who share common backgrounds are better suited as marriage partners than people who are very different in their backgrounds.
Having children first raises your chances of marrying.	Having a child out of wedlock reduces the chance of ever marrying. The only characteristic men and women rank as less desirable in a partner than having children is the inability to hold a steady job.
Educated women are less likely to marry than women with lower levels of education.	Although the first generation of college-educated women (those who earned baccalaureate degrees in the 1920s) married less frequently than their less-educated peers, the reverse is true today. College-educated women's chances of marrying are better than the chances of less well-educated women.
Living together before marriage has proved useful as a "trial marriage."	People who have multiple cohabiting relationships before marriage are more likely to experience marital conflict, marital unhappiness, and eventual divorce than people who do not cohabit before marriage.

(Continues)

Myths *and* Facts

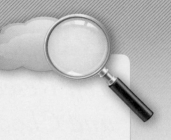

Ten Research Findings on Marriage and Choosing a Marriage Partner (Cont.)

MYTH	FACT
Marriage is expensive.	Marriage helps people to generate wealth. Compared with those who merely live together, people who marry become economically better off. Men become more productive after marriage; they earn between 10% and 40% more than do single men with similar education and job histories. Marital social norms that encourage healthy, productive behavior and wealth accumulation play a role. Some of the greater wealth of married couples results from their more efficient specialization and pooling of resources; also, they have been shown to save more.
People who are married are less likely to have satisfying sex lives than single people or cohabiting people.	Contrary to the popular belief that married sex is boring and infrequent, married people report higher levels of sexual satisfaction than both sexually active singles and cohabiting couples. The higher level of commitment in marriage is probably the reason for the high level of reported sexual satisfaction. Marital commitment also contributes to a greater sense of trust and security, less drug- and alcohol-infused sex, and better communication between the couple.
A person who grew up in a family broken by divorce will do best marrying someone with a similar background—someone who understands how painful divorce can be.	According to one study, the divorce risk nearly triples if one marries someone who also comes from a broken home. The increased risk is much lower, however, if the marital partner is someone who grew up in a happy, intact family.
People getting married today are just as likely to get divorced as stay married.	Although the overall divorce rate in America remains close to 50% of all marriages, it has been dropping gradually over the past two decades. Also, the risk of divorce is far below 50% for educated people going into their first marriage, and lower still for people who wait to marry at least until their mid-twenties, who haven't lived with many different partners prior to marriage, or who are strongly religious and marry someone of the same faith.

REPRODUCED FROM: Popenoe, D. and Whitehead, B. D. *Ten Important Research Findings on Marriage and Choosing A Marriage Partner: Helpful Facts for Young Adults*. The National Marriage Project. 2004. Available at: http://www.virginia.edu/marriageproject/pdfs/pubTenThingsYoungAdults.pdf.

partner's religious and political views, values, and life goals similar? Where do you want to live?

■ *Accept each other just as you are.* Do not enter a life partnership expecting to change your partner. If you cannot accept him or her, warts and all, the relationship will most likely be short-lived. And, do not expect yourself to change either. People come to life partnerships after many years of experiences that shape them, and it is unlikely they can change who they are; a life partner should not be asked or expected to change.

■ *Recognize that liking is as important as loving.* Over the years, love changes from a romantic type of love to a more companionate one. Therefore, it is important that partners like each other as well as love each other. There may be many people with whom you could fall in love, but only a select few with whom you could live compatibly. Life partnerships in which partners describe themselves as best friends are the most successful.

To determine your readiness for marriage, complete Health Check Up 10.3 (see Health Check Up 10.3 on the companion website). Once completed, place Health Check Up 10.3 in your Health Decision Portfolio. Then, determine what your ideal mate is like by completing Health Check Up 10.4 (see Health Check Up 10.4 on the companion website). Once completed, place Health Check Up 10.4 in your Health Decision Portfolio.

Parenting

One of the most fulfilling relationships of all is that between parent and child. At the same time, being a parent requires more responsibility than that for any other relationship. For a myriad of reasons, many people decide that parenthood is not for them. They believe they can enjoy meaningful and fulfilling lives without having children. In fact, 55% of American marriages do not include children (U.S. Census Bureau, 2011). Some of these married couples and other life partners plan on having children in the future, whereas others purposely do not. Do you want children at some point in your life? Are you ready to be a parent? Complete Health Check Up 10.5 to find out (see Health Check Up 10.5 on the companion website). Once completed, place Health Check Up 10.5 in your Health Decision Portfolio.

Single-Parent Families

My wife Karen and I have two children, a boy and a girl. The typical American family, right? Wrong. In fact, only 71% of children 18 years of age and under live in a household with two parents. Twenty-six percent live in single-parent households, and 4% live with neither parent. Eighty-eight percent of single-parent households are headed by mothers and 12% by fathers. The increase in the number of single-parent families is a function of divorce, out-of-wedlock births (52% of all U.S. births), and unmarried cohabitation.

There are negative effects as well as positive outcomes associated with growing up in a single-parent family. On average, children in single-parent households have higher rates of antisocial behavior, aggression, anxiety, and school problems than those of children in two-parent families. They also have higher absentee rates at school,

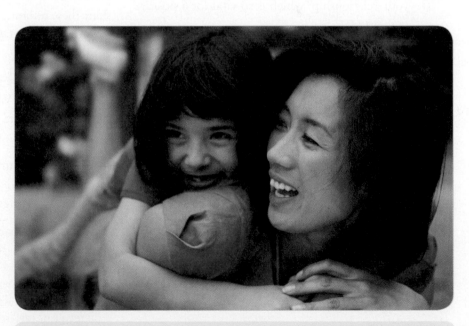

Some couples want to have children, whereas others are perfectly content to live without the responsibility of raising a child.

lower levels of education, higher dropout rates, and are more likely to experience alcohol and drug addiction. In contrast, there are some positive outcomes for children in single-parent families. The single parent often develops a strong bond with his or her children, and friends and family members may contribute more to the children's up-bringing, thereby creating a community of care. Children tend to develop a sense of responsibility by having to help the single parent with chores.

Four factors appear to be related to children's healthy adjustment to living in a single-parent household: the passage of time, the quality of the children's relationships with their parents, the level of conflict between their parents, and the economic condition of the single-parent family. Here are some strategies you can use to enhance the likelihood of positive outcomes if you are from a single-parent family:

1. *Wait it out.* Recognize the truth in the saying, "Time heals all wounds." Things will get better, and you will become more accepting of what you have and what you are missing as time goes by.

2. *Learn to accept the situation.* Strive to accept the strengths and weaknesses of the parent who raised you, and appreciate the challenges and obstacles he or she faces. This will help improve your relationship, which is so vital for a positive outcome.

3. *Help your family's economic situation.* Taking a job, even a part-time one, and limiting your expenses can help your family. For example, you might give up big purchases while you are still dependent on your parent's money.

4. *Choose your life partner carefully.* Because your own parents didn't role-model a strong partnership for you, you should take extra care in choosing your own spouse or life partner. This will increase the strength of your partnership and the likelihood that any children you may have will grow up in a two-parent household.

Blended Families

Separate families sometimes unite as a result of remarriage after divorce or the death of a spouse. These families blend their members into a new arrangement and are therefore called **blended families**, or stepfamilies. Given that 12% of men and 13% of women have married twice, and 3% of them have married three times, it is not surprising that the number of blended families has risen in recent years. The latest U.S. Census Bureau report estimated that in the year 2000, there were more stepfamilies than original families. Further, by 2004, 17% of American children under age 18 (12.2 million) lived in stepfamilies (Kreider, 2007).

One issue facing blended families is what role the stepparent should have in raising and disciplining his or her stepchild. Stepparents have no legal standing as regards the stepchild, unless they go through an official adoption process. Therefore, when discipline comes up, disagreement and disharmony between stepparents and stepchildren may occur. Yet, in spite of the adjustment required, when stepchildren are asked to describe their relationship with their stepparents, 54% rate the relationship a 6 or higher on a scale from 1 to 10; 69% either *strongly agree* or *agree* that the stepparent is loving and affectionate to them; and 74% either *disagreed* or *strongly disagreed* they felt tense or on edge when with their stepparent (National Survey of Families and Households, 2005).

If you are part of a blended family, there are several things you can do to help your family function well. You can also share these recommendations with other family members so you can work together on making the family a successful one.

- Try to limit the number of changes family members need to make. With as little adjustment as necessary, family members will feel more at ease in the family, and sooner.

- Do not adopt unrealistic expectations. Recognize it takes time to develop a positive/loving relationship with new siblings and stepparents.

- Make time to participate in activities together to build bonds more readily.

> **Blended families:** separate families that unite as a result of remarriage, after divorce, or after the death of a spouse.

- Require respectful interaction, even when arguing or disagreeing.

- Involve all family members in setting family rules, regulations, and expectations. When discipline is necessary, the biological parent should do the disciplining.

- Initially, show affection verbally rather than physically, especially for girls who may be uncomfortable with physical contact from their stepfather.

- Seek support from others such as stepparenting organizations or friends who are living in blended families.

SUMMARY

The goal of this chapter is to provide you with the tools you need to develop satisfying relationships. To help you do that, a summary of important information included in this chapter is provided.

- Studies have found a low quantity or quality of social relationships is associated with a host of conditions, including development and progression of cardiovascular disease, recurrent heart attacks, atherosclerosis, high blood pressure, cancer and delayed cancer recovery, slower wound healing, impaired immune function, and mortality.

- Friendships can be developed by spending more time with people, joining organizations, participating in sports activities, and volunteering. One strategy for maintaining friendships is to share intimacy.

- There are different types of love and different types of lovers. Erotic love (eros) is a passionate, all-enveloping love. Ludic love (ludus) is a playful, flirtatious love. Storgic love (storge) is a calm, companionate love. Manic love (mania) is a combination of erotic and ludic love.

- Research shows that physical contact, such as hugging, is good for your health. Between loving partners, between parents and children, or even between close friends, physical affection can help the brain, the heart, and other body systems to be healthier.

- One of the needs found to be very important in maintaining of love relationships is attachment anxiety: being dependent on one's partner to affirm one's worthiness of having his or her needs met. People with high attachment anxiety seem to be less psychologically willing or able to break up a relationship even when their partners fail to meet their psychological needs.

- Two strategies are especially important in working through a breakup. The first is sharing feelings and thoughts with friends and family. The second is making a conscious decision to interact with friends, go out socially, and open oneself up to new relationships.

- Emotionally abusive and controlling relationships compose relationship abuse. Relationship abuse is a pattern of abusive and coercive behaviors used to maintain power and control over a former or current intimate partner. If you are in an emotionally abusive or controlling relationship, consider ending the relationship.

- Relationship violence may occur in unhealthy relationships. If your relationship is susceptible to violence or sexual assault, consider ending the relationship, speaking with someone for advice, and, in extreme circumstances, reporting violence to the police and/or obtaining a restraining order.

- More than 5 million Americans are cohabiting with someone of the opposite sex, and another 779,867 have same-sex cohabiting partners. The cohabitation effect refers to the consistent finding that couples who cohabit premaritally are at greater risk for marital distress and divorce.

- The probability of adults getting married at some point during their lifetime is nearly 90%. Marriage is associated with good health. Married people are the least likely to be in poor or fair health, to have limitations in work activity or in activities of daily living, to develop cardiovascular disease, and to have depressive symptoms.

- To choose a life partner, look past the looks, identify traits that are important to you, agree on important issues, accept each other as you are, and like the other person. Marrying as a teenager is the highest known risk factor for divorce, and the more similar people are in their values, backgrounds, and life goals, the more likely they are to have a successful marriage or life partnership.

- Children in single-parent households have higher rates of antisocial behavior, aggression, anxiety, school problems, absenteeism, and lower levels of education than those of children in two-parent families. In contrast, they often develop a strong bond with their parent, a sense of a community of care as friends and family members help out, and a sense of responsibility as a result of having to help the single parent with chores. Children's healthy adjustment to living in a single-parent household are related the passage of time, the quality of the children's relationships with their parents, the level of conflict between parents, and the economic condition of the single-parent family.

■ As a result of divorce, death of a spouse, or out-of-wedlock birth, families sometimes get together to form larger families. These families blend their members into a new arrangement called blended families.

■ There are several things stepfamilies can do to help the family function well. Among these are limiting of the number of changes required, not expecting to fall in love with stepbrothers, stepsisters, or stepparent overnight, spending time together, insisting family members treat each other with civility and respect, showing affection verbally rather than physically, and finding support through a local stepparenting organization.

REFERENCES

American College Health Association. *American College Health Association—National College Health Assessment II: Reference Group Data Report, Fall 2008*. Baltimore, MD: American College Health Association, 2009.

Baldino, R. G. Excessively controlling behavior in love relationships: What to do when only one partner sets all the parameters. *SixWise.com*. 2011. Available at: http://www.sixwise.com/newsletters/06/11/01/excessively-controlling-behavior-in-love-relationships.htm.

Bumpass, L. and Hsien-Hen, L. Trends in cohabitation and implications for children's family contexts in the U.S. *Population Studies* 54 (2000): 29–41.

Bumpass, L. L. and Lu, H. H. Trends in cohabitation and implications for children's family contexts in the United States. *Population Studies* 54 (2000): 29–41.

Center for Relationship Abuse Awareness. *Verbal Abuse*. 2010a. Available at: http://stoprelationshipabuse.org/educated/types-of-abuse/verbal-abuse/#impact.

Center for Relationship Abuse Awareness. *Warning Signs of Abuse*. 2010b. Available at: http://stoprelationshipabuse.org/educated/warning-signs-of-abuse/.

Center for Relationship Abuse Awareness. *What Is Relationship Abuse*. 2010c. Available at: http://stoprelationshipabuse.org/educated/what-is-relationship-abus/.

Cohan, C. L. and Kleinbaum, S. Toward a greater understanding of the cohabitation effect: Premarital cohabitation and marital communication. *Journal of Marriage and Family* 64 (2002): 180–192.

Ertel, K. A., Glymour, M., and Berkman, L. F. Social networks and health: A life course perspective integrating observational and experimental evidence. *Journal of Social and Personal Relationships* 26 (2009): 73–92.

Everson-Rose, S. A. and Lewis, T. T. Psychosocial factors and cardiovascular diseases. *Annual Review of Public Health* 26 (2005): 469–500.

Giles, L. C., Glonek, F. V., Luszcz, M. A., and Andrews, G. R. Effect of social networks on 10 year survival in very old Australians: The Australian longitudinal study of aging. *Journal of Epidemiology and Community Health* 59 (2005): 574–579.

Holt-Lunstad, J., Smith, T. B., and Layton, J. B. Social relationships and mortality risk: A meta-analytic review. *PLoS Medicine* 7 (2010): e1000316. Available at: http://www.ncbi.nlm.nih.gov/pmc/articles/PMC2910600/.

Hughes, M. E. and Waite, L. J. 2009. Marital biography and health at midlife. *Journal of Health and Social Behavior* 50 (2009): 344–358.

Kamp Dush, C. M., Cohan, C. L., and Amato, P. R. The relationship between cohabitation and marital quality and stability: Change across cohorts? *Journal of Marriage and Family* 65 (2003): 539–549.

Kiecolt-Glaser, J. K., McGuire, L., Robles, T. F., and Glaser, R. Emotions, morbidity, and mortality: New perspectives from psychoneuroimmunology. *Annual Review of Psychology* 53 (2002): 83–107.

Kline, G. H., Stanley, S. M., Markman, H. J., Olmos-Gallo, P. A., St. Peters, M., Whitton, S. W., et al. Timing is everything: Pre-engagement cohabitation and increased risk for poor marital outcomes. *Journal of Family Psychology* 18 (2004): 311–318.

Kreider, R. M. Living arrangements of children: 2004. *Current Population Reports*. P70-114. Washington, DC: U.S. Census Bureau, 2007.

Mather, M. and Lavery, D. In U.S., proportion married at lowest recorded levels. *Population Reference Bureau*. 2011. Available at: http://www.prb.org/Articles/2010/usmarriagedecline.aspx.

Mikulincer M. and Shaver, P. R. *Attachment in Adulthood: Structure, Dynamics, and Change*. New York: Guilford, 2007.

National Crime Prevention Council. *Dating Violence*. 2006. Available at: http://www.ncpc.org/programs/teens-crime-and-the-community/monthly-article/dating-violence/?searchterm=sexual%20Assault.

National Survey of Families and Households. Center for Demography, University of Wisconsin. 2005. Available at: http://www.ssc.wisc.edu/nsfh/content3.htm.

Online Dating Magazine. Online dating magazine media center: Abbreviated online dating facts and stats. *Onlinedatingmagazine.com*. 2007. Available at: http://www.onlinedatingmagazine.com/mediacenter/onlinedatingfacts.html.

Patrick, H. C., Knee, R., Canevello, A., and Lonsbary, C. The role of need fulfillment in relationship functioning and well-being: A self-determination theory perspective. *Journal of Personality and Social Psychology* 92 (2007): 434–456.

Pew Research Center. *As Marriage and Parenthood Drift Apart, Public is Concerned about Social Impact.*

2007. Available at: http:pewresearch.org/pubs/526/marriage-parenthood.

Popenoe, D. and Whitehead, B. D. *The State of Our Unions, 2006.* The National Marriage Project, Rutgers, The State University of New Jersey. 2006. Available at: http://marriage.rutgers.edu.

Rhoades, G. K., Stanley, S. M., and Markman, H. J. Couples' reasons for cohabitation: Associations with individual well-being and relationship quality. *Journal of Family Issues* 30 (2009): 233–258.

Robles, T. F. and Kiecolt-Glaser, J. K. The physiology of marriage: Pathways to health. *Physiology and Behavior* 79 (2003): 409–416.

Schoenborn, C. A. Marital status and health: United States, 1999–2002. *Advance Data From Vital and Health Statistics*, Number 351, December 15, 2004.

Slotter, E. B. and Finkel, E. J. The strange case of sustained dedication to an unfulfilling relationship: Predicting commitment and breakup from attachment anxiety and need fulfillment within relationships. *Personality and Social Psychology Bulletin* 35 (2009): 85–100.

Sprecher, S. Two sides of the breakup of dating relationship. *Personal Relationships* 1 (1994): 199–222.

Sprecher, S., Felmlee, D., Metts, S., Fehr, B., and Vanni, D. Factors associated with distress following the breakup of a close relationship. *Journal of Social and Personal Relationships* 15 (1998): 791–809.

Stanley, S. M., Whitton, S. W., and Markman, H. J. Maybe I do: Interpersonal commitment and premarital or nonmarital cohabitation. *Journal of Family Issues* 25 (2004): 496–519.

Teachman, J. Premarital sex, premarital cohabitation, and the risk of subsequent marital disruption among women. *Journal of Marriage and the Family* 65 (2003): 444–455.

U.S. Census Bureau. *Statistical Abstract of the United States 2009.* Washington, DC: U.S. Government Printing Office, 2008.

U.S. Census Bureau. *Statistical Abstract of the United States 2011.* Washington, DC: U.S. Government Printing Office, 2011.

Uchino, B. N. *Social Support and Physical Health: Understanding the Health Consequences of Relationships.* New Haven, CT: Yale University Press, 2004.

Wood, R. G., Goesling, B., and Avellar, S. *The Effects of Marriage on Health: A Synthesis of Recent Research Evidence.* Washington, DC: U.S. Department of Health and Human Services, 2007.

Zhang, Z. and Hayward, M. D. Gender, the marital life course, and cardiovascular disease in late midlife. *Journal of Marriage and Family* 68 (2006): 639–657.

INTERNET RESOURCES

Marriage Builders
  http://www.marriagebuilders.com/
Mind Tools: Introduction to Communication Skills
  http://www.mindtools.com/CommSkll/
  CommunicationIntro.htm
Growth Central: Relationship Conflict Skills and
  Concepts
  http://www.growthcentral.com/RelationshipSkills
  .htm

Selfcreation.com: Problems in Love Relationships
  http://www.selfcreation.com/love/love_problems.
  htm
MedlinePlus: U.S. National Library of Medicine
  http://www.nlm.nih.gov/medlineplus/domesticvio-
  lence.html

Being Sexual and Responsible

 Access Health Check Ups and Health Behavior Change activities on the Companion Website: **go.jblearning.com/Empowering.**

Learning Objectives

- Describe the male and female reproductive systems and how to maintain their health.

- Summarize the recommended health screenings for reproductive health.

- Discuss different ways in which people sexually express themselves.

- Describe how conception occurs relative to the menstrual cycle.

- List and discuss methods of contraception, including their effectiveness, benefits, and disadvantages.

- Describe the options available if an unintended pregnancy occurs.

- List sexually transmitted infections, their causes and means of prevention, their symptoms, and their treatment.

- Explain how to protect and express one's sexual rights.

As a professor teaching health, I often have students come to my office to discuss issues raised in class. Sometimes the issues relate to their sexuality and are very personal. (I have changed their names here to protect identities.) I recall Seth, whose parents were so upset when he divulged his homosexuality that they threatened to stop paying his tuition. And Kelly, so joyful about getting married at the end of the semester—she wanted to discuss contraception options. And Kirk, who developed herpes from a sexual encounter and wondered if it was treatable. Then there was Lydia, a senior just accepted to medical school, who recently learned she was pregnant. She and her boyfriend decided to keep the baby and raise it together; she would be the one to work to earn money while he attended graduate school, meaning she would have to delay medical school. She worried whether they were making the right choice.

As you can see from these situations, concerns involving sexuality are varied and can have an enormous impact on emotional, spiritual, and physical health. This chapter acknowledges your existence as a sexual person and provides you with the tools to make responsible sexual decisions. The goal is to help you be a sexually healthy person.

Maintain Your Sexual Health

In general, how do you stay healthy? Perhaps you go to the gym to keep your body strong or avoid fatty foods to keep your arteries clear. When you feel the flu coming on, you probably visit your doctor or campus health center. Perhaps you regularly meditate for stress management.

The same diligence is needed to maintain sexual health. Part of maintaining your sexual health is being able to tell when something is wrong. This chapter begins with an overview of the anatomy of the male and female reproductive systems; it also discusses health screenings that identify reproductive system health problems early enough so they can be treated effectively and with minimum intervention.

Know Your Reproductive System and How It Functions

In their earliest moments, your sexual organs were neither male nor female. Right after conception, the **zygote,**

Zygote: a fertilized ovum.

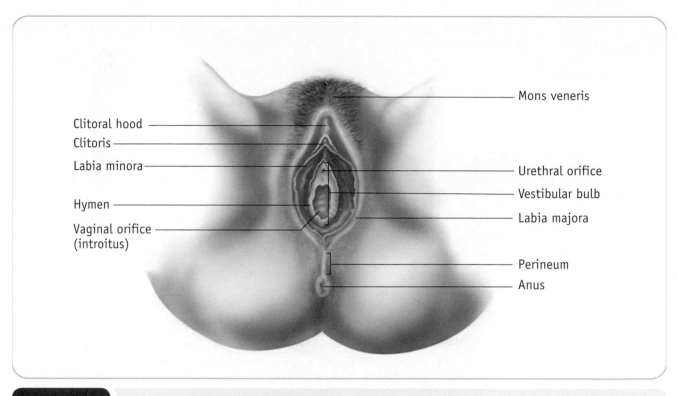

Clitoral hood
Clitoris
Labia minora
Hymen
Vaginal orifice (introitus)

Mons veneris
Urethral orifice
Vestibular bulb
Labia majora
Perineum
Anus

FIGURE 11.1   The external female genitalia.

or fertilized egg, has the potential to become either male or female. The sex of the embryo is determined during development based on the presence or absence of the Y chromosome. If the Y chromosome is present, the embryo develops into a baby boy, with a penis, scrotum, and so on. If no Y chromosome is present, a baby girl with a clitoris, labia majora, and other female sex organs develops. The term **genitalia** refers to the external reproductive structures of either sex; additionally, there are internal reproductive organs that differ between the two sexes.

Male and female structures that originate from the same type of embryonic tissue, such as the penis and the clitoris, are termed **homologous**. As you read about the male and female reproductive organs in the following sections,

Genitalia: structures of the reproductive system, some of which are external and some internal.

Homologous: developing from the same tissue.

keep in mind that most structures have a counterpart in the organ system of the opposite sex. This will help you recognize that although males and females differ sexually, they have common origins.

The Female Reproductive System

On the outside, an MP3 player has buttons and a screen, and, on the inside, it has circuits and a battery and other structures vital to its functioning. Likewise, the female reproductive system is composed of external and internal structures. Collectively, the external female genitalia are called the *vulva*, and they include the mons pubis, labia majora, labia minora, clitoris, vestibule, and the urethral opening. See **FIG. 11.1 ▲** for an illustration of these structures.

The internal female genitalia, the structures involved in fertilization and pregnancy, include the vagina, cervix, uterus, fallopian tubes, and the ovaries. See **FIG. 11.2 ▶** for an illustration of these structures.

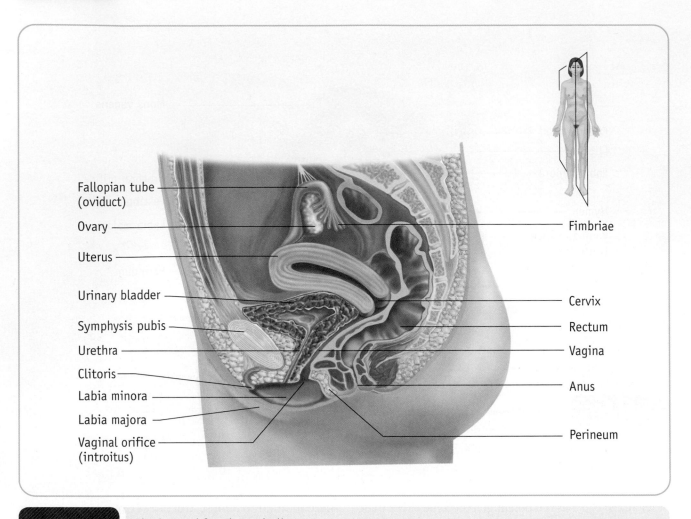

Fallopian tube
(oviduct)

Ovary

Uterus

Urinary bladder

Symphysis pubis

Urethra

Clitoris

Labia minora

Labia majora

Vaginal orifice
(introitus)

Fimbriae

Cervix

Rectum

Vagina

Anus

Perineum

FIGURE 11.2   The internal female genitalia.

The External Female Genitalia

The hair-covered mound immediately above the pubic bone is called the **mons pubis**, or *mons veneris* (*mount of Venus*). Below the mons are two sets of skins folds, the **labia majora** and the **labia minora**, which surround and protect the **clitoris**. These three structures also contain numerous nerve endings and are very sensitive to stimulation. Within the labia minora are the Bartholin glands that help lubricate the labia during sexual intercourse.

The clitoris is the most sensitive structure in the female body and, like its brother organ, the penis, becomes engorged with blood and erect when sexually aroused. The

Mons pubis: the rounded, soft area above the pubic bone in a female.

Labia majora: two large folds of skin that protect the external genitalia in a female.

Labia minora: two folds of skin that lie within the labia majora.

Clitoris: external female sex organ that holds the highest concentration of nerves in the female body; during sexual arousal, the clitoris becomes erect and engorged with blood, similar to the male penis.

clitoris is covered by the *clitoral hood*, which protects it much like the foreskin protects the penis. When the clitoris is erect and the labia minora spread open, the urethral opening and vaginal opening (called the *vestibule*) are visible.

The *urethral opening* allows urine to pass out of the body and is not generally considered to be part of the reproductive system in females. Behind the urethral opening is the vaginal opening, the entrance to the vagina.

The Internal Female Genitalia

The **vagina** is a muscular, tube-like structure that leads from the vaginal opening up to the uterus. During vaginal intercourse, the penis enters the vagina. The vagina also channels menstrual blood out of the body and serves as the birth canal during childbirth.

A baby emerging from the birth canal would have just spent about 9 months in the **uterus**, which has the function of holding, nurturing, and expanding to accommodate a developing fetus. The lower end of the uterus, the **cervix**, extends into the vagina, and the upper end connects to two **fallopian tubes**, which deliver eggs from the **ovaries** to the uterus during a normal menstrual cycle. Usually only one egg makes the journey each month, but sometimes two or more eggs are released by the ovaries. The union of a sperm cell and an egg cell, or fertilization, occurs in the fallopian tube.

After bursting from an ovary, an egg (or **ovum**) makes its way through the fallopian tube to the uterus. If an egg becomes fertilized during the course of its journey, it attaches to the uterine wall and, if all goes well, grows into an embryo, then a fetus, and eventually is born a baby. Any unfertilized eggs also make their way through the fallopian tube but deteriorate in the uterus and exit the body, along with sloughed off tissue from the uterine wall, through the vaginal opening with the menstrual flow.

If a fertilized egg attaches to the abdominal cavity or to the fallopian tube itself rather than in the uterus, an *ectopic pregnancy* can result. An ectopic pregnancy is not viable—the embryo cannot develop properly—and the pregnancy may endanger the woman's life. Consequently, when an ectopic pregnancy is detected, the embryo is surgically removed.

The Male Reproductive System

As with the female reproductive system, the male reproductive system includes external and internal structures. The external male genitalia include the penis and scrotum.

The internal male genitalia include the urethra, corpora cavernosa and corpus spongiosum, testes, epididymis, vas deferens, seminal vesicles, prostate gland, and Cowper's gland. See **FIG. 11.3 ▶** for an illustration of the male reproductive system.

The External Male Genitalia

The **penis** contains numerous nerve endings and, as a result, is the most sensitive part of the male anatomy. The penis is covered by a *foreskin* that protects the head of the penis (the *glans*) and that produces a cheesy-textured substance called *smegma*. Smegma can irritate the glans and should, therefore, be washed away regularly. Sometimes, for religious or hygienic reasons, the foreskin is surgically removed—typically in early infancy—in a procedure called **circumcision**.

Vagina: a hollow, tube-like structure that runs from the vaginal opening to the uterus.

Uterus: a pear-shaped organ to which a fertilized egg attaches to grow and develop until birth.

Cervix: where the uterus opens into the vagina.

Fallopian tubes: tubes that connect the ovaries to the uterus. After being released from an ovary, an egg travels through a fallopian tube to the uterus. Fertilization usually takes place in the fallopian tube.

Ovaries: the female organ that produces and stores eggs and from which an egg ruptures each menstrual cycle.

Ovum: an egg; one ruptures from an ovary each menstrual cycle.

Penis: the external male sex organ through which urine and semen are passed out of the body.

Circumcision: the surgical removal of the foreskin of the penis.

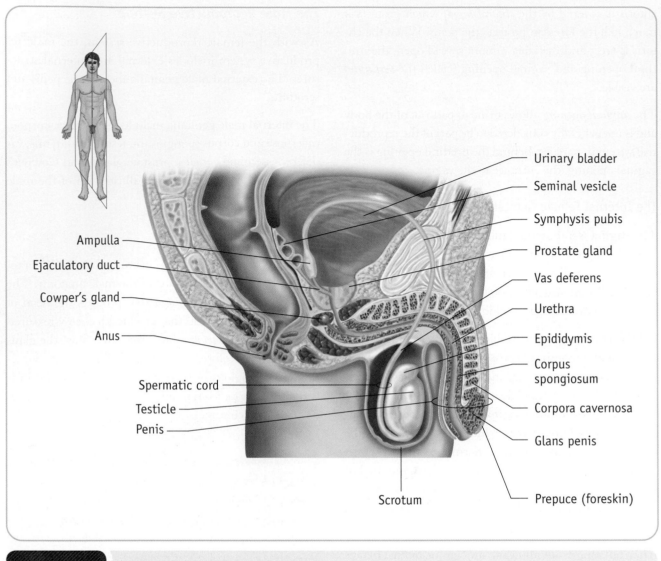

Ampulla

Ejaculatory duct

Cowper's gland

Anus

Spermatic cord

Testicle

Penis

Urinary bladder

Seminal vesicle

Symphysis pubis

Prostate gland

Vas deferens

Urethra

Epididymis

Corpus spongiosum

Corpora cavernosa

Glans penis

Prepuce (foreskin)

Scrotum

FIGURE 11.3   The male reproductive system.

Sometimes a man is concerned about the size of his penis and is embarrassed if his penis is shorter than what he perceives to be normal. This concern is unnecessary. In fact, a penis that is short when flaccid (nonerect) gains more size during erection than one that is longer when flaccid. It is also interesting to note that the outermost third of the vagina is where the nerve receptors are located and is therefore the part of the vagina that is most sensitive. Consequently, a man with a shorter penis will still be able to stimulate his partner effectively during vaginal intercourse.

The **scrotum** is a sac of skin that contains the testes and regulates their temperature so as to maintain the viability of sperm. This is accomplished by the cremasteric muscle. When this muscle contracts, it brings the testes closer to the body's core, thereby raising their temperature. When the cremasteric muscle relaxes, the testes hang lower,

Scrotum: a sac of skin containing the testes.

where they can maintain a cooler temperature than that of the body's core.

The Internal Male Genitalia

Sperm is produced within the *seminiferous tubules* in the **testes**. The testes also produce the male sex hormone *testosterone* in the *interstitial cells*, the cells between the seminiferous tubules.

After production in the seminiferous tubules, sperm travel to the *epididymis*, where they are nourished before proceeding through the **vas deferens**, the tube through which sperm travel to the penis. The **seminal vesicles** secrete a substance that allows them to move spontaneously.

When ejaculation begins, the **prostate gland** secretes an alkaline (higher than neutral pH) fluid that combines with the seminal vesicle secretions and sperm. The **Cowper's glands**, two small glands adjacent to the urethra, also secrete a small amount of alkaline fluid. (The evolutionary explanation for this is that alkaline fluids offset the acidity in the vagina that would otherwise kill the sperm.) Sperm, seminal vesicle fluids, prostate gland fluids, and Cowper's gland secretions combine to compose **semen**.

Semen may be forcibly expelled, or ejaculated, from the penis at the height of sexual arousal, called *climax*. Prior to ejaculation, the **corpora cavernosa** and the **corpus spongiosum** in the penis fill with blood and the penis becomes erect. Semen is ejaculated through the **urethra**, the tube through which urine is also secreted (but never at the same time). Semen that is not secreted through ejaculation, such as for celibate men, is absorbed in the body tissue and expelled as waste.

Check to see how well you know the reproductive systems by completing Health Check Ups 11.1 and 11.2 (see Health Check Ups 11.1 and 11.2 on the companion website). Once completed, place these in your Health Decision Portfolio. If you find you need a refresher on the reproductive systems, re-read this section or ask your instructor to recommend an anatomy or sexuality textbook.

Have Regular Screenings

What usually prompts people to see their doctors for reproductive system concerns is pain. If it hurts when you urinate or if you have severe menstrual discomfort, you need to get yourself to a doctor's office or your campus health center. Other reasons to seek medical advice are itching that does not resolve after a day or two, any swelling, the presence or sores or pus, or any unusual discharge from your genitals. However, you should also go to the doctor for regular physical examinations, even if you do not have any symptoms. Various sexually transmitted infections and some reproductive cancers can be detected by preventive tests and exams.

Female Screenings

In the recent past, women were instructed to perform breast self-exams regularly. However, in 2009, the U.S. Preventive Services Task Force recommended against women being taught how to do breast self-exams (U.S. Preventive Services Task Force, 2009). The task force concluded that the potential harms from performance of breast exams (whether conducted by oneself or by one's healthcare provider) outweigh the potential benefits. The

---

Testes: structures that produce sperm and the male sex hormone testosterone.

Vas deferens: the tube through which sperm from the epididymis travel to the penis.

Seminal vesicles: two sacs that secrete a substance believed to activate the ability of sperm to move spontaneously.

Prostate gland: a gland that secretes an alkaline medium that neutralizes the acidity in the vagina.

Cowper's glands: small glands adjacent to the urethra that secrete small amounts of an alkaline fluid.

Semen: sperm and the secretions of the seminal vesicles, prostate gland, and Cowper's gland.

Corpora cavernosa: a structure in the penis that fills with blood during sexual arousal resulting in penile erection.

Corpus spongiosum: a structure in the penis that fills with blood during sexual arousal resulting in penile erection.

Urethra: a tube that runs through the penis providing a route for urine and semen to exit the body.

potential harms cited, although thought to be small, "include false-positive test results, which can lead to anxiety and breast cancer worry, as well as repeated visits and unwarranted imaging and biopsies" (U.S. Preventive Services Task Force, 2009, p. 718). These potential harms were judged against the small number of new cancers that would be detected by breast self-exams or clinical breast exams.

The U.S. Preventive Services Task Force also recommends that women wait until age 50 before having biennial (every 2 years) x-rays of the breasts, called a **mammogram**, to check for signs of breast cancer. The task force cites evidence that biennial mammograms are likely to decrease the radiation harm by half while still maintaining the preventive benefit of the mammogram results. However, the task force also states that patient or physician preferences or medical history can influence the age at which to begin mammograms and their frequency thereafter.

The recommendations of the task force differ from those of several other health organizations. For example, the American Cancer Society recommends mammograms every year for women over age 40, and the American College of Obstetricians and Gynecologists recommends mammograms every 1 to 2 years for women between the ages of 40 and 49 and every 2 years after age 50.

Women also need to see a healthcare provider annually for a gynecological exam. The examination should include an inspection of the genitalia to identify any irritation, discoloration, unusual discharge, or other abnormalities. The healthcare provider should also examine the vagina and cervix with a speculum (an instrument inserted into the vagina to hold the walls apart during the inspection) and the breasts for discharge.

In addition, women should have a regular Pap smear. In a **Pap smear**, some cells are gently scraped from the tissue of the cervix and tested for signs of cervical cancer. The first Pap smear should start 3 years after a woman first has vaginal intercourse, but no later than 21 years of age, whether she is sexually active or not. Thereafter, Pap smears should be done every 2 years. For women more than 30 years of age who have had three normal Pap smears in a row, screening can be scheduled every 2 to 3 years. For women more than 70 years of age who

have had three normal Pap smears in a row within the past 10 years, further screening is not required (American Cancer Society, 2010).

Female Concerns

Among other sexual concerns for women are toxic shock syndrome and yeast and bacterial infections. Caused by the bacteria *Staphylococcus aureus*, *toxic shock syndrome* occurs when the bacteria grow in the vagina and are absorbed by the body. These toxins enter the bloodstream and cause fever, nausea, vomiting, diarrhea, a rapid drop in blood pressure, sometimes aching muscles and peeling skin on the palms and feet, and even death. The syndrome appears to be linked to the use of tampons, particularly those made of superabsorbent materials. For this reason, superabsorbent tampons should not be used. In addition, tampons should not be left in place for longer than 2 hours.

Vaginal infections occur in many women. The most common form is a bacterial infection called *trichomoniasis*, or trick, caused by *Trichomonas vaginalis*. The common mode of transmission is through sexual intercourse, but it can also be contracted by prolonged exposure to moisture (e.g., wet bathing suits, towels, or other clothing). The main symptom is an odorous, foamy, white or yellow-green discharge that irritates the vagina and vulva. If symptoms appear, a medical care provider should be consulted for a medication regimen effective in treating the infection.

The second most common vaginal infection is a yeast infection called *candidiasis*, which is caused by the fungus *Candida albicans*. Candidiasis occurs when the vagina's bacteria that prevent infection is reduced by too frequent douching or the use of antibiotics, thereby allowing the naturally occurring yeast to multiply. Wearing tight jeans, nonabsorbent nylon underwear, and wet, synthetic

Mammogram: an x-ray of the breast to detect lumps.

Pap smear: a screening test for cervical cancer that involves scraping tissue off the cervix and examining it.

bathing suits can also result in yeast infection. The result is itching, a rash or redness on the vulva, and a white and curdy vaginal discharge. Treatment entails medication inserted in the vagina by tablet, suppositories, or creams.

Male Screenings

College-aged men are at the age most prone to *testicular cancer*. This rare form of cancer is highly curable when caught early but much less curable in its later stages. To catch the disease early, men are encouraged to conduct monthly self-examination of their testes. They need to look for any swelling, pain, or lumps, and should report these abnormalities to their healthcare provider. Instructions for doing a testicular self-exam are found in Health Check Up 11.3 (see Health Check Up 11.3 on the companion website).

Older males are more likely to develop *prostate cancer*, and some experts recommend they have a test to identify the level of prostate specific antigen (PSA) in their blood. PSA increases when prostate cancer exists (Grunkemeier and Vollmer, 2006). There has been recent controversy over the usefulness of PSA screening after men have reached a certain age. Recognizing this, most major medical organizations recommend that clinicians discuss the potential benefits and known harms of PSA screening with their patients and consider their patients' preferences rather than routinely ordering PSA screening. However, older men should still have regular digital rectal exams, which allow their physicians to determine the size and texture of the prostate gland.

Men should also be periodically examined by a healthcare provider. Referrals to specialists can be made if the healthcare provider identifies a need for consultation. If any signs or symptoms of reproductive health issues arise (such as swelling, pain, pus, sores) between regular examinations, these should be reported to the healthcare provider.

Decide How to Express Yourself Sexually

A comedian once lamented, "If sex is so dirty, why are we supposed to save it for a loved one?" Well, sex is not *dirty*. It is fun and pleasurable and can be a beautiful thing.

Each of us is born a sexual person. At birth, we have sexual organs, the need for touch, and the desire to be loved by another person. Even infants experience penile and clitoral erections. Note that the genitalia of both sexes contain the highest concentration of nerve endings in the whole body. It seems the human body is hard-wired to enjoy sex!

To deny our sexuality is to deny the existence of a significant part of ourselves.

But sex is also serious business with important consequences. Those who decide to engage in sexual activities need to be aware of potential negative consequences and how to avoid them. Deciding how to express your sexuality is a personal choice, and it needs to be made responsibly.

What Does It Mean to Be Sexually Active?

Being *sexually active* does not necessarily mean engaging in vaginal intercourse, or *coitus*. Coitus is merely one means of sexual expression. Hugging, kissing, and touching that are sexually arousing are also forms of sexual expression. So are masturbation, oral–genital sex, and anal intercourse.

Sexual Orientation

Sexual orientation refers to one's erotic, romantic, and affectional attraction to the opposite sex, the same sex, or to both. People who identify themselves as heterosexual, or *straight*, are attracted to the opposite sex. People who identify themselves as homosexual, or *gay*, are attracted to the same sex. Gay women may also use the term *lesbian* to identify themselves. People who identify themselves as bisexual, or *bi*, are attracted to both sexes.

How people develop their sexual orientation is not known. There is some evidence that both nature and nurture are involved. That is, some research implicates differences in parts of the brain influencing sexual orientation

> **Sexual orientation:** one's erotic, romantic, and affectional attraction to the same sex, the opposite sex, or to both sexes.

(Berglund, Lindstrom, and Savic, 2006). Other research concludes that genetics determines sexual orientation (Rahman and Wilson, 2003). And still other research finds childhood and family interactions to be the key factors.

Identifying the percentage of people of different sexual orientations is extremely difficult. Some people may not admit to their sexual orientation, and others may be in their developmental years and not have fully determined their sexual preferences. In addition, many potential research subjects may shy away from participating in studies concerning sex. However, in the most comprehensive study of sexual behavior to date, it was found that approximately 1.4% of American women and 2.8% of American men identify themselves as homosexual. Yet, 9.1% of men and 4.3% of women report having engaged in same-sex activity since puberty (Laumann, Gagnon, Michael, and Michaels, 1994). Less than 1% of males and females (0.8% of males and 0.5% of females) reported a bisexual sexual identity. In a more recent study of people who were sexually active in the previous 12 months, 3.3% of men had sex with men, 2.6% of women had sex with women, and 0.4% of men and 1.6% of women had sex with both sexes. Further, 96.3% of men and 97.8% of women had sex with the opposite sex (Smith, 2003).

Another problem in determining the prevalence of various sexual orientations relates to the definitions of gay, bisexual, and straight. If someone engages in sex with someone of the same sex once, is that person gay? If a person engages in *situational* homosexual activity—that is, when the opposite sex is not available, such as in prison—is that person a homosexual? Or, if someone engages in homosexual behavior when young but does not when older, is that person gay or lesbian? To clarify these issues, many years ago renowned sex researcher Alfred Kinsey developed a continuum of homosexuality that is still referred to today. The Kinsey scale differentiates between sexual behavior and sexual orientation. It ranges from exclusively heterosexual to exclusively homosexual, with gradations in between (see **FIG. 11.4 ▼**).

Discrimination is often a very real problem for gays and lesbians. In a study of the experiences of gays, lesbians, and bisexuals on college campuses, 36% of these undergraduate students reported experiencing harassment on campus during the past 12 months due to their sexual orientation. In addition, 20% feared for their safety, and 51% concealed their sexual orientation to avoid intimidation (Rankin, 2003). To combat discrimination and its consequences, about two dozen college campuses have established fraternities for gay students (DeQuine, 2003). There are other organizations on most campuses that serve gay and lesbian students. If you are gay, lesbian, or bisexual or questioning whether you might be, you should consider joining one of these organizations and benefiting from the social support they provide.

Types of Sexual Behaviors

Is giving someone a seductive glance a sexual behavior? Sure. Is flirting a sexual behavior? Sure. There are many expressions of sexual behavior that do not involve intimate touch. And, of course, there are many forms of sexual behavior that do.

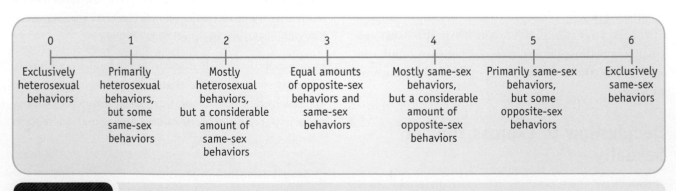

FIGURE 11.4 Kinsey sexual orientation continuum.

Some of the more intimate forms of sexual behavior—coitus, oral–genital sex, and anal sex—all introduce the risk of sexually transmitted infection (STI); coitus introduces the additional risk of pregnancy. There are also emotional and psychological risks to sex, which depend in part on your personal morals and beliefs. When considering which sexual activities are right for you, you should determine what steps you will take to minimize any risks to you and your partner. Also consider how you are likely to feel in a few months or years about your behavior today. Thinking about these things now is part of being a responsible sexual being.

Abstinence and Celibacy

Whether or not you engage in sexual activity is a choice you make. Unless you are raped, or coerced into having sex, you are the one who decides what to do with your body. Some people choose to remain sexually abstinent at a certain stage in their lives—in their teens or before marriage, for example. In theory, **sexual abstinence** refers to refraining from all sexual activity, although for some people it means not engaging in vaginal or anal intercourse, specifically. **Celibacy** refers to a lifestyle in which one remains abstinent.

What might lead college students to embrace abstinence? They may feel that the risks associated with sexual intimacy are not worth the pleasure or other benefits. Fear of pregnancy or contracting an STI may lead them to refrain from sex. Others choose sexual abstinence because they believe that sex should only happen between people who are committed to or married to their partner.

Another perspective embraced by some college students is that sex is a gift from a higher being or a natural phenomenon and should be enjoyed as such. They argue that by using certain precautions, sex can be enjoyed with a minimum of risk of pregnancy or of contracting an STI.

There are several perplexing questions regarding abstinence, however. Should you remain abstinent from all sexual activities or just sexual intercourse? Should your age matter—15 years old versus 28 years or older? What if a person is divorced or his or her spouse dies? If you are gay or lesbian should you remain abstinent from all sexual activity as well? How you answer these questions will influence your sexual choices.

Autoerotic Behaviors

If you sexually stimulate yourself through images or self-touch, you engage in **autoerotic behavior**. The most common forms of autoerotic behavior are sexual fantasy and masturbation. Autoerotic behaviors do not result in pregnancy or STIs.

Sexual fantasies involve sexually stimulating images. These images can be from dreams, wishes, magazines, videos, or the internet. Fantasizing about something does not necessarily mean you want the fantasy to come true. For instance, in a study of university students and employees, 98% of men and 80% of women reported having sexual fantasies about someone other than their current sexual partner during the past 2 months (Hicks and Leitenberg, 2001). But it is not likely that all these people wanted to cheat on their partners.

The internet has become an increasing source of fantasy images. Several studies have explored the prevalence of college students' use of the internet to view sexually explicit material. Although the results are fraught with caveats and questions (such as whether students are being truthful), they are still interesting. In one study of 506 college students, 44% reported accessing sexually explicit material online (Goodson, McCormick, and Evans, 2001). In another study of 985 university students, 38% reported they used the internet to view sexually explicit images (Rumbough, 2001).

Female fantasies are more likely to involve emotional attachment, whereas male fantasies are more detailed in terms of sexual image, often without romantic or emotional context (Leitenberg and Henning, 1995). One researcher puts the difference between male and female sexual fantasies this way: more men than women imagine doing something to a partner, whereas more women

Sexual abstinence: refraining from engaging in sexual activity; usually refers to vaginal intercourse.

Celibacy: a lifestyle of sexual abstinence.

Autoerotic behavior: sexually stimulating oneself with images or fantasies or by masturbating.

imagine something sexual being done to them (Christensen, 1990).

Masturbation is the self-stimulation of the genitals (or, as the comedian Woody Allen once described it, making love to the one you love the most). Studies over the years have concluded that approximately 90% of adults have masturbated at one time or another, somewhat fewer females than males. Sexual fantasies are usually used as stimulation when masturbating. No physical harm is associated with masturbation, although psychological harm can occur if someone feels shameful, guilty, or embarrassed about masturbating.

Outercourse

Many sexual behaviors do not involve direct, or skin-on-skin, stimulation of the genitals. As opposed to *intercourse*, these activities are classified as **outercourse**. Examples include sensual hugging, massage, or caressing and rubbing of clothed bodies together. Discussion of sexual fantasies together is another outercourse behavior that can be quite sexually stimulating. Outercourse provides sexual pleasure without the risk of contracting an STI or becoming pregnant.

Mutual Manual Stimulation of the Genitals

Mutual manual sexual stimulation of the genitals (sometimes called *mutual masturbation*) involves the erotic touching of a partner's genitals. Both men and women may reach sexual climax from manual stimulation. There is no risk of contracting an STI or becoming pregnant as long as body fluids (such as semen and vaginal fluids) are not transferred on the hands to a partner's genitals or mouth.

Oral–Genital Stimulation

Oral–genital sexual behavior involves contact between the mouth, lips, and tongue of one partner and the genitals of another. When a female's genitals are stimulated, the act is called *cunnilingus*. When the male's genitals are stimulated, it is called *fellatio*. When partners orally stimulate one another simultaneously, the act is referred to as *69* because their body positions resemble the numbers 6 and

9. In the most comprehensive study of Americans' sexual behaviors to date, Michael, Gagnon, Laumann, and Kolata (1994) found that 77% of men and 68% of women reported having given oral sex *to* a partner, and 79% of men and 73% of women had received oral sex *from* a partner.

Although there is no risk of pregnancy during oral–genital sex, the risk of contracting an STI is very real. Disease-causing organisms can be transmitted from the genitals to the mouth, and vice versa. To minimize these risks, it is recommended that males wear condoms during fellatio, and females use dental dams. (These barrier methods of "safer sex" will be discussed further later in this chapter.) Whereas these behaviors decrease the risk of contracting an STI, they do not eliminate the risk.

Vaginal Intercourse

When the penis penetrates the vagina, the act is called *vaginal intercourse*, or *coitus*. Vaginal intercourse is *always* associated with some risk of pregnancy and of contracting an STI, even when using some form of protection. There are strategies (discussed later in this chapter) that can minimize the risks of pregnancy and of contracting an STI.

Anal Stimulation

There are different forms of anus stimulation, one of which is anal penetration, or the insertion of a finger or penis into the anus. Some people find the activity is sexually arousing, and this is due to the numerous nerve endings in that area. *Anal intercourse*, which specifically involves the penis entering the anus, carries the risk of spreading an STI, as it can result in tiny tears or fissures in the anal canal through which disease-causing organisms can enter the body. Using a condom can lessen the risk but not eliminate it. Condoms can break or leak. There is often greater stress and friction imposed on a condom during anal sex compared with vaginal sex, increasing the risk of a tear in the condom. The HIV virus is also more readily spread via anal sex than vaginal sex.

Outercourse: sexual activities that do not involve penetration, such as hugging, massage, caressing, and rubbing clothed bodies together.

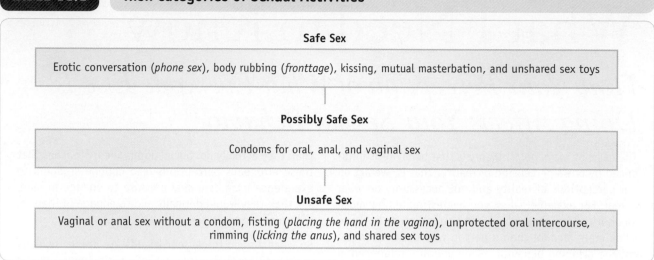

| **TABLE 11.1** | **Risk Categories of Sexual Activities** |

Safe Sex

Erotic conversation (*phone sex*), body rubbing (*fronttage*), kissing, mutual masterbation, and unshared sex toys

Possibly Safe Sex

Condoms for oral, anal, and vaginal sex

Unsafe Sex

Vaginal or anal sex without a condom, fisting (*placing the hand in the vagina*), unprotected oral intercourse, rimming (*licking the anus*), and shared sex toys

Licking the anus, or *analingus*, is an especially health-threatening behavior. Intestinal infections such as *Escherichia coli*, as well as hepatitis and other STIs, can be spread from the anus to the mouth through analingus, even if the anus is carefully washed (Table 11.1).

Whether you are engaging in it already or not, are you ready for sex? Is it a good thing to have in your life at this point? To help you answer this question, complete Health Check Up 11.4 (see Health Check Up 11.4 on the companion website). Once completed, place Health Check Up 11.4 in your Health Decision Portfolio. In making this decision, remember the various factors that should be considered: religious teachings, ethics and morality, cultural influences, family values, and relationship issues. Return to Health Check Up 11.4 after you have finished reading this chapter to see if any of your feelings about sex have changed.

Understanding Fertility and Conception

If you engage in vaginal intercourse, use of a contraceptive strategy (or strategies in combination) can lessen the chances of a pregnancy occurring. Before choosing a strategy, you should understand how conception occurs and how it can be prevented.

The Menstrual Cycle

One key to understanding conception is **fertility**: In females, fertility is all about the menstrual cycle. A female's first period, termed **menarche**, usually happens between the ages of 11 and 14 years. After menarche, a menstrual cycle will occur regularly. The perception is that the average menstrual cycle is 28 days long, but it is common for women to have shorter or longer cycles. The menstrual cycle can be divided into four phases: the menstrual phase, the follicular phase, the ovulatory phase, and the luteal phase (Hatcher et al., 2008) (**FIG. 11.5 ▶**).

During the menstrual phase, the unimpregnated uterus lining—the endometrium—is sloughed off through the vaginal opening. Menstruation lasts an average of 3–5 days, but some women's periods are as short as 2 days or as long as 7 days, and these are considered normal.

After menstruation, the follicular phase occurs, during which *follicle-stimulating hormone* (FSH) is produced by the pituitary gland. FSH stimulates the ripening of follicles in an ovary. The follicles then produce the hormone

Fertility: the ability to conceive a child.

Menarche: a female's first menstrual period; usually occurs between the ages of 11 and 14 years.

What I Need to Know

How Your Perception of What Everyone Else Is Doing Affects Your Sexual Behavior

The basis of *social norms theory* is that behavior is influenced by one's perception of reality. That is, we act on our perceptions of reality and not necessarily on what is real. For example, when you overestimate how much alcohol college students drink, you are more likely to drink more alcohol than a person who underestimates college drinking behavior. When you are influenced in this way, it is called *imaginary peer pressure*.

Sexual behavior is no exception. A study of 20,869 U.S. college students found that 77% believed college students have more sexual partners than they actually do (Adams and Rust, 2006). Ninety-eight percent also believed that college students engage in sex more often

than they actually do. Social norms theory teaches that these erroneous perceptions lead college students to experience *imaginary peer pressure* to engage in more sex than they would normally and to engage in that sex with more partners.

So what do you think your friends are doing, sexually speaking? Are their behaviors influencing yours? Would you behave differently if you knew that those in your social circle did not reflect the national norm? Why or why not?

ADAPTED FROM: Adams, T. and Rust, D. "Normative gaps" in sexual behaviors among a national sample of college students. *American Journal of Health Education* 37 (2006): 27–34.

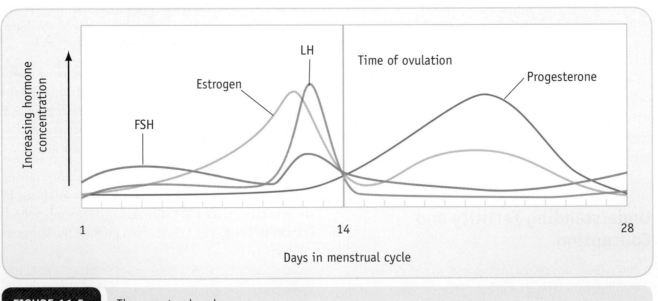

FIGURE 11.5 The menstrual cycle.

estrogen, which causes the lining of the uterus to thicken in preparation for the implantation of a fertilized egg. An increased level of estrogen in the bloodstream signals the pituitary to slow down production of FSH. The pituitary also increases production of the hormone *luteinizing hormone* (LH). LH prepares the ovary to release an egg.

Ovulation is the release of an egg from a follicle in the ovary, which occurs in the ovulatory phase of the cycle. After ovulation, an egg is available to be impregnated by a sperm. In some months, two or more eggs may be ovulated. (If these multiple eggs are then fertilized, fraternal twins—or triplets, or more—may result.)

The luteal phase begins after ovulation occurs. Continued secretions of LH transform the follicle into a yellow body called the *corpus luteum*, from which the hormone progesterone is produced. Progesterone causes further thickening of the endometrium. If a fertilized egg is implanted on the endometrium, cells surrounding the developing embryo release a hormone, *human chorionic gonadotropin* (HCG), which increases estrogen and progesterone secretions, maintaining the endometrium so the embryo can be nurtured and develop. HCG also signals the pituitary gland not to start a new menstrual cycle. If implantation does not occur, the pituitary shuts down production of FSH and LH, causing degeneration of the corpus luteum resulting in a decrease in estrogen and progesterone. The menstrual cycle then begins anew.

Male Fertility

At some time during puberty, males mature sexually and begin producing sperm. They are then fertile, meaning capable of reproduction. If they engage in vaginal intercourse, their sperm can penetrate an egg and result in a pregnancy. The cause of male reproductive maturity is the increased secretions of hormones from the pituitary gland. These hormones, called *gonadotropins*, stimulate the testes to produce the hormone *testosterone*. Increased levels of testosterone result in the growth of the penis, prostate, seminal vesicles, and epididymis. Before development of this increased level of testosterone, males cannot ejaculate because the prostate and seminal vesicles are not functional.

Conception

The moment when a sperm and an egg unite is called **conception**, and it occurs in the fallopian tubes. **FIG. 11.6 ▼** shows an ovum being impregnated by a sperm. There are only 6 days of the menstrual cycle during which vaginal intercourse carries the risk of conception (Hatcher et al., 2008). After ovulation, an egg lives for approximately 1 day, and sperm live in the female's genital tract for approximately 5 days (Hatcher et al., 2008). So, if sperm enter the genital tract on any of the 4 days before ovulation, on the day of, or on the day after (a total of 6 days), they may successfully fertilize the egg.

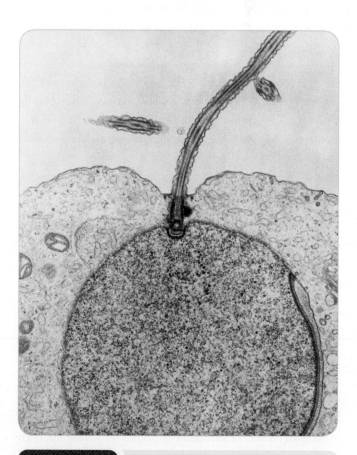

FIGURE 11.6 This is how you started. An egg was fertilized by a sperm.

> **Ovulation:** the rupturing of an ovum (egg) from an ovary, which occurs cyclically.
>
> **Conception:** when a sperm penetrates an egg; the beginning of a pregnancy.

Prevent Unintentional Pregnancy: Methods of Contraception

Abstinence is the only 100% effective means of preventing conception. However, there are methods of contraception that minimize the likelihood of pregnancy for those who engage in vaginal intercourse (Table 11.2). Some of these methods are more effective than others, reported as *perfectly used* (such as in the laboratory) and as *typically used* by people. Some of these methods are more convenient and less expensive than others.

Methods of contraception typically work in one of the following ways:

- By preventing the sperm from getting to the egg.

- By preventing the ovary from releasing eggs so none is available to be fertilized.

- By identifying fertile days in the menstrual cycle during which partners refrain from coitus.

Nonprescription Methods

Several methods of contraception can be bought over the counter and do not require a prescription. They can be purchased at a pharmacy or other retail store. These can be used safely and effectively if instructions are followed carefully.

Male and Female Condoms

There are condoms for both males and females. The **male condom** is a sheath that covers the penis and collects ejaculated semen. If the condom is placed on the penis properly and removed as recommended, it prevents sperm from entering the woman's body and fertilizing an egg. Condoms are generally made of latex, a synthetic form of rubber, "lambskin" (made from sheep intestine), or from polyurethane or other synthetics. Latex condoms are recommended over lambskin, as lambskin contains tiny pores through which STI-causing organisms can pass. Polyurethane condoms are less resistant to deterioration than latex condoms and, although they have not been well researched for protection against STIs, it is believed they offer protection similar to that of latex condoms. As

noted in **FIG. 11.7A ▶**, there should be a place left at the tip of the condom for semen to collect, otherwise it might spill out into the vagina.

Condoms should not be kept in wallets or glove compartments where they will become brittle and be more likely to break. Also, condoms should not be used beyond the expiration date printed on their packets. Immediately after ejaculation, the rim at the base of the condom should be grasped between the fingers as the penis is slowly withdrawn from the vagina; care must be taken that no semen is spilled. As typically used, the male condom is 85% effective in preventing pregnancy (Hatcher et al., 2008). In addition, latex condoms, and probably polyurethane condoms, provide protection against organisms that cause STIs.

The **female condom**, shown in **FIG. 11.7B ▶**, is a loose-fitting sheath made of polyurethane with rings on both ends. One ring covers the cervix and the other covers the vaginal opening. As with the male condom, it should be removed immediately after ejaculation and a new condom used for each act of sexual intercourse. Female and male condoms should not be used at the same time because they can stick together and dislodge each other. As typically used, the female condom is 79% effective against pregnancy (Hatcher et al., 2008).

Spermicidal Agents

Spermicides are chemical agents that kill sperm. They come in different forms: foams, creams, films, suppositories, or gels. Spermicidal foams and creams are placed against the cervix by means of a plastic applicator, whereas

---

Male condom: a latex, polyurethane, or lambskin sheath that covers the penis and collects semen thereby preventing it from entering the vagina.

Female condom: a loose-fitting sheath made of polyurethane that is placed in the vagina to collect the ejaculate.

Spermicides: chemical agents that kill sperm; can be foams, creams, suppositories, films, or gels.

TABLE 11.2 **Percentage of Women Experiencing an Unintended Pregnancy During the First Year of Typical Use and the First Year of Perfect Use of Contraception: United States**

Method	Typical Use (Failure Rate, %)	Perfect Use (Failure Rate, %)	Cost
Periodic abstinence	25	NA	0
Male condom	15	2	50-plus cents each
Female condom	21	5	$2.50 each
Spermicidal agents	29	18	$4 to $8
Contraceptive sponge			$7.50 to $9 for three
Women who have given birth	32	20	
Women who have not given birth	16	9	
Withdrawal	27	4	0
Natural family planning			$5 to $8-plus for a temperature kit
Calendar method	NA	9	
Basal body temperature method	NA	2	
Cervical secretions method	NA	3	
Contraceptive pill	8	0.3	$35 to $175 exam; $20 to $35 per month
Depo-Provera	3	0.3	$20 to $40 exam; $30 to $75 per injection
Ortho Evra (the Patch)	8	0.3	$35 to $175 exam; $30 to $35 per month
Nuva Ring	8	0.3	$35 to $175 exam; $30 to $35 per month
Intrauterine devices			$175 to $500
ParaGard (copper T)	0.8	0.6	
Mirena (LNG-IUS)	0.1	0.1	
Diaphragm	16	6	$50 to $200 exam; $15 to $75
Cervical cap			$50 to $200 exam; $15 to $75
Women who have given birth	32	26	
Women who have not given birth	16	9	
Emergency contraception	Reduces risk of pregnancy by at least 75% if taken within 72 hours		

Note: Typical use refers to the failure rate when the method of contraception is typically used by men and women. *Perfect use* refers to the failure rate when the method of contraception is used perfectly, as when tested in a laboratory. NA, not available.

Reproduced from: Hatcher, R. et al. *Contraceptive Technology*, 19th ed. New York: Ardent Media, 2008, p. 792; Planned Parenthood Federation of America. *Your Contraceptive Choices*. New York: Planned Parenthood Federation of America, 2006. Available at: http://www.plannedparenthood.org/pp2/portal/files/portal/medicalinfo/birthcontrol/pub-contraception-choices.xml.

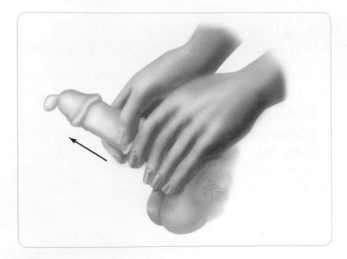

(a)

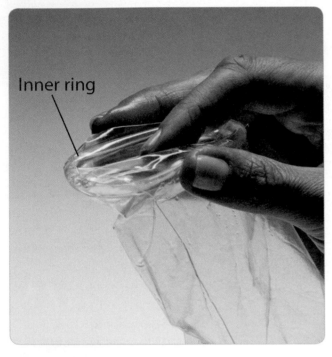

Inner ring

(b)

FIGURE 11.7   Male and female condoms.

protection against organisms that cause STIs. Spermicides are 71% effective as typically used.

Contraceptive Sponge

The **contraceptive sponge** looks like a small pillow. It is made of polyurethane and contains a spermicidal agent. To use the sponge effectively requires moistening it first per package instructions. Then, the concave side of the sponge is placed over the cervix. It can be removed by pulling the loop on its other side. One of the advantages of the sponge is that it protects against conception up to 24 hours, regardless of the number of times intercourse occurs. However, the sponge must be left in place for at least 6 hours after the last intercourse. As typically used, the sponge is 84% effective for women who have not given birth and 68% effective for women who have given birth. This discrepancy is due to the stretching of the cervix that occurs during childbirth, which makes it more difficult for the sponge completely to cover the cervix. The sponge does not offer protection against organisms that cause STIs.

Withdrawal

Withdrawal (or coitus interruptus) is a method of contraception requiring removal of the penis from the vagina prior to ejaculation so that no semen enters the woman's body. Typically, this is not a reliable form of birth control for young couples, as young men often have difficulty withdrawing the penis in time or overcoming the powerful urge to ejaculate.

One of the concerns with withdrawal is that the pre-ejaculate fluid, the drop of fluid at the tip of the penis that occurs prior to ejaculation, may contain sperm. Although that fluid comes from the Cowper's gland, which does not

suppositories and films are manually inserted deep into the vagina. The packet insert accompanying the spermicide should be read carefully before use. Some spermicides require 15 or so minutes before they are effective, and most must be inserted within 1 hour of intercourse. Spermicides can be purchased over the counter and do not need to involve the sexual partner. However, they offer no

Contraceptive sponge: a sponge containing a spermicidal agent that is placed over the cervix to prevent live sperm from entering the uterus.

Withdrawal: a method of birth control that requires removing the penis from the vagina just prior to ejaculation.

include sperm, a previous ejaculation could leave a small number of sperm within the male urethra that could pose a risk of fertilization. Although this is possible, and should be a concern, it is highly unlikely because normal urination removes any such sperm.

The advantages of withdrawal are that it is free, always available, easy to use, and has no medical side effects. The major disadvantages are that men may not recognize when ejaculation is imminent or may not have the will power to withdraw in time. Another major disadvantage is that it does not protect against STIs. Withdrawal may also diminish sexual pleasure because instead of simply enjoying the experience, males must monitor their reactions during coitus and females are concerned their male partners might not withdraw in time. As typically used, withdrawal is 73% effective. With perfect use, it can be up to 96% effective (Hatcher et al., 2008).

Natural Family Planning

There is a riddle you may have heard pertaining to **natural family planning**, which is abstinence from intercourse during the fertile period in a woman's cycle. Question: *What do you call people who practice rhythm?* Answer: *Parents.* Well, that need not be the case if those using this method learn how to determine fertility signs and patterns and adhere closely to recommendations. Using natural family planning effectively requires a good deal of education and practice and a large commitment to refrain from intercourse during fertile periods. An additional challenge to use of this technique is that many women have irregular menstrual cycles, meaning that their cycles vary in length from one cycle to another, making the timing of ovulation difficult to predict accurately.

Because it is a birth control method requiring planning and commitment by both partners and because it does not protect from STIs, it is a method best used by committed couples in a monogamous relationship. Natural family planning provides alternative birth control methods for those for whom other methods of contraception go against their religious or personal beliefs or are not appropriate for other reasons.

There are several natural family planning methods. If these methods are used in conjunction, success is more likely, as the couple will gain a clearer understanding of the woman's fertility.

- *Calendar method.* A chart is kept—preferably for a year—of the length of a woman's menstrual cycles. The first day of menstruation is day 1, and the last day of the cycle is the day before the next menstruation begins. To determine the fertile days, 18 is subtracted from the number of days of the previously recorded shortest cycle. For example, if the shortest cycle was 25 days, day 7 would be the start of the fertile period. Next, 10 is subtracted from the number of days of the previously recorded *longest cycle*. For example, if the longest cycle was 32 days, day 22 would be the end of the fertile period. Intercourse would then be avoided on days 7 through 22 of each new menstrual cycle.

- *Basal body temperature method.* Just before ovulation, a woman's basal body temperature—the body temperature upon awakening—drops slightly (0.2°F). If basal body temperature is recorded daily, it can be determined when ovulation occurs. Intercourse is unlikely to result in pregnancy if it is avoided from the beginning of the menstrual cycle until at least 24 hours after the drop in temperature. (The egg is still able to be fertilized for about a day after ovulation.)

- *Cervical secretions method.* Cervical secretions change throughout the menstrual cycle, and monitoring these changes can help determine the time of ovulation. At the beginning of the cycle, there are few secretions. As estrogen levels increase, cervical mucus becomes thick and cloudy. At midcycle, secretions become clearer, stretchy, and slippery. In fact, at ovulation, the mucus can be stretched 2 to 3 inches between the thumb and forefinger. After ovulation, the mucus becomes thick again. At that point, the fertile period has ended and intercourse is not likely to result in pregnancy.

As typically used, natural family planning has a 75% effectiveness rate (Hatcher et al., 2008). **FIG. 11.9 ▶**

> **Natural family planning:** a method of birth control that involves abstaining from intercourse during the fertile period in the menstrual cycle.

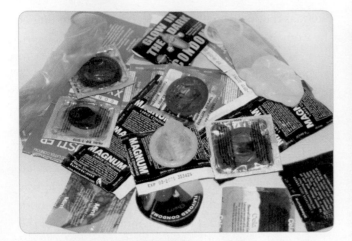

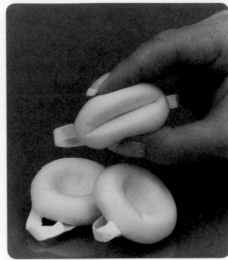

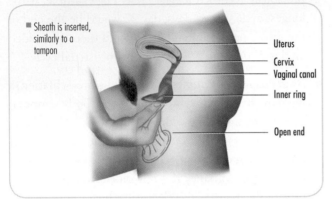

■ Sheath is inserted, similarly to a tampon

- Uterus
- Cervix
- Vaginal canal
- Inner ring
- Open end

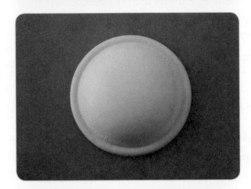

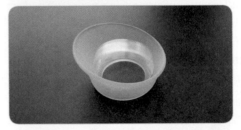

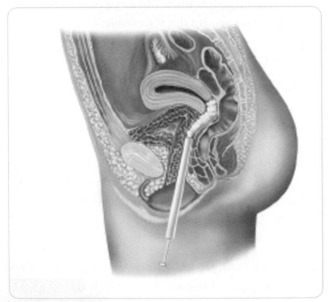

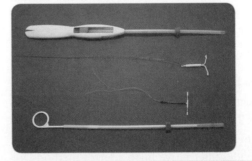

FIGURE 11.8 Methods of contraception.

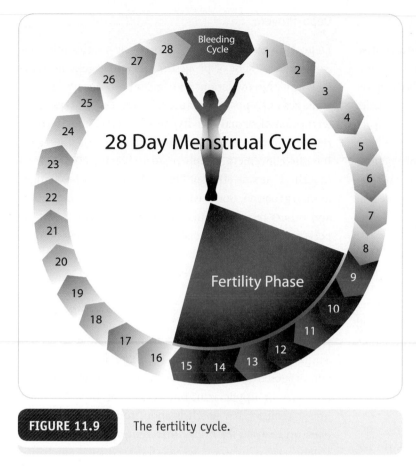

28 Day Menstrual Cycle

Bleeding Cycle

Fertility Phase

FIGURE 11.9 The fertility cycle.

method works by reducing the likelihood of successful implantation of a fertilized egg in the uterus or by preventing sperm from fertilizing the egg. It reduces the risk of pregnancy by 75% (Hatcher et al., 2008).

Emergency contraception is dispensed at pharmacies to women or men 18 years of age and older without a prescription required; those younger than 18 need a prescription to obtain emergency contraception. Some people are opposed to emergency contraception, arguing that because the method may prevent the development of an already-fertilized egg, it may act *after* conception (and therefore is viewed by some people as being effectively a form of abortion). The abortion controversy will be covered at length later in this chapter.

Prescription Methods

Some methods of birth control require a prescription. This is because they either need to be fit to the individual or have serious potential side effects. Consequently, their use needs to be monitored by a healthcare provider. Among these methods are oral contraceptives, Depo-Provera, intrauterine devices, the diaphragm, and the cervical cap.

depicts the fertility cycle and identifies the days in which conception is more likely to occur and the days on which it is less likely to occur.

Emergency Contraception

Trina knows that she needs to be sexually responsible, so she insists her partner use a condom to protect against conception and STIs. In spite of her precautions, she gets the shock of her life when the condom tears. When she seeks advice from the campus health center, she is advised to take emergency contraception. What's that all about?

Oral contraceptives can be effective in preventing pregnancy after unprotected sex or after a condom breaks, as in Trina's case. Use of oral contraceptives in this manner is called **emergency contraception**, also commonly known as the *morning-after pill*. Emergency contraception involves taking two oral contraceptive pills within 72 hours of unprotected intercourse. One of these pills is taken as soon as possible and the other 12 hours later. This

Hormonal Methods

Several methods of contraception use hormones to prevent ovulation, meaning there is no egg available to be fertilized. Among these hormonal methods are the contraceptive pill, Depo-Provera, Ortho-Evra (the patch), and the Nuva Ring. Emergency contraception (essentially a high-dose contraceptive pill) also uses hormones to prevent pregnancy but sometimes does so after ovulation or fertilization occurs.

> **Emergency contraception:** a method of using oral contraceptives to prevent pregnancy after unprotected sex, commonly referred to as the morning-after pill.

Contraceptive Pill

Although there are different types of oral **contraceptive pills,** the most common form combines estrogen with progestin (a synthetic progesterone). The pill signals the brain to prevent the pituitary gland from producing follicle-stimulating hormone and luteinizing hormone. As a result, ovulation does not occur, and an egg is not available to be fertilized. Because of health concerns, contraceptive pills now contain less estrogen than they used to, only between 0.20 and 0.35 milligrams of estrogen, but are still effective (Schwartz and Gabelnick, 2002).

Most packets contain 28 pills: 21 of which contain estrogen and progestin and 7 of which are "dummy" or sugar pills that allow for the woman to have her period. One pill is taken each day. In this way, women need not remember to take the pill for 21 days, stop taking it for 7 days, and then resume taking it again. (Some packets, however, only contain 21 pills.) Usually, menstruation occurs on the 23rd or 24th day, 2 or 3 days after the last pill containing hormones is taken.

The advantages of oral contraceptives are that they are highly effective in preventing pregnancy (92%), do not require interruption of sexual activity, and help regulate the menstrual cycle. They also lower a woman's risk of ovarian cancer, uterine cancer, breast masses, and ovarian cysts. However, oral contraceptives have been associated with greater risk of circulatory diseases, including heart attacks and stroke. They may also produce side effects such as abdominal and chest pain, headaches, eye problems, and severe leg pain.

These risks and side effects are particularly acute for women who smoke. For that reason, smokers should not use oral contraceptives. In addition, women with liver function problems, hypertension, circulatory problems, heart disease, breast cancer, asthma, varicose veins, or migraine headaches should not use the pill. There is also a slightly greater risk of development of breast cancer among pill users. However, as use of the pill results in fewer cases of ovarian and uterine cancer, fewer users die of cancer than do nonusers.

Contraceptive pills provide no protection against STIs and therefore usually need to be used with a condom.

Depo-Provera

Depo-Provera is an injected form of progestin-only contraception. A shot of progestin every 12 weeks prevents ovulation. No ovulation, no egg, and no conception. Advantages of Depo-Provera are that it does not require interruption of sexual activity, and it is reversible (fertility returns approximately 13 weeks after the last injection). It is also convenient, simply requiring an injection every 3 months. One side effect of Depo-Provera may be changes in menstruation. Some women report having no periods, and others report frequent bleeding. Spotting between periods is common, especially during the first few months of use. Some women also report minor weight gain. As typically used, Depo-Provera is 97% effective.

Ortho Evra (the Patch)

Ortho Evra is a patch worn on the skin that functions similar to oral contraceptives, steadily releasing estrogen and progesterone. It can be worn on the lower abdomen, buttocks, or upper arm, but not on the breast or near breast tissue. Each patch is about the size of a matchbook and is used for 7 days, then removed and discarded. Patches are worn for 3 weeks, followed by a patch-free week to allow menstruation to occur. Advantages of the Ortho Evra contraceptive patch are that it is safe, rapidly reversible, convenient (as it requires attention only once a week), and can easily be checked to see if it is still attached to the skin. Disadvantages include the patch not providing protection against STIs, possible local skin irritation or rash, and the typical disadvantages common to

---

Contraceptive pills: birth control method that involves taking a daily dose of hormones in pill form; the hormones, usually estrogen and progestin, prevent ovulation, and therefore no egg is available to be fertilized.

Depo-Provera: birth control method that involves receiving an injection of progestin every 12 weeks to prevent ovulation.

Ortho Evra: birth control method that involves wearing a patch on the skin that steadily releases estrogen and progesterone.

forms of birth control that combine hormones (e.g., heart attack, stroke, hypertension, and diabetes). The patch is approximately as effective as oral contraceptives. It is 92% effective as typically used (Hatcher et al., 2008).

Nuva Ring

The **Nuva Ring** is a ring manually inserted into the vagina by a woman. It emits a form of estrogen and progesterone daily for 21 days. One advantage of the Nuva Ring is that it need not be inserted correctly to be effective. Unlike the pill, the Nuva Ring does not require daily attention. It is also reversible.

Disadvantages of using the Nuva Ring include the risks associated with all synthetic estrogens, so smokers and women susceptible to blood clots are advised not to use it. In addition, the Nuva Ring does not offer any protection against STIs, and it is more expensive than oral contraceptives. As typically used, the Nuva Ring is 92% effective.

Intrauterine Devices

Intrauterine devices (IUDs) are plastic or copper objects of different shapes and sizes that are inserted by a medical provider into the uterus (see **FIG. 11.8** ◀). One type of IUD can remain in place for up to 10 years, whereas another has to be replaced every year (SIECUS, 2003). IUDs prevent pregnancy in a number of ways:

- They prevent sperm from fertilizing ova.

- They immobilize sperm.

- They change the environment in the fallopian tubes and in the uterus; for example, by suppressing the thickening of the uterine lining.

- In some women, they prevent ovulation.

IUDs have several advantages. They remain in place, so no action has to be taken prior to intercourse. Also, once removed, their effects are reversible. Disadvantages include increased chances of contracting STIs and pelvic infection, especially in women with multiple sex partners. Consequently, they are not recommended for women who have not had children and who plan to do so. In addition, IUDs can be discharged. Two to ten percent of first-time users find their IUDs expelled from their bodies. Lastly, if a woman becomes pregnant with an IUD in place, the result is likely to be a miscarriage or ectopic pregnancy, infection, blood poisoning, bleeding, or premature labor.

IUDs are one of the most effective birth control methods on the market, being 99% effective as typically used.

Diaphragm and Cervical Cap

There are two contraceptive devices that work by covering the cervix and blocking sperm from entering the fallopian tubes: the **diaphragm** and the **cervical cap**. Both need to be sized correctly by a healthcare provider. They are then inserted manually into the vagina prior to intercourse. They should be coated with a spermicide before insertion and must be removed to allow for menstruation and to prevent bacterial growth that could lead to toxic shock syndrome.

The diaphragm is a shallow, rubber or synthetic rubber cap surrounding a flexible metal ring. The diaphragm must remain in place for at least 6 hours after intercourse, and spermicide should be added for each act of intercourse. It should be removed at least once every 24 hours to prevent the risk of toxic shock syndrome. As typically used, the diaphragm is 84% effective.

The cervical cap is made of rubber, plastic, or metal and is smaller than the diaphragm. The cervical cap also needs

---

Nuva Ring: birth control method that involves the insertion of a vaginal ring that releases a form of estrogen and progesterone.

Intrauterine devices: synthetic objects inserted by a medical provider into the uterus for the purpose of contraception.

Diaphragm: a shallow, rubber or synthetic rubber cap surrounding a flexible metal ring that covers the cervix to prevent sperm from entering the uterus.

Cervical cap: a rubber, plastic, or metal cap containing a spermicidal agent that covers the cervix; similar to, but smaller than, the diaphragm.

What I Need to Know

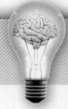

Using Behavior Change Theory to Help Prevent Pregnancy

If you decide to be sexually active, you can use *stages of change* theory to ensure your use of practices that will reduce the risk of pregnancy. (Be aware that you will also want to adopt practices, discussed later in this chapter, that can help protect you from sexually transmitted infections.)

- At the *precontemplation stage*, you can research statistics regarding the pregnancy risk of unprotected sexual intercourse. This will get you thinking about protecting yourself.

- At the *contemplation stage*, you can discuss with a friend whether you should consider using contraception with a current or future partner.

- At the *planning stage*, you can develop a plan to use contraception. Include topics you will discuss with a sexual partner and the steps you will need to take (e.g., getting a prescription for contraceptive pills and buying condoms).

- At the *action stage*, you can, for example, buy a package of condoms with the intent to use them if you engage in sexual activity. This way you will be prepared and will be more likely to follow through.

- At the *maintenance stage*, you can keep an adequate supply of materials necessary to use practices that reduce pregnancy risk. For example, you might have a supply of condoms or a diaphragm and spermicides readily available.

---

to be coated with a spermicide and manually inserted before intercourse (see Figure 11.8). The cervical cap can be left in place for up to 48 hours. The advantages of the cervical cap are that it is reversible, easy to use, and has no side effects. Disadvantages include increased risk of precancerous cervical abnormalities (found in some studies but not in others). For this reason, women interested in using the cap are advised to obtain a Pap smear; if the results are abnormal, they should not use it.

In addition, the cervical cap may occasionally irritate the cervix and may cause an unpleasant odor, vaginal dryness, and may be dislodged during coitus. As typically used, the cervical cap is 84% effective for women who have never given birth and 68% effective for women who have previously given birth.

Surgical Methods

Surgical methods of contraception include *tubal ligation* for women and *vasectomy* for men. Tubal ligation cuts or closes off the fallopian tubes so that eggs cannot travel to the uterus, and a vasectomy cuts or closes off the vas deferens so that sperm cannot travel into the male reproductive tract. These methods are highly successful at preventing pregnancy, but because they are usually permanent and not easily reversible, they are unlikely choices for college students.

Deciding Which Contraception to Use

Choosing a method of contraception to protect against pregnancy is a matter of personal preference. However, note that use of a latex or polyurethane male or female condom is the best method to protect against STIs. Remember: Even if you choose another method as your primary means of contraception, you can also use a condom.

In choosing contraception, you need to consider the effectiveness and advantages and disadvantages of each method, as well as factors like convenience and cost. Personal morals or beliefs may also factor into your decision. To find out how to evaluate your contraceptive needs and to determine which method(s) of birth control is right for you, complete Health Check Up 11.5 (see Health Check Up 11.5 on the companion website). Once completed, place Health Check Up 11.5 in your Health Decision Portfolio.

How might you use other behavior change theories to encourage the use of practices that reduce the risk of pregnancy and STIs? Complete the Applying Behavior Change Theory activity for this chapter (see the companion website) using a different theory than stages of change theory. Once completed, place it in your Health Decision Portfolio.

Unintended Pregnancy: Know Your Options

Even when used as prescribed, contraceptive methods are not foolproof. And given that people often use them incorrectly or not at all, it is not surprising that there are approximately 3 million unintended pregnancies in the United States each year (Finer and Henshaw, 2006). When an unintended pregnancy occurs, many decisions need to be made. Among these are whether or not to have the baby and, if the decision is to have the baby, whether to raise the child or give him or her up for adoption.

Choosing Adoption

Couples or women who decide they do not want to end a pregnancy but are not able or ready to raise a child—perhaps because they are too young, financially insecure, or emotionally unprepared—have adoption as an option. **Adoption** is when a woman or a couple assigns the responsibility of parenting a child to others, the adoptive

parents. Adoption is a particularly attractive alternative for women or couples who oppose abortion or do not want to terminate the pregnancy for other reasons.

Types of Adoptions

There are two basic types of adoption: *closed adoption* and *open adoption*. With a closed adoption, the birth parents and the adoptive parents have no contact with each other and do not know the identity of one another. With open adoptions, the birth parents may know the adoptive parents and may have contact with them. In open adoptions, the birth parents may even select the adoptive parents.

In spite of some highly publicized cases in which the rights of adoptive parents were challenged, it is far more typical that, after a short time, adoptions are legally binding and irreversible. Birth parents sign *relinquishment papers*.

Adoptions can be arranged through agencies, independently, or by relatives. *Agency adoptions* have several advantages. Agencies handle legal matters, make hospital arrangement for the birth, screen and choose adoptive parents, arrange for financial assistance, and provide counseling for the birth parents.

Independent adoptions involve the birth parents choosing the adoptive parents. Physicians, lawyers, and independent adoption centers often arrange independent adoptions. Adoptive parents often pay any medical costs and, sometimes, living expenses during the pregnancy. When the baby is born, the adoptive parents sign a *take into care* form that allows them to take the baby to their home. The state, meanwhile, investigates their ability to raise the child. At any time while this investigation is occurring, either set of parents can change their minds. At the end of the investigation, the birth parents sign *relinquishment papers*, and the adoption is finalized.

Sometimes the birth parents want the child to stay in the family—to be raised by a grandparent or other relative.

> **Adoption:** a legal arrangement in which birth parents turn over responsibility of parenting the child to others, the adoptive parents.

What I Need to Know

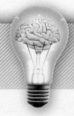

Abortion Rates Around the World

Data comparing abortion rates in different countries indicate significant variation from country to country:

Abortion Rates by Country

Country	Rate*
Germany	0.17
Finland	0.31
Italy	0.33
France	0.37
Norway	0.46
Denmark	0.48
Canada	0.49
Sweden	0.56
Australia	0.67
United States	0.73

*Rate is the number of abortions that an average woman will have in her lifetime.

Data from: Bankole, A., Singh, S., and Taylor, H. Characteristics of women who obtain induced abortion: A worldwide review. *International Family Planning Perspectives* 25 (1999): 68–77.

There are many reasons for these differences in abortion rates, but unintended pregnancy is the key. Forty percent of the 210 million pregnancies that occur annually around the world are unintended, with about half of those pregnancies ending in abortion (Guttmacher Institute, 2005). Therefore, when the number of unintended pregnancies in a country is low, its abortion rate is correspondingly lower.

Education about and the availability of contraception is the most effective strategy to decrease the number of unintended pregnancies and, therefore, the number of abortions (Boonstra, Gold, Richards, and Finer, 2006). Studies have concluded that the levels of sexual activity and the age at which teenagers initiate sex do not vary appreciably across countries. Yet, the pregnancy rate among U.S. teens is higher than that in other Western industrialized countries. It is nearly twice as high as in Canada and Great Britain and approximately four times as high as in France and Sweden (Guttmacher Institute, 2005). What is the reason for the higher U.S. teen pregnancy rate? Teens in other countries use contraceptive methods more often and more consistently. Experts recommend that sexuality education in the schools and personal health courses, such as the one in which you are now enrolled, are important strategies to decrease unintended pregnancies and abortions in this country and around the world.

ADAPTED FROM: Boonstra, H., Gold, R. B., Richards, C. L., and Finer, L. B. *Abortion in Women' Lives*. New York: Guttmacher Institute, 2006; Guttmacher Institute. *Teen Pregnancy: Trends and Lessons Learned*. *Issues in Brief*. New York: Guttmacher Institute, 2005.

In this case, *adoption by relative* is used. Even though the baby is kept in the extended family, approval of the courts is required. The state investigates the relatives to determine their suitability to raise the child. Once the state approves the adoption, the birth parents relinquish all parental rights to the child.

Choosing Abortion

Sometimes pregnant women choose not to maintain their pregnancies. In these cases, the woman (or the couple together) intentionally terminate the pregnancy with an **abortion**. In most cases the pregnancy is unwanted, but in some, the pregnancy seriously endangers the woman's health or even her life. Of all unintended pregnancies,

> **Abortion:** the termination of a pregnancy; *induced abortion* is the purposeful termination of a pregnancy.

47% end in abortion. In 2007, about 1.21 million pregnancies were terminated by abortion (Jones and Kooistra, 2011; see Tables 11.3 and 11.4).

The Controversy

Abortion was an issue debated in our society even before it became legal in 1973. It remains one of the most contentiously debated issues in our society today. Abortion opponents (those on the *pro life* side of the debate) believe that life begins at conception and equate a developing embryo or fetus with a human life. They believe the rights of this unborn being need to be protected. On the other side, advocates of abortion choice (the *pro choice* side of the debate) contend that carrying a pregnancy to term is something that happens exclusively within a woman's body; therefore, abortion should be a personal health decision that the government and courts should leave to individuals. As you can imagine, the issue elicits very emotional reactions from both sides.

There are also many opinions about how far into a pregnancy abortion should be legal. Some who are pro life oppose abortion in all instances. Others believe abortion ought to be permitted under certain extenuating circumstances; for example, if the woman's life is in danger or if the pregnancy is a result of incest or rape. Some people consider themselves pro choice but do not believe abortions should be performed during the third trimester of pregnancy, when the fetus could potentially survive outside the womb.

Aside from the basic issue of whether abortion is right or wrong, heated debate also occurs regarding regulations associated with legal abortion. For example, some people believe that minors (individuals under 18 years of age) ought to be required to have parental permission before being allowed an abortion. Others believe that requiring such permission might discourage a minor from considering an abortion. And, what about cases where a pregnant woman's parents are abusive? (What if they might physically harm their child if she told them she was pregnant?) Another regulation issue under debate is whether there ought to be a required waiting period between when one seeks an abortion and when it occurs. The reasoning is that the waiting period would allow thought as to whether this is the best decision under the circumstances.

These issues have been considered by the courts, and their decisions are described in the following section. Periodically these issues are reconsidered by the courts and, depending on the view of the justices, either reinforced or changed.

The Law

Before 1973, abortion was illegal. Women who wanted to terminate their pregnancies had to go to other countries where abortion was legal or have someone who was willing in the United States perform an illegal abortion. The former was only an option for women who could afford the cost of the trip and the medical services. The latter often took place under unsterile or unprofessional conditions, leading to infection, permanent sterility, or the perforation of the uterus or other kinds of tissue damage resulting in profuse bleeding and, sometimes, the woman's death. In 1973, the U.S. Supreme Court, in *Roe v. Wade*, ruled that abortion should be available to women during the first trimester and that the decision ought to be between the woman and her physician. The court ruled that during the second trimester, abortion should also be available and that states could develop regulations they deem necessary to maintain the woman's health. The court ruled that during the third trimester, the states can limit or prohibit abortions if the mother's health is not in jeopardy. *Roe v. Wade* is the basis for current abortion regulations. However, case rulings since then have refined abortion practice.

In 1983, the Supreme Court determined that medical practice had improved over the decade such that the states cannot interfere with abortion even in the second trimester. This ruling invalidated state laws that required second-term abortions to be performed in hospitals rather than clinics.

Several cases have challenged the parental notification requirement. Rulings have concluded that as long as there is a judicial bypass in the state law, such requirements are constitutional. That is, if there are abusive parents or other valid reason parents should not be notified, a judge must approve the abortion before it can be performed.

Some states have passed laws requiring a woman to have counseling before being allowed to have an abortion. The courts have ruled this requirement to be constitutional, as well as the requirement by some states for a 24-hour waiting period.

Another controversy associated with abortion pertains to a specific type of abortion called *intact dilation and evacuation* (intact D&E). Intact D&E is used late in the second trimester or early during the third trimester. Intact D&E usually involves procedures to gradually dilate the cervix over two to three days. When the cervix is sufficiently dilated, an ultrasound and forceps are used to grasp the fetus's leg. Then one or both legs are pulled out of the cervix. Next, the rest of the fetus is extracted, leaving only the head still inside the uterus. An incision is made at the base of the skull, and an instrument inserted in the incision to widen the opening. Then a catheter is inserted into the opening and the brain is suctioned out.

Intact D&E is used when the fetus is too large for other abortion procedures to be performed safely and effectively. Those opposed to intact D&E argue the fetus is far enough developed that the procedure constitutes interference with the birth of a live baby, rather than the termination of a pregnancy. In fact, they call intact D&E *partial birth abortion*. In 2000, the Supreme Court ruled that bans on intact D&E abortions were unconstitutional and, in spite of various attempts to reinstitute a ban at both the state and federal levels, it still remains a legal method of abortion.

Abortion Procedures

Depending on the stage of pregnancy and the wishes of pregnant women, different methods of abortion are performed. Still, approximately 90% of abortions are performed during the first trimester. And, 95% of abortions performed use *vacuum aspiration*. This method involves inserting a tube through the cervix into the uterus and suctioning out the products of conception.

During the second trimester, *dilation and evacuation* (D&E) is the abortion procedure used. D&E involves dilating the cervix, scraping the walls of the uterus, and removing the endometrial lining with suction. A variation of D&E is used late in the second trimester or early in the third trimester. (This is the procedure discussed earlier, called *intact D&E*.)

TABLE 11.3 **Pregnancy Outcome Statistics for the United States**

Outcome of All Unintended Pregnancies (%)

Births	57
Abortion	43

Data from: Guttmacher Institute. *An Overview of Abortion in the United States, 2011*. Available at: http:www.guttmacher.org/presentations/ab_slides.html, accessed 2012.

There are also *medical abortions*, which are procedures that use drugs to induce abortion. Among these drugs are *mifepristone* (formerly known as RU 486) or *methotrexate* in combination with *misoprostol*. Mifepristone blocks the hormone progesterone, which is needed to maintain a pregnancy. A woman who is no more than 49 days past her last missed period takes mifepristone at a clinic visit. She returns to the clinic 2 days later and takes misoprostol, a drug that causes uterine contractions. In 92% of cases, the pregnancy is terminated. Methotrexate, in contrast, blocks folic acid and prevents cell division. A woman who is no more than 49 days past her last missed period receives an injection of methotrexate at a clinic and swallows misoprostol pills 2 to 7 days later. This combination is 92–94% effective in terminating pregnancy.

Choosing Parenthood

Deciding to become a parent is an important decision under the best of circumstances. When the pregnancy is unintended, however, that decision becomes even more complex. Examples of questions that need consideration are the following:

- Does having and raising a child fit the lifestyle I want?

- Can I afford to raise a child?

- Am I emotionally able to raise a child?

- Will my partner and family be supportive?

To determine your readiness for parenthood, complete Health Check Up 11.6 (see Health Check Up 11.6 on

TABLE 11.4	Abortion Rates (Number of Abortions per 1,000 Women Aged 15–44 Years) in Industrialized Countries: 2008

Country	Abortion Rate (%)
China	24.2
United States	20.8
Sweden	20.2
Australia	19.7
United Kingdom	17.0
France	16.9
Canada	15.2
Denmark	14.3
Israel	13.9
Netherlands	10.4
Germany	7.8

Note: In 2008, 1.21 million pregnancies in the United States were terminated by abortion. Almost 2% of all U.S. women aged 15–44 years had an abortion in 2008.

Data from: United Nations Statistics Division. *Abortion Rate. 2008.* Available at: http://data.un.org/Data.aspx?d=GenderStat&f=inID%3A12.

TABLE 11.5	Reasons for Terminating an Unwanted Pregnancy

Concern for/responsibility to other individuals	74%
Cannot afford a baby now	73%
A baby would interfere with school/employment/ability to care for dependents	69%
Would be a single parent/having relationship problems	48%
Has completed childbearing	38%

Reproduced from: Guttmacher Institute. *An Overview of Abortion in the United States, 2011.* Available at: http:www.guttmacher.org/presentations/ab_slides.html, accessed 2012.

the companion website). Once completed, place Health Check Up 11.6 in your Health Decision Portfolio.

Weighing All the Options

At the opening of this chapter, Lydia's story was presented. Lydia became pregnant unintentionally and had to decide whether to have the child, place the child for adoption, or seek an abortion. She chose parenthood and married her boyfriend, thereby postponing medical school. An unintended pregnancy requires a very careful evaluation of many issues. Sometimes a woman makes this evaluation alone, but often her partner is involved. She or they must confront their views of values and morality and must also consider (see Table 11.5):

■ The quality of the relationship that led to the pregnancy (is there a future between the parents?).

■ Future goals and the impact giving birth would have on that future.

■ The physical and emotional health of the pregnant woman.

■ The financial ability to raise a child.

TABLE 11.6 **Abortion Demographics: United States**

Parameter	Percentage (%)
Age (years)	
<15	0
15–17	6
17–18	11
20–24	33
25–29	24
30–34	14
35–39	8
40–44	3
Gestational age (weeks since last menstrual period)	
<9	62
9–10	17
11–12	9
First trimester total	88
13–15	7
16–20	3
21+	2
Second trimester total	12
Marital status	
Married	15
Separated/divorced/widowed	11
Never married	74
Race/ethnicity	
White	36
African American	30
Hispanic	25
Other	9
Religion	
Protestant	37
Catholic	28
Other	7
None	28

Data from: Guttmacher Institute. *An Overview of Abortion in the United States, 2011.* Available at: http:www.guttmacher.org/presentations/ab_slides.html, accessed 2012.

- The number of children the pregnant woman already has.

- The capacity to provide a good life for the child.

Planned Parenthood Association of Edmonton (2002) recommends that a woman facing an unintended pregnancy make a list of her options (parenthood, adoption, abortion) and identify the short-term and long-term anticipated effects of each option. Then, she should imagine herself 1 year later and guess what her biggest fears versus best outcome would be for each option. Lastly, she should list the important people in her life and the advice and opinions each has provided regarding this decision. After these steps, the decision will be made more systematically and, therefore, more likely to be the right one for the woman.

Avoid Sexually Transmitted Infections

Jessica was enrolled in a course I taught. One day after class, she asked if she could discuss something "private." In Jessica's case, "private" meant her concern that she might have an STI. After a sexual encounter with a man she recently met, Jessica noticed a rash on her inner thighs and became alarmed. After scheduling an appointment for Jessica at the University Health Center, I took advantage of our private time together to talk about the wisdom of coitus without the use of a condom and/or any other method of birth control; I also explored with her the decision to engage in coitus with someone she had only recently met.

It turned out that all Jessica had was a rash from some nylon underpants she wore during her weekly jog. The relief on her face said it all, and I doubt that Jessica forgot that scare the next time she was faced with a decision to have sex. That is not to say she will refrain or become abstinent, although those are certainly possibilities and are decisions others have made. Rather, I think she will now more fully understand that any choice to engage in sexual activity is accompanied by risk (even if she practices "safer sex"). The risk of contracting an STI is always a possibility.

Although Jessica did not have an STI, some of my other students have been infected with an STI. Fortunately, most of these students were diagnosed early enough and treated successfully. But sadly, some are still suffering the long-term health consequences. In the sections that follow, you will learn how STIs are transmitted, how they can be prevented, common symptoms, and how they are treated.

STIs and Their Transmission

Some STIs are caused by *bacteria*. Among these are *gonorrhea*, *non-gonococcal urethritis*, *chlamydia*, and *syphilis*. Others are caused by *viruses*. Among these are *herpes* *genitalis*, *genital warts*, and *HIV/AIDS*. Still other STIs are caused by *fungi*, such as *candidiasis* (commonly referred to as *yeast infection*). There are also STIs caused by *parasites*. These include *pubic lice* and *scabies*.

For bacteria and viruses to cause infection, there needs to be an entry into the body. Possible sites of entry include the vagina, anus, mouth, and urethral opening in the glans penis. If there are cuts on the body, entry can occur through the skin. Sometimes friction that takes place in the vagina or anus during sex creates tiny fissures through which disease-causing organisms gain entry into the body.

For fungi to cause disease, there needs to be a conducive environment. For example, if the vagina's normal alkalinity is changed to be more acidic, fungi can grow and cause disease. Oral contraceptives and vaginal deodorant sprays are two substances that can alter the vaginal environment in this way.

For parasitic infection to occur, one has to come in skin contact with the disease-causing agents. Examples include contraction of pubic lice when a sexual partner is infested with lice and contraction of scabies when engaging in sexual activity with a partner who has the disease-causing mite on his or her skin.

Contrary to popular myth, STIs are not contracted from toilet seats. The disease-causing organisms do not live long enough outside the body to thrive on toilet seats and cause disease. They also generally require a moist environment in which to live.

Protecting Yourself from STIs

Because STIs are caused by organisms that enter into the body or by contact with a sexual partner who is infested with lice or mites, it stands to reason that preventing transmission of the organism will prevent an STI. Engaging in **safer sex** means the use of strategies to minimize

> **Safer sex:** sexual behaviors performed in a way that offer some protection against contraction of sexually transmitted infections, such as using a condom and limiting the number of sexual partners.

the risks of contracting an STI. Note there is no truly *safe sex*; if you have sex, there is always some risk. Here is a list of safer sex strategies:

- *Practice abstinence.* Abstain from sexual activity, meaning coitus (vaginal sex), oral sex, and anal sex.

- *Be monogamous.* If your sexual partner is STI free and is the only person with whom you engage in sexual activity, then you will not contract an STI. For this method to work, you must trust that your partner is also committed to monogamy and has told the truth about his or her sexual history.

- *Reduce the number of sexual partners.* Decreasing the number of sexual partners will lessen your odds of contracting an STI (and using latex condoms with each of your partners will lessen it much further). The more sexual partners you have, the greater your likelihood of becoming infected.

- *Use latex condoms.* The organisms that cause STIs cannot penetrate the small pores of a latex condom. Therefore, the use of a latex condom during coitus, oral sex, and anal sex is effective in reducing the risk of contracting an STI.

- *Avoid high-risk behaviors.* Because organisms that cause STIs are present in semen and vaginal secretions, the goal is to prevent them from being transmitted from an infected person to an uninfected person. Coitus without the use of a condom can result in disease-causing organisms carried in the semen to enter a woman's body and vaginal secretions to enter the man's body through the urethra. Fellatio without a condom or cunnilingus without a dental dam can also transmit STIs. (A dental dam is a piece of latex used as a barrier between the mouth and a woman's genitals.) Anal sex is particularly high risk due to the fissures created in the anus that allow easy access by disease-causing organisms.

- *Get vaccinated.* There are several STIs for which there are vaccines that offer protection. For example, a vaccine that protects against several types of HPV (human papillomavirus) is available, as is a vaccine for hepatitis B virus. These vaccines should be obtained by all adults and, as regards the HPV vaccine, by males and females entering adolescence.

- *Refrain from abusing alcohol and other drugs.* Alcohol and other drugs can interfere with decision making by decreasing inhibitions and affecting judgment (which may lead, in some instances, to unprotected sex). Therefore, protecting yourself against STIs includes refraining from the abuse of alcohol and other mind-altering drugs. Furthermore, sharing of needles to inject drugs that may contain drops of blood from another person puts one at high risk for disease. The organisms that cause STIs reside in the bloodstream as well as in semen and vaginal secretions.

- *Adopt other protective measures.* There are other behaviors that can lessen the likelihood an STI will be contracted:

  - Wash the genitals before and after sex.

  - Do not share razors, toothbrushes, hypodermic needles, or grooming scissors with anyone.

  - Do not handle towels, wet bedding, or undergarments immediately after they have been in contact with another person.

  - Do not get tattoos or body piercings except from businesses that maintain the highest hygiene and safety standards.

Common Symptoms of STIs

Often, STIs can be recognized by their symptoms. Inspect the genitalia regularly for any abnormalities. Women can use a compact mirror to aid inspection. Also be especially wary of:

- Pain or a burning sensation while urinating

- Unusual discharge such as pus from the urethra

- Odorous, foamy, white or yellow-green discharge from the vagina

- Tenderness or irritation of the genitalia

- Abdominal pain

- Sores, lesions, bumps, or rashes on the skin and genitalia

- Intense itching

- Swelling and/or fever

- Skin turning a yellowish color (jaundice)

- Excessive fatigue, vomiting, and stomach and joint pain

Some STIs may be asymptomatic. That is, there are no noticeable symptoms. In these cases, the infection may cause significant damage before being detected. This is one of the reasons regular medical examinations are recommended, whether you feel fine or not. But do not wait for your regular physical examination to bring up any concerns. If any of the above symptoms occur, immediately seek medical advice. Early detection will usually means less invasive treatment methods and a greater likelihood the STI will be cured before serious bodily damage occurs.

Treatment for STIs

Although different treatments are available for different STIs, their effectiveness may vary depending on the stage of the STI. Some diseases are incurable by their later stages. Gonorrhea, syphilis, non-gonococcal urethritis, chlamydia, trichomoniasis (vaginal infections), candidiasis, pubic lice, and scabies can be cured with medication if treated early.

For some STIs there is no cure. These include genital herpes, genital warts, hepatitis B, and acquired immunodeficiency syndrome (AIDS). However, these STIs do have treatments or vaccines. For genital herpes and warts, there are treatments that can postpone reoccurrences (breakouts) so they are not as frequent. (But note that the viruses causing these STIs can still be transmitted to a sexual partner even when sores or warts are not present.) Hepatitis B virus (HBV) has a vaccine. And for HIV, there is a combination of drugs—called a "drug cocktail"—that may be taken to delay the onset of AIDS for many years.

Table 11.7 lists common STIs, how they are transmitted, their symptoms, and how they are treated.

Assert Your Sexual Rights: Rape and Sexual Harassment

Your sexual rights are obviously violated if you are forced to engage in sex against your will but also if you are subjected to sexual harassment at school or work. You need not tolerate these violations. They are against the law. There are effective ways to respond to these situations to prevent them from continuing and ways to react if these violations persist.

Rape: Nonconsensual Intercourse

Rick and Tricia know each other from a psychology class and have been flirting on and off for a few weeks. One Friday night, they happen to attend the same fraternity party. After they've both had a few beers and a shot or two of tequila, they find themselves chatting on the back porch and laughing at the same jokes.

Soon, he invites her up to his room so they can talk somewhere *quiet*. Tricia says okay, and Rick assumes that means she wants to have sex with him. Tricia assumes that Rick just likes her and wants to talk to her away from the surrounding noise and chaos. Before long, they're both sitting on the couch, listening to music. They start kissing.

Rick moves along quickly and Tricia thinks they're going too fast. She objects to his roaming hands, and asks, then yells, at him to stop. Rick insists on continuing, because he thinks she's just playing hard to get. (Note that at this point, according to the law, Rick has just become a sexual molester.) Rick then holds Tricia down and forces himself on her. His penis penetrates her vagina. (By law, Rick has just committed rape.)

Rape is forcible sexual intercourse. Although most rapes involve a male aggressor and a female victim, occurrences of females raping males and males raping males also happen. Rape is the fault of the rapist and not the victim. That last sentence seems obvious. Yet, women have been chastised for dressing in a particular way or putting

> **Rape:** forcible sexual intercourse.

TABLE 11.7	**Sexually Transmitted Infections**

STI	Caused by	Symptoms	Treatment	Photo
Gonorrhea	Bacteria: *Neisseria gonorrhoeae*	Frequent, painful urination, discharge of pus from the urethra, tenderness in groin, swollen lymph nodes; usually no noticeable symptoms in females although there may be yellowish discharge from vagina	Antibiotics: penicillin, tetracycline, ciprofloxacin	
Non-gonococcal urethritis	Bacteria: *Chlamydia trachomatis*, *Ureaplasma urealyticum*, *Mycoplasma hominis*, *Trichomonas vaginalis*, herpes simplex virus	Discharge from penis, burning sensation when urinating, mild vaginal irritation, discharge from vagina, as many as 70% of women may be asymptomatic	Antibiotics: doxycycline, azithromycin, erythromycin, or ofloxacin	
Chlamydia	Parasite: *Chlamydia trachomatis*	75% are asymptomatic, painful or burning sensation when urinating, white discharge from penis, vaginal discharge, abdominal pain	Antibiotics: azithromycin, doxycycline, erythromycin, or ofloxacin	Asymptomatic so there are no visible signs.

TABLE 11.7   **Sexually Transmitted Infections** *(Cont.)*

STI	Caused by	Symptoms	Treatment	Photo
Syphilis	Spirochete: *Treponema pallidum*	Chancre (sore), rash, fever, hair loss, blindness, paralysis, brain damage, or death	Antibiotics: penicillin	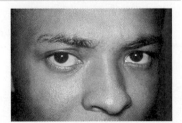
Herpes genitalis	Virus: herpes simplex virus	Painful lesions, sluggish feeling, fever, lymph node enlargement	No cure, but can manage symptoms and minimize recurrences with acyclovir, famciclovir, or valacyclovir (antiviral agents)	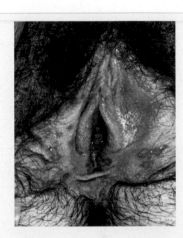
Hepatitis B	Virus: hepatitis B virus	30% are asymptomatic, eyes or skin turn yellow (jaundice), loss of appetite, nausea, vomiting, fever, stomach or joint pain, fatigue	No cure, bed rest, drinking fluids to prevent dehydration, if liver damage alpha-interferon or lamivudine (antiviral agents) are administered	

(Continues)

TABLE 11.7 Sexually Transmitted Infections *(Cont.)*

STI	Caused by	Symptoms	Treatment	Photo
Genital warts	Virus: human papillomavirus	Lesions on the genitalia	Podophyllin (a resin) or cryotherapy (freezing lesions with liquid nitrogen), surgery to remove large warts; vaccine available for ages 9–26 (Gardasil)	
Trichomoniasis	Bacteria: *Trichomonas vaginalis*	An odorous, foamy, white or yellow-green discharge that irritates the vagina and vulva	Antibiotics: metronidazole (brand name Flagyl)	
Candidiasis	Fungus: *Candida albicans*	White, curdy discharge, rash, itching, redness on vulva, may experience pain when urinating	Antifungals: mycostatin tablets	

TABLE 11.7	Sexually Transmitted Infections *(Cont.)*

STI	Caused by	Symptoms	Treatment	Photo
Pubic lice (pediculosis pubis)	Lice: *Phthirus pubis*	Skin irritation, itching, swelling of glands in the groin	A-200 pyrinate or gamma-benzene (Kwell)	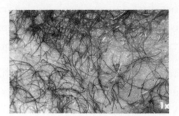
Scabies	Mite: *Sarcoptes scabies*	Itching and pus, raised lesions	Gamma-benzene (Kwell)	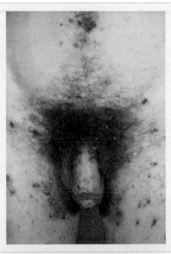
HIV/AIDS	Virus: human immuno-deficiency virus (HIV)	Swelling of glands in neck and arm pits, fatigue, weight loss, fever, diarrhea	Antiretroviral agents: triple drug therapy (zidovudine, indinavir, and delavirdine)	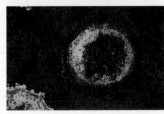

themselves in situations that place them at risk of rape. Although everyone should take precautions to ensure their safety, not doing so does not justify or excuse rape. For example, if a woman wearing a revealing blouse and short skirt dances closely with a man, that does not mean she wants to engage in sexual intercourse, and it does not excuse her partner's behavior if he acts against her will.

It might surprise you to learn that many rapists are either married or have a regular sexual partner. Many rapists are also known by their victim: the rapist may be a boyfriend or girlfriend, a date, a friend, or even a family member. Most experts agree that rape is designed to exert power over someone and is not necessarily for the sex. Aggression enhances the rapist's sense of power, masculinity, and self-esteem by expressing feelings of mastery and conquest.

Rape on College Campuses

Instances of rape among college-aged students often involve alcohol or other drugs. For example, one study found that in 75% of college rapes, the offender, the victim, or both had been drinking alcohol (Sampson, 2006). The use of "date-rape" drugs and/or alcohol can eliminate people's usual inhibitions or render them unconscious. Sexual intercourse that occurs in these scenarios, where a person is unable to give his or her consent, is also considered rape.

Date rape is not unfamiliar to college women. The U.S. Department of Justice found that 3% of college women reported experiencing a completed and/or attempted rape during the 2000–2001 academic year (Fisher, Cullen, and Turner, 2001). Nearly 90% of these women knew their rapist as a classmate, friend, ex-boyfriend, or acquaintance.

Preventing Date Rape

Later in this chapter, you will learn and practice resistance skills to respond to and prevent violations of your sexual rights. There are also some general means of preventing date rape, suggested by the American College Health Association (2011):

■ *Express your limits clearly.* If someone starts to offend you, tell them firmly and early. Polite approaches may be misunderstood or ignored.

■ *Be assertive.* Often, silence or passivity is interpreted as permission. State what you want—or don't want—and stick to your decision.

■ *Trust your instincts.* If you feel you are being pressured into unwanted sex, you probably are. If you feel uncomfortable, get out of the situation immediately.

■ *Listen carefully to what the other person is saying.* Are you getting mixed messages? Do you understand the other person? If not—ask. Yes only means yes when said clearly, not when your partner is drunk, high, asleep, or impaired in any way.

■ *Ask, rather than assume.* Be aware of the potential for misunderstanding. Talk with your partner about what you both find acceptable.

■ *Remember that effective communication may not always work.* Sometimes people don't listen. However, no one ever deserves to be a victim of sexual violence!

■ *Respond physically.* If someone is assaulting you and not responding to your objections, push the person away, scream "NO," and say that you consider what the person is doing to be an assault.

■ *Watch your drinks.* At a party or bar, accept drinks only from a bartender/server; do not leave drinks unattended, and do not accept open-container drinks from anyone.

■ *Get help if feeling intoxicated.* If you or a friend feel more intoxicated or disoriented than usual based on the amount of alcohol you consumed, get to a safe place with a trusted friend.

Sexual Harassment: Unwanted Sexual Advances

When younger and a high school teacher, as I walked through the school cafeteria, girls would whistle and make all sorts of lewd comments. I know—knowing me

> **Date rape:** rape that occurs between two people who date; this form can also occur in instances when the victim is unable to give consent because of intoxication or other altered states of consciousness.

Myths *and* Facts

Date Rape

MYTH	FACT
If she says *NO*, but I know she really wants to have sex with me, I can continue to try to excite her by touching and kissing her. Soon she will probably be urging me on.	If you pursue touching one's genitals against that person's will, this is a legal violation called *sexual molestation*; you can be prosecuted for that illegal behavior. If you persist to the point where you force sexual intercourse, this is called *rape*, which is punishable by time in prison. Take *NO* to mean just that. Do not continue unless given explicit permission. To prevent this kind of confusion, remember that it is everyone's responsibility to communicate their sexual intentions clearly. Do not say *NO* if you mean *YES* and, conversely, do not say *YES* when you mean *NO*. Be assertive and communicate honestly and forcefully. Let your partner know that you mean what you say, and assume what your partner says is what he or she means.
If she wears sexy, revealing clothes and comes to my apartment to be alone with me late at night, I can assume she wants to have sex with me.	Wearing revealing clothing may be someone's way of attracting attention. The person dressed in that manner may not want to participate in sexual activity at all. Perhaps she is mimicking a celebrity she admires. Likewise, agreeing to be alone with someone does not necessarily mean that person is agreeing to anything else. Perhaps the party or lounge is too noisy and the person just wants to get to know her partner better through quiet conversation.
We were both so drunk when we had sex, it can't possibly have been rape.	Forcing sexual intercourse on someone who is inebriated is rape.
Men cannot be raped because they are always in the mood for sex.	Men, just like women, may be forced to have sex against their will. A man—whether he is homosexual or not—may be raped by a man. Or he may be raped by a woman. Rape is as much about power over the victim as it is about sex. Rape is a violent, dehumanizing, and intimate invasion of the victim's privacy and integrity as a human being. Rape victims, whether men or women, experience intense psychological and sometimes physical trauma.

now, it is hard to believe. But remember, I was younger then (he pleads). I did not realize it then, but that was a form of **sexual harassment**.

Many of us have the misconception that there has to be some physical sexual behavior, such as groping, for sexual harassment to occur. This is not the case. Sexual harassment is defined as unwelcome sexual advances, requests for sexual favors (e.g., in return for a privilege or promotion at school or work), and other verbal and physical conduct of a sexual nature that negatively affects an individual's school or work performance or creates an intimidating, hostile, or offensive learning or working environment. Sexual harassment is illegal and need not be tolerated.

Sexual Harassment on College Campuses

The number of sexual harassment complaints more than doubled, from 6,000 to 13,000 between 1990 and 2004 (Equal Employment Opportunity Commission, 2005). Although most of these charged violations occurred in the workplace, sexual harassment also occurs on college campuses. Nearly two-thirds of college students experience sexual harassment at some point during college, including nearly one-third of first-year students (American Association of University Women, 2006). Examples of sexual harassment on college campuses include:

- Disturbing sexual comments or jokes that interfere with another student's ability to pay attention in class and to earn a good grade.

- Touching or groping another student sexually.

- Requiring sexual favors (such as oral sex or intercourse) for a good grade or good recommendation, to enroll in an oversubscribed course, or as a prerequisite to being hired on a research project or being kept on a project.

> **Sexual harassment:** unwelcome sexual advances, requests for sexual favors, and other verbal and physical conduct of a sexual nature that negatively affects an individual's school or work performance or creates an intimidating, hostile, or offensive learning or working environment.

Some campuses have policies prohibiting faculty from dating students, administrative assistants, and others over whom they have authority. This is because faculty are in a position of giving special privileges or advantages to their subordinates; if they are dating, it is hard to know if a sexual relationship might be influencing those privileges. Violation of this dating policy may lead to charges of sexual harassment. Faculty and others found guilty of sexual harassment can lose their jobs, be fined, or be sued.

What to Do if You Are Sexually Harassed

No one, male or female, needs to tolerate sexual harassment. Ways to avoid and respond to sexual harassment include the following:

- *Avoid placing yourself in a position where you can be harassed.* For example, do not meet in a classmate's home to work on a class project with no one else present. Bring a friend with you if necessary. Refrain from being alone with someone you suspect will try to harass you sexually.

- *Keep conversations professional.* If sexual innuendos or flirting occurs, turn the conversation back to academic and/or professional issues.

- *Keep a record of harassing behavior.* If you decide to report the harasser or to speak with the harasser about behaviors you find disturbing, it will help to be able to refer to specific occasions on which harassment occurred and to specific harassing behaviors. Record dates, times, the behavior, and your reactions and feelings at the time.

- *Speak with others for advice.* Friends and family members may provide insight regarding what to do. Professors and authorities on campus (e.g., department chairpersons or deans) may have dealt with previous cases of harassment and learned the best ways to respond.

- *Speak with the harasser.* Let the offender know that you object to the behavior and that you consider it sexual harassment. Be specific about the behavior and when it occurred. Be clear about what you will do if the behavior continues. Be sure to speak about the *behavior* to which you object and not about the character of the offender. You do not want the offender to become confrontational. Rather, you want the behavior to change.

- *Report the harasser.* If after speaking with the harasser the behavior continues, report it to someone of authority. Insist that the person of authority take action to have the objectionable behavior cease.

- *File a formal complaint.* Your state's human rights commission and/or the Equal Employment Opportunity Commission receive sexual harassment complaints regularly. If necessary, you may avail yourself of their assistance.

- *Take legal action.* Take the harasser to court and sue for damages and punitive awards. By definition, sexual harassment interferes with you being successful at work or in school. That means you are affected financially. You can recover damages from the harasser.

When responding to sexual harassment or to pressure to engage in sexual activity that you find objectionable, resistance skills can be helpful. These are described in the next section.

Using Resistance Skills

Kara loves Rich and wants to maintain their relationship. But lately, Rich has been pressuring her for sexual intercourse, and she does not feel comfortable with that. How could Kara resist this activity in the most effective way? One solution is to use **resistance skills**.

Resistance skills are delineated by the *SESS* formula:

- **S**tate the behavior that you want to resist.

- **E**xpress how you feel when being pressured to engage in the behavior to which you object.

- **S**pecify the reasons you choose not to engage in that behavior.

> **Resistance skills:** ways to resist pressure to engage in objectionable activities while still maintaining positive personal relationships.

- **S**uggest an alternative behavior that would be acceptable to you.

Using the SESS formula, Kara says, "When I am pressured into engaging in a sexual activity with which I am uncomfortable (**S**tate the behavior), I feel as though my interests are being neglected (**E**xpress how you feel). I do not want to do that activity because I don't want to move our relationship to that level. I'm also worried about pregnancy; it's always a possibility, even if we took every precaution (**S**pecify the reasons). I love you and want us to have a satisfying relationship, too. Can we achieve intimacy in other ways? I'm comfortable with intimate massage, are you? (**S**uggest an alternative.)

In this way, Kara is communicating her needs, explaining her views to Rich, and responding to his point of view without blaming him. Kara should not have to give in to pressure to behave in ways that violate her values or feelings. And, Kara need not if the SESS formula is used.

To practice using the SESS formula to assert your sexual rights, complete Health Check Up 11.7 (see Health Check Up 11.7 on the companion website). Once completed, place Health Check Up 11.7 in your Health Decision Portfolio. Remember, when you use SEES, be sure you are comfortable with any alternative you propose.

Your resistance will be more believable if you express it with assertive body language. Imagine you made an SESS verbal response but kept looking down the whole time or kept fidgeting with your fingers and speaking in such a low voice you were difficult to hear. Regardless of what you said, your resistance would not be taken seriously. Assertive body language includes:

- Standing tall and straight

- Facing the person to whom you are speaking straight on

- Maintaining eye contact

- Speaking in a steady, clear voice, loud enough to be heard

- Speaking without hesitation and with assurance and confidence

Combine the SESS formula with assertive body language and now you have something—your resistance is taken seriously.

SUMMARY

The goal of this chapter is to provide you with the tools you need to be sexually responsible. If we have succeeded, you will be better able to make healthy sexual decisions—now and in the future. To help you do that, a summary of important information included in this chapter is provided.

- Males produce sperm in the testes and may deposit them in the female vagina through the penis during vaginal intercourse. Females produce eggs (ova) in the ovaries, and the eggs travel through the fallopian tubes on their way to the uterus. An unfertilized egg will disintegrate and exit the body with the menstrual flow. A fertilized egg will implant in the lining of the uterus and result in a pregnancy.

- Females can maintain their sexual health by receiving annual screenings from a healthcare provider—such as a nurse practitioner or a gynecologist. The healthcare provider will inspect the external genitalia for irritations, discolorations, unusual discharge, and other abnormalities, as well as inspect the vagina and cervix, the internal reproductive organs, and breasts.

- Women should receive a Pap smear annually after age 18. The Pap smear tests tissue scraped from the cervix for cancerous cells. After three consecutive annual Pap smears report normal findings, the Pap smear can be performed less frequently at the discretion of the woman and her physician.

- By age 50, women should also have an annual mammogram—an x-ray of the breasts to inspect for tumors. Males should regularly perform testicular self-examinations and periodically receive screenings from a healthcare provider. In addition, some experts recommend that men have an annual PSA blood test that screens for prostate cancer, although some experts advise against PSA tests arguing that the potential harms of such tests exceed their potential benefits.

- Sexual abstinence is the only 100% effective method of preventing pregnancy or of preventing STIs.

Abstinence is a choice made by many, although others who choose to engage in sex can decrease their chances of pregnancy by using a contraceptive method and of contracting an STI by using safer sex techniques.

- As a result of changes in hormonal secretions, an egg is released from a woman's ovary every menstrual cycle—ovulation. Because the egg lives for approximately 1 day and sperm lives in the female's genital tract for approximately 5 days, there are only 6 days during the menstrual cycle that conception can occur.

- Methods of birth control prevent conception in a number of ways: by setting up a barrier to prevent sperm from getting to the egg, by preventing the ovary from releasing an egg so none is available to be fertilized, by preventing or limiting sperm production, by preventing a fertilized egg from implanting on the inner lining of the uterus, or by identifying fertile days in the menstrual cycle during which partners refrain from coitus.

- Several methods of birth control do not require a prescription. Among these are male and female condoms, spermicidal agents, the contraceptive sponge, withdrawal, natural family planning, and emergency contraception (for those over the age of 18).

- Several methods of birth control do require a prescription. Among these are contraceptive pills, Depo-Provera, Ortho Evra (the patch), the Nuva Ring, intrauterine devices, the diaphragm, and the cervical cap.

- Among the considerations when choosing a contraceptive method should be its side effects, whether it is effective, provides protection from STIs, is convenient to use, affordable, reversible, and is consistent with one's personal values.

- STIs are caused by microorganisms (bacteria, viruses, or fungi) or parasites that are transmitted during sexual contact. Routes of transmission include the mouth, fissures in the vaginal or anal canals, the opening in the glans penis, and cuts in the skin.

- "Safer sex" behaviors used to protect against contracting an STI are sexual abstinence, monogamy, reducing the number of sexual partners, using latex condoms, and refraining from abuse of alcohol and other drugs.

- Strategies for preventing date rape include not abusing alcohol and other drugs, keeping responses to social pressure consistent with values, assertively communicating limits, leaving a situation if threatened, asking rather than assuming a sexual activity is agreeable to your partner, and responding physically by pushing or screaming if necessary.

- Sexual harassment does not have to involve physical touching. It can also be verbal sexual comments that create a hostile environment interfering with work or school performance. To discourage sexual harassment, avoid placing yourself in a position where you can be harassed, keep conversations professional, speak with others seeking their advice, speak with the harasser, report the harasser, file a formal complaint, or sue the harasser in a court of law.

- The SESS formula is an effective way of using resistance skills to respond verbally to pressure to engage in an activity you find objectionable. The SESS formula consists of stating the behavior you want to resist, expressing how you feel when being pressured to engage in that behavior, specifying the reasons you choose not to engage in that behavior, and suggesting an alternative behavior. The SESS formula response should be accompanied by assertive body language that includes standing tall and straight, facing the other person, maintaining eye contact, speaking clearly and loudly, and speaking with confidence.

REFERENCES

Adams, T. and Rust, D. "Normative gaps" in sexual behaviors among a national sample of college students. *American Journal of Health Education* 37 (2006): 27–34.

American Association of University Women. *Drawing the Line: Sexual Harassment on Campus.* 2006. Available at: http://www.aauw.org/research/dtl.cfm.

American Cancer Society. *Chronological History of ACS Recommendations for the Early Detection of Cancer in Asymptomatic People.* Atlanta, GA: American Cancer Society, 2010. Available at: http://www.cancer.org/Healthy/FindCancerEarly/CancerScreeningGuidelines/chronological-history-of-acs-recommendations.

American College Health Association. *Sexual Violence: What Everyone Should Know.* Hanover, MD: American College Health Association, 2011.

Berglund, H., Lindstrom, P., and Savic, I. Brain response to putative pheromones in lesbian women. *Proceedings of the National Academy of Sciences* 103 (2006): 8269–8274.

Boonstra, H., Gold, R. B., Richards, C. L., and Finer, L. B. *Abortion in Women' Lives.* New York: Guttmacher Institute, 2006.

Christensen, F. M. *Pornography: The Other Side.* New York: Praeger, 1990.

DeQuine, J. Out of the closet and on to fraternity row. *Time* 161 (March 17, 2003): 8.

Equal Employment Opportunity Commission. *Sexual Harassment Charges: EEOC and FEPA Combined, FY 1992–2004.* 2005. Available at: http://www.eeoc.gov/stats/harass.html.

Finer, L. B. and Henshaw, S. K. Disparities in rates of unintended pregnancy in the United States, 1994–2001. *Perspectives on Sexual and Reproductive Health* 38 (2006): 90–96.

Fisher, B. S., Cullen, F. T., and Turner, M. G. *The Sexual Victimization of College Women.* Washington, DC: National Institute of Justice, U.S. Department of Justice, 2001.

Goodson, P., McCormick, D., and Evans, A. Searching for sexually explicit materials on the internet: An exploratory study of college students' behavior and attitudes. *Archives of Sexual Behavior* 30 (2001): 101–118.

Grunkemeier, M. N. and Vollmer, R. T. Predicting prostate biopsy results: The importance of PSA, age, and race. *American Journal of Clinical Pathology* 26 (2006): 1–3.

Guttmacher Institute. *Teen Pregnancy: Trends and Lessons Learned. Issues in Brief.* New York: Guttmacher Institute, 2005.

Hatcher, R. A., Trussell, J., Nelson, A. L., Cates, W., Stewart, F., and Kowal, D. *Contraceptive Technology, Nineteenth Revised Edition.* New York: Ardent Media, 2008.

Hicks, T. V. and Leitenberg, H. Sexual fantasies about one's partner versus someone else: Gender differences in incidence and frequency. *Journal of Sex Research* 38 (2001): 43–50.

Jones, R. K. and Kooistra, K. Abortion incidence and access to services in the United States, 2008. *Perspectives in Sexual and Reproductive Health* 43 (2011): 41–50.

Laumann, E. O., Gagnon, J. H., Michael, R. T., and Michaels, S. *The Social Organization of Sexuality: Sexual Practices in the United States.* Chicago: The University of Chicago, 1994.

Leitenberg, H. and Henning, K. Sexual fantasy. *Psychological Bulletin* 117 (1995): 469–496.

Michael, R., Gagnon, J., Laumann, E., and Kolata, G. *Sex in America.* Boston: Little, Brown, 1994.

Planned Parenthood Association of Edmonton. *Decision Making for Unplanned Pregnancy.* 2002. Available at: http://www.ppae.ab.ca/index.php?m=9&s=5&p=3.

Rahman, Q. and Wilson, G. D. Born gay? The psychobiology of human sexual orientation. *Personality and Individual Differences* 34 (2003): 1337–1382.

Rankin, S. R. *Campus Climate for Gay, Lesbian, Bisexual, and Transgender People: A National Perspective.* New York: National Gay and Lesbian Task Force Policy Institute, 2003.

Rumbough, T. B. Controversial uses of the internet by college students. 2001. Available at: http://www.eucuase.edu/ir/library/pdf/C5D1618.pdf.

Sampson, R. *Acquaintance Rape of College Students.* Washington, DC: U.S. Department of Justice, Office of Community Oriented Policing Services, 2006.

Schwartz, J. L. and Gabelnick, H. L. Special report: Current contraceptive research. *Perspectives on Sexual and Reproductive Health* 34 (2002): 310–316.

SIECUS. Protecting against unwanted pregnancy: An overview of standard contraceptives. *SIECUS Report* 31 (2003): 24–26.

Smith, T. W. *American Sexual Behavior: Trends, Socio-Demographic Differences, and Risk Behavior.* Chicago: University of Chicago, National Opinion Research Center, 2003.

U.S. Preventive Services Task Force. Screening for breast cancer: U.S. Preventive Services Task Force recommendation statement. *Annals of Internal Medicine* 151 (2009): 716–726.

INTERNET RESOURCES

Planned Parenthood Federation of America
http://www.plannedparenthood.org

Association of Reproductive Health Specialists
http://www.arhp.org/

Division of STD Prevention, Centers for Disease Control and Prevention
http://www.cdc.gov/std/

The Alan Guttmacher Institute
http://www.guttmacher.org/

Sexuality Information and Education Council of the United States
http://www.siecus.org/

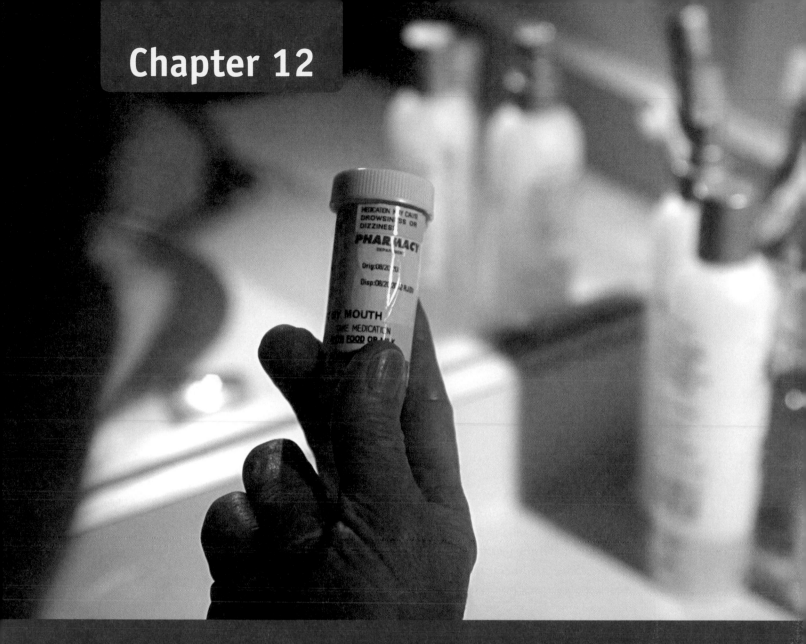

Chapter 12

Using Drugs Healthfully and Avoiding Drug Abuse and Misuse

 Access Health Check Ups and Health Behavior Change activities on the Companion Website: **go.jblearning.com/Empowering**.

Learning Objectives

- Describe how alcohol affects the brain and its effects on health.
- Explain why reactions to the ingestion of alcohol differ among people.
- Discuss how to drink alcohol responsibly and how to prevent alcohol-related problems.
- Explain the health effects of smoking and of secondhand smoke.
- Discuss why people use tobacco products, and list strategies for quitting.
- Distinguish between drug misuse versus abuse, and discuss the risks of commonly abused drugs.
- Define drug dependence, withdrawal, and tolerance.
- Define detoxification and the strategies used in drug treatment programs.

W hat do the actors Robert Downey, Jr., and Lindsay Lohan have in common? How about singers Britney Spears and Elton John? Or athletes Randy Moss and Mike Tyson? As you might have guessed, they have all been to rehab for alcohol and/or drug problems (DrugAlcohol-rehab.com, 2011). Anyone, regardless of social status, wealth, ethnicity, or age, can have alcohol or drug problems. This chapter describes the nature of those problems and the effects those problems have on the lives of those afflicted. This chapter also presents strategies you can use to avoid alcohol and drug problems.

Alcohol

A brightly colored cosmopolitan is the drink of choice for the glamorous characters in *Sex and the City*. James Bond depends on his famous martini—shaken, not stirred—to unwind after neutralizing a villain. And, weddings just wouldn't be the same without a champagne toast by the best man and the maid of honor. Alcohol holds a special and complicated place in our society. When used responsibly, alcohol can be an appropriate accompaniment to a healthy life, even helping to prevent heart disease. However, when abused, it can lead to a myriad of health and social problems.

Effects of Alcohol on the Brain

Chris is chatting with a friend at a party, and another friend comes by with bottles of beer. Chris drinks one bottle, then another, and then several more. Before he realizes

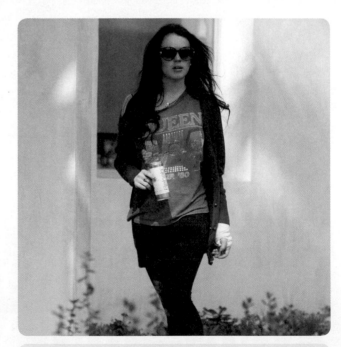

Alcohol and drug problems know no social, racial, ethnic, or educational boundaries. Some of the wealthiest and brightest people have been afflicted with these problems.

Myths *and* Facts

Misconceptions About Alcohol

MYTH	FACT
Beer will not get you as drunk as hard liquor will.	The alcohol is what is responsible for inebriation. It is true there is less alcohol per unit volume in beer; however, if you drink enough beers, you will ingest just as much alcohol as you will drinking hard liquor.
Drinking alcohol is relaxing.	A small amount of alcohol initially acts as a stimulant. Larger amounts depress the central nervous system. The feeling of relaxation, however, arises because the brain is deadened. The price paid is that other bodily functions are depressed as well, such as the ability to think clearly or perform coordinated actions. The result can be accidents or poor decisions that lead to injury or ill health.
The use of marijuana, cocaine, and similar drugs is the biggest drug problem on most college campuses.	Alcohol is both the most prevalent and frequently abused drug on college campuses, frequently leading to vandalism, fights, and other behaviors that can result in suspension or expulsion from school and/or criminal prosecution.

it, he is laughing more loudly than usual and swaying as he walks. By the end of the evening, Chris is too slow to move out of the way of other people and keeps bumping into them. The next morning, he wakes up feeling dizzy and his head hurts. Chris has a hard time remembering everything he did the night before.

These symptoms demonstrate the effects of alcohol on the brain. Using brain imaging and psychological tests, researchers have identified the regions of the brain most vulnerable to alcohol's effects (National Institute on Alcohol Abuse and Alcoholism, 2011):

■ *Cerebellum:* This area controls motor coordination. Damage to the cerebellum results in a loss of balance and stumbling and also may affect cognitive functions such as memory and emotional response.

■ *Limbic system:* This complex brain system monitors a variety of tasks including memory and emotion. Damage to this area impairs each of these functions.

■ *Cerebral cortex:* Our abilities to think, plan, behave intelligently, and interact socially stem from this brain region. In addition, this area connects the brain to the rest of the nervous system. Changes and damage to this area impair the ability to solve problems, remember, and learn.

Effects of Alcohol on Neurotransmitters

Neurotransmitters are chemicals produced by the nervous system that convey information between nerve cells. One neurotransmitter particularly susceptible to even small amounts of alcohol is called *glutamate*. Among other things, glutamate affects memory. Researchers

> **Neurotransmitters:** chemicals produced by the nervous system that convey information between nerve cells.

301

believe that alcohol interferes with glutamate action, and this may be what causes some people temporarily to "black out," or forget much of what happened during a bout of heavy drinking. Alcohol also causes an increased release of *serotonin*, another neurotransmitter, which helps regulate emotional expression, and *endorphins*, which are natural substances that may spark feelings of relaxation and euphoria as intoxication sets in.

When the brain tries to compensate for these disruptions, neurotransmitters adapt to create balance in the brain despite the presence of alcohol. These adaptations, however, can have negative long-term consequences. They build up an individual's alcohol tolerance, setting the stage for alcohol dependence.

Why Different People's Responses to Alcohol Are Varied

Because no two people are exactly alike, it is no surprise that different people react differently to alcohol. This is because of a variety of factors such as the following:

- *How much and how often one drinks.* The more often one drinks, the greater the quantity of alcohol that is required to achieve the desired effects.

- *The size of the person.* People who weigh more can ingest more alcohol before damage or impairment occurs than those of lesser weight.

- *The sex of the person.* Females have less body weight than males so it takes less alcohol for them to be affected than that for males.

- *Food in the stomach.* Food in the stomach will help absorb some alcohol and thereby diminish impairment.

- *How quickly one drinks.* The shorter the period of time during which alcohol is ingested, the more impairment is likely. This is because the body does not have the time to metabolize the alcohol and eliminate it from the body before more alcohol is ingested, thus a cumulative effect occurs.

- *One's genetic background and family history of alcoholism.* Certain ethnic populations can have stronger reactions to alcohol, and children of alcoholics are more likely to become alcoholics themselves.

- *One's physical health.* If you have liver or nutrition problems, the effects of alcohol will take longer to wear off.

How to Drink Responsibly

Some college students decide to abstain from drinking alcohol altogether. Others decide they want to drink sometimes, and for those ages 21 and older, that is a legal choice. If you choose to drink, doing so responsibly can prevent many of the negative consequences. Below are hints for drinking responsibly (National Institutes of Health, 2011):

- *Drink in moderation.* Moderation means the drinking is not getting you intoxicated, or drunk, and you are drinking no more than one drink per day if you are a woman and no more than two drinks per day if you are a man. One standard drink is 12 fluid ounces of regular beer, 8–9 fluid ounces of malt liquor, 5 fluid

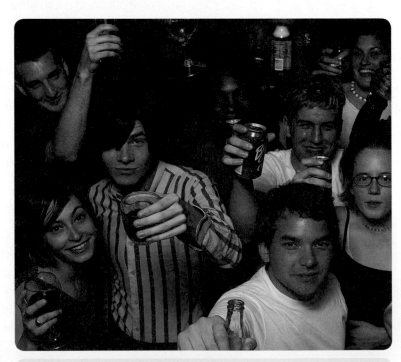

Alcohol can affect people differently based on their size, sex, experience drinking, and the amount of food and nonalcoholic drinks they ingest.

What I Need to Know

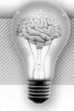

A Snapshot of Annual High-Risk College Drinking Consequences

The consequences of excessive and underage drinking affect virtually all college campuses and college communities. Individual college students may be affected whether they choose to drink or not. The following data refer to *annual* nationwide statistics.

- *Death:* 1,825 college students between the ages of 18 and 24 die from alcohol-related unintentional injuries, including motor vehicle crashes.

- *Injury:* 599,000 students between the ages of 18 and 24 are unintentionally injured under the influence of alcohol.

- *Assault:* 696,000 students between the ages of 18 and 24 are assaulted by another student who has been drinking.

- *Sexual abuse:* 97,000 students between the ages of 18 and 24 are victims of alcohol-related sexual assault or date rape.

- *Unsafe sex:* 400,000 students between the ages of 18 and 24 had unprotected sex while under the influence of drugs and alcohol, and more than 100,000 students between the ages of 18 and 24 report having been too intoxicated to know if they consented to having sex.

- *Academic problems:* About 25% of college students report academic consequences of their drinking including missing class, falling behind, doing poorly on exams or papers, and receiving lower grades overall.

- *Health problems/suicide attempts:* More than 150,000 students develop an alcohol-related health problem, and between 1.2% and 1.5% of students report that they tried to commit suicide within the past year due to drinking or drug use.

- *Drunk driving:* 3,360,000 students between the ages of 18 and 24 drive under the influence of alcohol.

- *Vandalism:* About 11% of college student drinkers report that they have damaged property while under the influence of alcohol.

- *Property damage:* More than 25% of administrators from schools with relatively low drinking levels and more than 50% from schools with high drinking levels say their campuses have a "moderate" or "major" problem with alcohol-related property damage.

- *Police involvement:* About 5% of 4-year college students are involved with the police or campus security as a result of their drinking, and 110,000 students between the ages of 18 and 24 are arrested for an alcohol-related violation such as public drunkenness or driving under the influence.

- *Alcohol abuse and dependence:* 31% of college students met criteria for a diagnosis of alcohol abuse and 6% for a diagnosis of alcohol dependence in the past 12 months, according to questionnaire-based self-reports about their drinking.

DATA FROM: National Institute on Alcohol Abuse and Alcoholism. *A Snapshot of Annual High-Risk College Drinking Consequences.* 2010. Available at: http://www.collegedrinkingprevention.gov/StatsSummaries/snapshot.aspx.

ounces of table wine, or 1.5 fluid ounces of 80-proof spirits (see **FIG. 12.1 ▼**).

■ *NEVER drink alcohol and drive a car.* If you are going to drink, have a designated driver (a friend who promises not to drink) or plan an alternative way home, such as a taxi or bus.

■ *Do not drink on an empty stomach.* Snack before and while drinking alcohol.

■ *Be wary of drug interactions.* If you are taking medication, including over-the-counter drugs, check with your doctor before drinking alcohol. Alcohol can intensify the effects of many drugs and can interact with other drugs, making them ineffective or dangerous.

■ *Alternate your drinks.* Drink a glass of water or other nonalcoholic drink for every alcoholic drink.

■ *Drink slowly.* Do not guzzle drinks. A good rule to live by is to consume no more than one drink an hour.

■ *Don't leave your drink unattended.* To prevent someone from putting something in your drink, such as the "date rape drug" Rohypnol, never leave it unattended. Also, to make sure you know what you are ingesting, do not drink out of punch bowls, and do not accept a drink from anyone else. Make a plan for getting safely home *before* you go out. Travel with friends to and from parties and clubs, with one of you being the designated driver.

■ *In some cases, refuse alcohol entirely.* If you are pregnant, do not drink at all, as you could severely harm the developing embryo or fetus. Do not drink if you have a history of alcohol abuse or alcoholism. If alcoholism runs in your family, you may be at increased risk of development of alcoholism yourself and may want to avoid drinking of alcohol altogether.

Signs of Problems with Alcohol

You may or may not think you have a problem with alcohol. Some problem drinkers rationalize their behavior and deny a problem exists. Drinking becomes **problem drinking** if it causes trouble in your relationships,

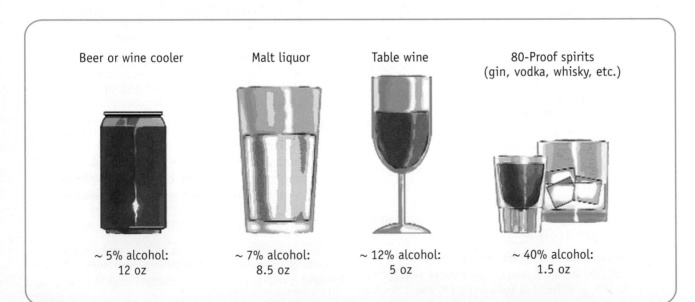

Beer or wine cooler	Malt liquor	Table wine	80-Proof spirits (gin, vodka, whisky, etc.)
~ 5% alcohol: 12 oz	~ 7% alcohol: 8.5 oz	~ 12% alcohol: 5 oz	~ 40% alcohol: 1.5 oz

FIGURE 12.1 What is a standard drink? In the United States, a standard drink is any drink that contains about 14 grams of pure alcohol (about 0.6 fluid ounces, or 1.2 tablespoons). The illustration demonstrates U.S. standard drink equivalents. These are approximate, as different brands and types of beverages vary in their actual alcohol content. Reproduced from: National Institute on Alcohol Abuse and Alcoholism. *Tips for Cutting Down on Drinking.* 2008. Available at: http://pubs.niaaa.nih.gov/publications/Tips/tips.htm.

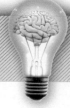

What I Need to Know

What Colleges Are Doing to Reduce the Alcohol Consumption of Their Students

Concerned about alcohol drinking and the health and safety of their students, colleges have adopted a number of strategies to reduce alcohol consumption. Among these are the following:

- Reinstating Friday classes and exams to reduce Thursday night partying; possibly scheduling Saturday morning classes.

- Implementing alcohol-free, expanded late-night student activities.

- Eliminating keg parties on campus where underage drinking is prevalent.

- Establishing alcohol-free dormitories.

- Employing older, salaried resident assistants or hiring adults to fulfill that role.

- Further controlling or eliminating alcohol at sports events and prohibiting tailgating parties that model heavy alcohol use.

- Refusing sponsorship gifts from the alcohol industry to avoid any perception that underage drinking is acceptable.

- Banning alcohol on campus, including at faculty and alumni events.

ADAPTED FROM: National Institute on Alcohol Abuse and Alcoholism. *College Drinking: Four Tiers*. 2007. Available at: http://www .collegedrinkingprevention.gov/statssummaries/4tier.aspx.

---

in school, in social activities, or in how you think and feel. The more severe these problems, the more problematic is the drinking. To determine if you have a problem with alcohol, complete Health Check Up 12.1 (see Health Check Up 12.1 on the companion website). Once completed, place Health Check Up 12.1 in your Health Decision Portfolio.

Strategies to Overcome Alcohol-Related Problems

If you experience alcohol-related problems or if you are just trying to take charge of your drinking, the National Institute on Alcohol Abuse and Alcoholism (2008) recommends trying the strategies in the list that follows, in addition to the strategies presented earlier on how to drink responsibly. Some should be tried the first week and others added next.

- *Keep track.* Keep track of how much you drink. Find a way that works for you, such as a card in your wallet, check marks on a calendar, or a personal digital assistant. If you make note of each drink before you drink it, this will help you slow down when needed.

- *Count and measure.* Know the standard drink sizes so you can count your drinks accurately (see Figure 12.1). Keep in mind that, especially with mixed drinks, it can be hard to keep track; at times you may be getting more alcohol than you think. If you are drinking wine at a restaurant or party, you will be better able to keep track if you ask the host or server not to "top off" a partially filled glass.

- *Set goals.* Decide how many days a week you want to allow yourself to drink and how many drinks you will have on those days. It is a good idea to have some days when you do not drink at all. Drinking within certain limits reduces your chances of developing an alcohol use disorder and related health problems.

Problem drinking: when alcohol causes trouble in relationships, in school, in social activities, or in how one thinks and feels.

- *Avoid "triggers."* What triggers your urge to drink? If certain people or places make you drink even when you do not want to, try to avoid them. If certain activities, times of day, or feelings trigger the urge, plan what you will do instead of drinking. If drinking at home is a problem, keep little or no alcohol there.

- *Plan to handle urges.* When an urge hits, consider these options: Remind yourself of your reasons for changing; talk it through with someone you trust; get involved with a healthy, distracting activity; or "urge surf"— that is, instead of fighting the feeling, accept it and ride it out, knowing that it will soon crest like a wave and pass.

- *Know your "no."* You are likely to be offered a drink at times when you do not want one. Have a polite, convincing "no, thanks" ready. The faster you can say no to these offers, the less likely you are to give in. If you hesitate, it allows time to think of excuses to go along.

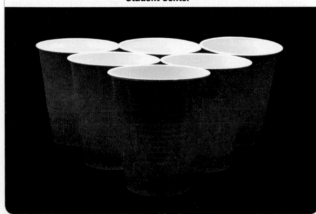

To accommodate students who do not drink alcohol, colleges offer alcohol-free events such as parties and dances.

If you want to change your drinking behavior, following a systematic plan can help you be successful. Use Health Check Up 12.2 to create a personalized plan. Once completed, place Health Check Up 12.2 in your Health Decision Portfolio.

The Hangover

A **hangover** is a combination of unpleasant physical and mental symptoms that occur after heavy alcohol drinking. Symptoms of hangover include fatigue and weakness; thirst; headache and muscle aches; nausea, vomiting, and stomach pain; decreased sleep; vertigo and sensitivity to light and sound; decreased attention and concentration; depression, anxiety, and irritability; and tremor, sweating, and increased pulse and systolic blood pressure. For the most part, the more alcohol consumed and the longer the duration of alcohol drinking, the more prevalent and severe the hangover. Notably, however, some people experience a hangover after drinking small amounts of alcohol—for example, one to three drinks; furthermore, some heavy drinkers do not experience hangovers at all.

Although ways to prevent hangovers and "remedies" for hangovers abound (see the accompanying What I Need to Know box), the best strategy is to prevent a hangover in the first place. To do so, when drinking alcoholic beverages:

- Pace yourself. Drink alcoholic beverages slowly. Intersperse water or other nonalcoholic drinks with the alcoholic drinks to keep your body hydrated.

- Munch on snacks to slow the absorption of alcohol thereby keeping your blood alcohol level low.

- Eat fruits and drink fruit juices to decrease the intensity of hangovers.

- Snack on crackers. Bland foods such as toast and crackers can raise low blood sugar and help with nausea.

Binge Drinking

Binge drinking is a pattern of drinking of alcohol that brings blood alcohol concentration (BAC) to 0.08 gram-percent or above. For a typical adult, this pattern corresponds to consumption of five or more drinks (male) or

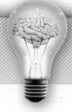

What I Need to Know

Hangover Prevention and Treatment

Many treatments have been tried to prevent hangover, shorten its duration, or reduce the severity of its symptoms. Among suggested treatments are the following:

- Consumption of fruits, fruit juices, or other fructose-containing foods is reported to decrease hangover intensity.

- Consumption of bland foods containing complex carbohydrates, such as toast or crackers, may relieve nausea.

- Sleep may relieve the feeling of fatigue.

- Drinking of nonalcoholic beverages may reduce dehydration.

- Antacids may alleviate nausea and gastritis.

- Aspirin and other nonsteroidal anti-inflammatory medications—such as ibuprofen or naproxen—may reduce the headache and muscle aches. However, if upper abdominal pain or nausea is present, these medications should not be used because anti-inflammatory medications are themselves gastric irritants.

- Caffeine may counteract the fatigue and malaise associated with a hangover.

- Having an alcoholic drink—the "hair of the dog that bit you" remedy—has been suggested to cure a hangover. However, further alcohol use should be avoided. Additional drinking will enhance the existing toxicity of the alcohol consumed during the previous bout and may lead to even further drinking.

Whereas these and other numerous hangover cures have been suggested, only a few of them have been scientifically investigated, and none of them prevents or relieves hangovers in a significant way. The best cure for a hangover is time. Symptoms usually subside after 8–24 hours as the liver metabolizes the alcohol in the body.

DATA FROM: Binns, C. Alcohol and hangover myths revealed. *Life Science*, December 29, 2006. Available at: http://www.livescience.com/9477-alcohol-hangover-myths-revealed.html; Data from: Pittler, M. H., Verster, J. C., and Ernst, E. Interventions for preventing or treating alcohol hangover: Systematic review of randomized trials. *British Medical Journal* 331 (2005): 1515–1518; Data from: Swift, R. and Davidson, D. Alcohol hangover mechanisms and mediators. *Alcohol Health & Research World* 22 (1998): 54–60.

---

four or more drinks (female) in about 2 hours (Centers for Disease Control and Prevention, 2010a). Binge drinking is common among college students who are more likely to participate in binge drinking than their noncollege peers (Dawson, D. A., Grant, B. F., Stinson, F. S., 2004). Forty-four percent of students attending 4-year colleges drink alcohol at the binge level or greater (Weschler and Nelson, 2008). Notably, current college students are less likely to have been binge drinkers prior to their college years compared with their peers who never attend college but are more likely to binge drink once they enter college—probably as a result of the college environment (Timberlake et al., 2007). That is, college students see their peers binge drink and perceive that as normal. To fit in, they, too, binge drink. Among other consequences, binge drinking is the major cause of alcohol poisoning, which can be fatal.

Alcohol Poisoning

Ingesting toxic amounts of alcohol can lead to **alcohol poisoning**. Symptoms of alcohol poisoning include

Hangover: a combination of unpleasant physical and mental symptoms that occur after heavy alcohol drinking.

Binge drinking: a pattern of drinking of alcohol that brings blood alcohol concentration (BAC) to 0.08 gram-percent or above; for a typical adult, this pattern corresponds to consumption of five or more drinks (male) or four or more drinks (female) in about 2 hours.

Alcohol poisoning: ingestion of a toxic amount of alcohol.

(Mayo Foundation for Medical Education and Research, 2010):

- Confusion, stupor

- Vomiting

- Seizures

- Slow breathing (less than eight breaths a minute)

- Irregular breathing (a gap of more than 10 seconds between breaths)

- Blue-tinged skin or pale skin

- Low body temperature (hypothermia)

- Unconsciousness ("passing out") and cannot be roused

If you suspect that someone has alcohol poisoning—even if you do not see the classic signs and symptoms—seek immediate medical care. In an emergency, follow these suggestions (Mayo Clinic Staff, 2010):

- *If the person is unconscious.* If the person is breathing less than eight times a minute or has repeated, uncontrolled vomiting, call 911 or your local emergency number immediately. Keep in mind that even when someone is unconscious or has stopped drinking, alcohol continues to be released into the bloodstream, and the level of alcohol in the body continues to rise. Never assume that a person will "sleep off" alcohol poisoning.

- *If the person is conscious.* Call 800-222-1222 (in the United States), and you will automatically be routed to your local poison control center. The staff at the poison control center or emergency call center can instruct you as to whether you should take the person directly to a hospital. All calls to poison control centers are confidential.

- *Be prepared to provide information.* If you know, be sure to tell hospital or emergency personnel the kind and amount of alcohol the person drank, and when.

- *Do not leave an unconscious person alone.* While waiting for help, do not try to make the person vomit. Alcohol poisoning affects the way your gag reflex works. That means someone with alcohol poisoning may choke on his or her own vomit or accidentally inhale vomit into the lungs, which could cause a fatal lung injury (Mayo Foundation for Medical Education and Research, 2010).

Fetal Alcohol Syndrome

Fetal alcohol syndrome refers to growth, mental, and physical problems that may occur in a baby or child whose mother drank alcohol during pregnancy. When a pregnant woman drinks alcohol, it easily passes across the placenta to the fetus. A pregnant woman who drinks any amount of alcohol is at risk, as no *safe* level of alcohol use during pregnancy has been established. However, consumption of larger amounts appears to increase the problems. A baby with fetal alcohol syndrome may have the following symptoms (PubMed Health, 2009):

- Poor growth while in the womb and after birth.

- Decreased muscle tone and poor coordination.

- Delayed development and significant functional problems in three or more major areas: thinking, speech, movement, or social skills (as expected for the baby's age).

- Heart defects.

- Structural problems with the face including narrow and small eyes, small head, small upper jaw, smooth groove in upper lip, and smooth and thin upper lip.

There is no cure for fetal alcohol syndrome: it lasts a lifetime. However, early intervention treatment services can improve a child's development (Centers for Disease Control and Prevention, 2010b).

In addition to fetal alcohol syndrome, drinking of alcohol during pregnancy may result in miscarriage, stillbirth, or premature delivery.

Tobacco Use

Have I got a deal for you! How would you like to get your teeth brown; your breath to smell; subject yourself to heart disease, cancer, and stroke; and pay only $8.30 for the privilege? Of course, I'm referring to cigarette

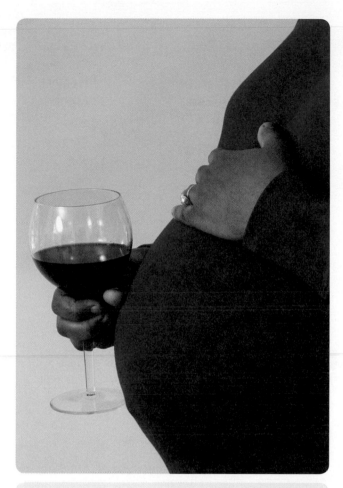

There is no safe amount of drinking that can prevent pregnant women from having babies born with fetal alcohol syndrome.

TABLE 12.1	Percentage of Current Adult Cigarette Smokers in the United States: 2011

Category	Percentage (%)
Total population	20.6
Gender	
Male	23.5
Female	17.9
Age (years)	
18–24	21.8
25–44	24.0
45–64	21.9
65 and older	9.5
Race/ethnicity	
American Indian/Alaska Native	23.2
African American	21.3
Hispanic	14.5
White	22.1
Education	
9–11 years of education	33.6
GED diploma	49.1
Undergraduate college degree	11.1
Graduate college degree	5.6
Poverty status	
Below poverty level	31.1
Above poverty level	19.4

Data from: Centers for Disease Control and Prevention. Vital signs: Current cigarette smoking among adults aged ≥ 18 years—United States, 2009. *Morbidity and Mortality Weekly Report* 59 (2010): 1135–1140.

smoking, although use of other tobacco products (such as cigar smoking or tobacco chewing) presents comparable risks. Most people know the risks associated with tobacco use. I'm sure you do as well. How can you miss them? Frightening pictures and statistics appear in public service ads depicting these risks, educating all of us to the harmful effects of tobacco use. And yet, many Americans still light up or chew tobacco (see Table 12.1). What's going on here?

The Center for Tobacco Research and Intervention conducted more than 6,000 interviews to determine why people smoke. The findings of this study appear in Table 12.2. As you can see, there are many reasons why people smoke. If you smoke, complete Health Check Up 12.3 to identify why you smoke (see Health Check Up 12.3 on the companion website). If you do not smoke, ask someone you know who does smoke to complete Health Check Up 12.3 to identify why he or she smokes. Once completed, place Health Check Up 12.3 in your Health Decision Portfolio.

Fetal alcohol syndrome: growth, mental, and physical problems that may occur in a baby when a mother drinks alcohol during pregnancy.

TABLE 12.2 Reasons Why People Smoke

Reason	Light Smokers (%)	Moderate Smokers (%)	Heavy Smokers (%)
It's a habit	79	94	97
I'm addicted	65	86	95
It relaxes me	75	79	80
I enjoy it	70	77	77
Something to do with my hands	47	52	63
It helps me cope	39	48	56
Keeps me going	21	31	35
An excuse to take a break	38	41	34
For social reasons	50	31	28
Helps me concentrate	17	21	27
It wakes me up	17	19	23
Keeps weight down	19	21	19

DATA FROM: Center for Tobacco Research and Intervention. *Why People Smoke: Action Paper Number 1*. Madison, WI: University of Wisconsin Comprehensive Cancer Center, 2002.

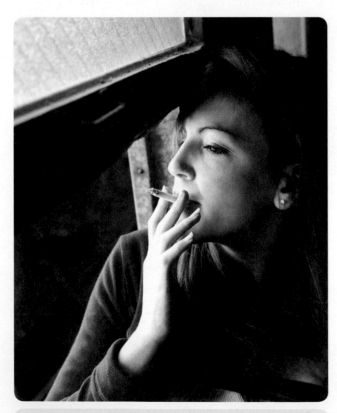

There are many reasons why people risk their health by smoking.

Health Effects of Smoking

The adverse health effects from cigarette smoking account for an estimated 443,000 deaths, or nearly one of every five deaths, each year in the United States. More deaths are caused each year by tobacco use than by all deaths from human immunodeficiency virus (HIV), illegal drug use, alcohol use, motor vehicle injuries, suicides, and murders combined.

Smokers are two to four times more likely to develop coronary heart disease, two to four times more likely to develop stroke, and 12–13 times more likely to die from chronic obstructive lung diseases (such as chronic bronchitis and emphysema). Furthermore, men who smoke are 23 times more likely and women who smoke are 13 times more likely to develop lung cancer compared with nonsmokers. In addition to lung cancer, smoking is also associated with bladder cancer, cancer of the cervix, cancer of the esophagus, kidney cancer, cancer of the larynx (voice box), cancer of the oral cavity (mouth), cancer of the pharynx (throat), stomach cancer, and cancer of the uterus (Centers for Disease Control and Prevention, 2011).

Smoking is also known to increase the risk of infertility, preterm delivery, stillbirth, low birth weight, and sudden infant death syndrome (SIDS). Also, smoking is associated with post-menopausal women having lower bone density and an increased risk for hip fracture.

Secondhand Smoke

Nonsmokers may suffer ill effects of tobacco smoke, too—if they are in proximity to smokers—by breathing secondhand smoke. **Secondhand smoke** is the combination of smoke from the burning end of a cigarette and the smoke breathed out by smokers. Secondhand smoke contains more than 7,000 chemicals, hundreds of which are toxic and 70 of which can cause cancer. Secondhand smoke causes numerous health problems in infants and children, including severe asthma attacks, respiratory infections, ear infections, and SIDS. Among the health conditions associated with secondhand smoke in adults are heart disease and lung cancer. In fact, secondhand smoke causes an estimated 46,000 premature deaths from heart disease each year in the United States among nonsmokers and an estimated 3,400 lung cancer deaths (Centers for Disease Control and Prevention, 2008). To prevent the inhalation of secondhand smoke, smoking is prohibited in many indoor public places such as workplaces, schools, restaurants, hospitals, and shopping centers. Some localities have even banned smoking in outdoor public places such as in parks, near schools, and on crowded streets.

Withdrawal Symptoms

Tobacco use creates a dependence on nicotine. One of the reasons it is so difficult for many people to quit is that when nicotine is taken away, intense withdrawal symptoms occur, including (Medline Plus, 2010):

- An intense craving for nicotine

- Anxiety, tension, restlessness, frustration, or impatience

- Difficulty concentrating

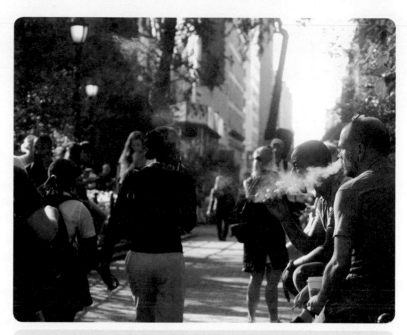

Secondhand smoke subjects nonsmokers to many of the same risks as those experienced by smokers.

- Drowsiness or trouble sleeping, as well as bad dreams and nightmares

- Headaches

- Increased appetite and weight gain

- Irritability or depression

Almost all people who try to quit have some form of nicotine withdrawal. Generally, people who have smoked the longest or smoked a greater number of cigarettes each day are more likely to have withdrawal symptoms. Withdrawal symptoms generally start within 2–3 hours after the last cigarette and peak about 2–3 days later. These symptoms occur even when a nicotine-dependent person merely cuts back on the number of cigarettes smoked instead of quitting altogether.

There exist several medications to treat nicotine withdrawal. Some of these medications replace the nicotine in less harmful ways; that is, by not drawing smoke into

Secondhand smoke: the combination of smoke from the burning end of a cigarette and the smoke breathed out by smokers.

What I Need to Know

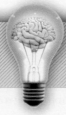

The Economics of Tobacco

- Tobacco companies spend billions of dollars each year to market their products. In 2006, cigarette companies spent $12.4 billion on advertising and promotional expenses in the United States alone, down from $13.1 billion in 2005, but more than double what was spent in 1997.[1]

- The money cigarette companies spent on U.S. marketing in 2006 amounted to approximately $34 million per day.[1]

- U.S. consumers spent an estimated $90 billion in 2006 on tobacco products.[2] Approximately $83.6 billion was spent on cigarettes.[2] Approximately $3.2 billion was spent on cigars.[2] Approximately $2.6 billion was spent on smokeless tobacco (e.g., chewing tobacco and snuff).[3]

- More than 315 billion cigarettes were purchased in the United States in 2009, with three companies selling nearly 85% of them.[4] Philip Morris alone accounted for more than 47% of sales.

- Approximately 121.4 million pounds of smokeless tobacco were purchased in the United States in 2009 (down from 124.7 million pounds in 2008).[5] Approximately 12 billion cigars (i.e., 9.7 billion large cigars and cigarillos; 2.3 billion little cigars) were purchased in the United States in 2009.

- During the period 2000–2004, cigarette smoking was estimated to be responsible for $193 billion in annual health-related economic losses in the United States ($96 billion in direct medical costs and approximately $97 billion in lost productivity).[6]

- The total economic costs (direct medical costs and lost productivity) associated with cigarette smoking are estimated at $10.47 per pack of cigarettes sold in the United States.[7]

- Cigarette smoking results in 5.1 million years of potential life lost in the United States annually.[6]

- In early 2010, the average retail price of a pack of cigarettes in the United States was approximately $4.80 (including federal, state, and municipal excise taxes), but prices vary widely across states.[8]

- Increases in cigarette prices lead to significant reductions in cigarette smoking.[9,10] A 10% increase in price has been estimated to reduce overall cigarette consumption among adolescents and young adults by about 4%.

[1]Data from: Federal Trade Commission. *Cigarette Report for 2006*. Washington, DC: Federal Trade Commission, 2009.

[2]Data from: U.S. Department of Agriculture. *Table 21: Expenditures for Tobacco Products and Disposable Personal Income, 1989–2006*. Washington, DC: U.S. Department of Agriculture, Economic Research Service, 2007.

[3]Data from: Federal Trade Commission. *Smokeless Tobacco Report for the Year 2006*. Washington, DC: Federal Trade Commission, 2009.

[4]Data from: Maxwell J. C. *The Maxwell Report: Year End & Fourth Quarter 2009 Sales Estimates for the Cigarette Industry*. Richmond, VA: John C. Maxwell, Jr., 2010.

[5]Data from: Maxwell J. C. *The Maxwell Report: The Smokeless Tobacco Industry in 2009*. Richmond, VA: John C. Maxwell, Jr., 2010.

[6]Data From: Maxwell J. C. *The Maxwell Report: Cigar Industry in 2009*. Richmond, VA: John C. Maxwell, Jr., 2010.

[7]Data From: Centers for Disease Control and Prevention. Smoking-attributable mortality, years of potential life lost, and productivity losses—United States, 2000–2004. *Morbidity and Mortality Weekly Report* 57 (2008): 1226–1228.

[8]Data From: Centers for Disease Control and Prevention. *Sustaining State Programs for Tobacco Control: Data Highlights 2006*. Atlanta, GA: U.S. Department of Health and Human Services, Centers for Disease Control and Prevention, National Center for Chronic Disease Prevention and Health Promotion, Office on Smoking and Health, 2006.

[9]Data From: U.S. Department of Health and Human Services. *Reducing Tobacco Use: A Report of the Surgeon General*. Atlanta, GA: U.S. Department of Health and Human Services, Centers for Disease Control and Prevention, National Center for Chronic Disease Prevention and Health Promotion, Office on Smoking and Health, 2000.

[10]Data From: Task Force on Community Preventive Services. Tobacco. In Zaza, S., Briss, P. A., and Harris, K. W., eds. *The Guide to Community Preventive Services: What Works to Promote Health?* New York: Oxford University Press, 2005, 3–79.

the lungs. For example, nicotine replacement therapy may include patches, gum, and lozenges and may be available over the counter. If thinking of using over-the-counter replacement therapy medications, it is a good idea to check with one's physician to make sure there are no anticipated adverse reactions with other medications one may be taking and considering one's personal health. Nicotine nasal sprays and nicotine inhalers are available by prescription. Other prescription medications include bupropion (Zyban), which controls nicotine cravings, or varenicline (Chantix), which reduces both the pleasurable effects of smoking and any nicotine withdrawal symptoms.

Strategies to Quit Smoking

More than 38 million people in the United States have successfully quit smoking. Yet there are still around 50 million Americans who smoke. Most say they would like to quit (Medline Plus, 2010). Someone once said that the best method to quit smoking is the last one tried. That is, people usually try several different means of quitting, only to relapse, and then try again. Still, there are several strategies that have been found effective in helping people quit (Mayo Foundation for Medical Education and Research, 2011; Smokefree.gov, 2011):

- *Put it on paper.* Write on a sheet of paper what you do not like about smoking and why you want to quit. Then carry that paper around with you and each time you have an urge to smoke, read that paper to remind yourself why you want to quit.

- *Enlist support.* Tell your family, friends, classmates, and coworkers that you are trying to quit smoking. Ask them to remind you why it is important to quit smoking if they see you pick up a cigarette. You might also ask your friends or anyone in your household who smokes to quit smoking, too. That way you will have support for your efforts from someone who can empathize with you. You will also reduce your exposure to secondhand smoke, which might undermine your intention to stop smoking.

- *Take it slow.* Although some people can quit smoking by setting a date to do so and stopping then, many others find that approach unsuccessful. Gradual

withdrawal is suggested. Ways that you can cut back gradually include delaying your first cigarette of the day, smoking only half of each cigarette, buying only one pack of cigarettes at a time, and trading one smoking break a day for physical activity.

- *Avoid smoking triggers.* Smoking is usually associated with certain places, situations, or people. For example, smoking might occur after meals, or when out with friends, or when stressed. Recognize the places and situations that trigger your smoking and, as best as possible, avoid them. In addition, hang out with people who do not smoke, and make it difficult to get at cigarettes. For example, don't keep cigarettes in your pocket or purse. This way it will be more bothersome to get a cigarette to smoke. To identify your triggers or the triggers of someone else you know who smokes, complete Health Check Up 12.4 (see Health Check Up 12.4 on the companion website). Once completed, place Health Check Up 12.4 in your Health Decision Portfolio.

- *Try a stop-smoking product.* As discussed earlier, quitting smoking results in nicotine withdrawal symptoms. For some people, these symptoms are severe enough to drive them back to smoking. In these instances, medications that can alleviate or diminish the effects of these symptoms can be prescribed or purchased over the counter.

- *Manage stress.* It is well known that stress and anxiety can increase the urge to smoke. Therefore, an important component of a quit-smoking program is to better manage stress and anxiety. For example, practice a relaxation technique such as meditation or imagery or focus attention on something other than the urge to smoke.

- *Keep busy.* Keeping active is a good way to avoid thinking about smoking. Go to a movie, exercise, take long walks, or go bike riding. It may also help to spend as much free time as possible where smoking is prohibited—such as in malls, libraries, museums, theaters, department stores, and places of worship. If you miss the feeling of holding a cigarette, you might hold something else, such as a pencil, a paper clip, a marble, or a water bottle. If you miss having something in your mouth, try toothpicks, cinnamon sticks, sugar-free candy, sugar-free gum, or carrot sticks.

- *Reward not smoking.* You will have more spending money available if you are not buying as many cigarettes. Start a "money jar" in which the cigarette money that would have been spent each day is set aside. Soon, you will have saved enough money to purchase a significant reward that will reinforce not smoking. (Mayo Foundation for Medical Education and Research, 2011.)

Other Drugs

We all use drugs as some point in our lives. We take prescribed antibiotics, we buy over-the-counter cold remedies, and we ingest aspirin or ibuprofen when our muscles ache. The key is to use safe drugs safely, in the way they were intended to be used. Whereas these over-the-counter drugs, alcohol, and tobacco are legal substances, other drugs are used illegally. Some of these drugs are prescribed medications, whereas others are termed recreational drugs. Tables 12.3 and 12.4 list these drugs, their

| TABLE 12.3 | Commonly Abused Prescription Drugs |

Substance (by Category)	Examples of Commercial and Street Names	U.S. DEA Schedule*/ How Administered†	Intoxication Effects/Potential Health Consequences
Depressants			
Barbiturates	Amytal, Nembutal, Seconal, phenobarbital; barbs, reds, red birds, phennies, tooies, yellows, yellow jackets	II, III, V/ injected, swallowed	Reduced pain and anxiety; feeling of well-being; lowered inhibitions; slowed pulse and breathing; lowered blood pressure; poor concentration/confusion, fatigue; impaired coordination, memory, judgment; respiratory depression and arrest; addiction.
Benzodiazepines (other than flunitrazepam)	Ativan, Halcion, Librium, Valium, Xanax; candy, downers, sleeping pills, tranks	IV/swallowed	Also: For barbiturates: sedation, drowsiness/depression, unusual excitement, fever, irritability, poor judgment, slurred speech, dizziness.
Flunitrazepam‡,§	Rohypnol; forget-me pill, Mexican Valium, R2, Roche, roofies, roofinol, rope, rophies	IV/swallowed, snorted	For benzodiazepines: sedation, drowsiness/dizziness. For flunitrazepam: visual and gastrointestinal disturbances, urinary retention, memory loss for the time under the drug's effects.
Dissociative Anesthetics			
Ketamine	Ketalar SV; cat Valium, K, Special K, vitamin K	III/injected, snorted, smoked	Increased heart rate and blood pressure, impaired motor function/memory loss; numbness; nausea/vomiting. Also for ketamine: at high doses, delirium, depression, respiratory depression and arrest.

TABLE 12.3	Commonly Abused Prescription Drugs *(Continued)*

Substance (by Category)	Examples of Commercial and Street Names	U.S. DEA Schedule*/ How Administered†	Intoxication Effects/Potential Health Consequences
Opioids and Morphine Derivatives			
Codeine	Empirin with Codeine, Fiorinal with Codeine, Robitussin A-C, Tylenol with Codeine; Captain Cody, Cody, schoolboy; (with glutethimide) doors & fours, loads, pancakes and syrup	II, III, IV/ injected, swallowed	Pain relief, euphoria, drowsiness/ respiratory depression and arrest, nausea, confusion, constipation, sedation, unconsciousness, coma, tolerance, addiction. Also for codeine: less analgesia, sedation, and respiratory depression than morphine.
Fentanyl	Actiq, Duragesic, Sublimaze; Apache, China girl, China white, dance fever, friend, goodfella, jackpot, murder 8, TNT, Tango and Cash	II/injected, smoked, snorted	
Morphine	Roxanol, Duramorph; M, Miss Emma, monkey, white stuff	II, III/injected, swallowed, smoked	
Opium	Laudanum, paregoric; big O, black stuff, block, gum, hop	II, III, V/ swallowed, smoked	
Other opioid pain relievers: oxycodone, meperidine, hydromorphone, hydrocodone, propoxyphene	Tylox, OxyContin, Percodan, Percocet; oxy 80s, oxycotton, oxycet, hillbilly heroin, percs Demerol, meperidine hydrochloride; demmies, pain killer Dilaudid; juice, dillies. Vicodin, Lortab, Lorcet, Darvon, Darvocet	II, III, IV/ swallowed, injected, suppositories, chewed, crushed, snorted	
Stimulants			
Amphetamines	Biphetamine, Dexedrine; bennies, black beauties, crosses, hearts, LA turnaround, speed, truck drivers, uppers	II/injected, swallowed, smoked, snorted	Increased heart rate, blood pressure, metabolism; feelings of exhilaration, energy, increased mental alertness/rapid or irregular heart-beat; reduced appetite, weight loss, heart failure.
Cocaine	Cocaine hydrochloride; blow, bump, C, candy, Charlie, coke, crack, flake, rock, snow, toot	II/injected, smoked, snorted	

(Continues)

TABLE 12.3   **Commonly Abused Prescription Drugs** *(Continued)*

Substance (by Category)	Examples of Commercial and Street Names	U.S. DEA Schedule*/ How Administered†	Intoxication Effects/Potential Health Consequences
Stimulants *(continued)*			
Methamphetamine	Desoxyn; chalk, crank, crystal, fire, glass, go fast, ice, meth, speed	II/injected, swallowed, smoked, snorted	Also: For amphetamines: rapid breathing; hallucinations/tremor, loss of coordination; irritability, anxiousness, restlessness, delirium, panic, paranoia, impulsive behavior, aggressiveness, tolerance, addiction.
Methylphenidate	Ritalin; JIF, MPH, R-ball, Skippy, the smart drug, vitamin R	II/injected, swallowed, snorted	For cocaine: increased temperature/chest pain, respiratory failure, nausea, abdominal pain, strokes, seizures, headaches, malnutrition.
			For methamphetamine: aggression, violence, psychotic behavior/memory loss, cardiac and neurologic damage; impaired memory and learning, tolerance, addiction.
			For methylphenidate: increase or decrease in blood pressure, psychotic episodes/digestive problems, loss of appetite, weight loss.
Other Compounds			
Anabolic steroids	Anadrol, Oxandrin, Durabolin, Depo-Testosterone, Equipoise; roids, juice	III/injected, swallowed, applied to skin	No intoxication effects.
			Hypertension, blood clotting and cholesterol changes, liver cysts and cancer, kidney cancer, hostility and aggression, acne.
			Adolescents: premature stoppage of growth.
			In males: prostate cancer, reduced sperm production, shrunken testicles, breast enlargement.
			In females: menstrual irregularities, development of beard and other masculine characteristics.

DEA, Drug Enforcement Agency.

*Schedule I and II drugs have a high potential for abuse. They require greater storage security and have a quota on manufacturing, among other restrictions. Schedule I drugs are available for research only and have no approved medical use. Schedule II drugs are available only by prescription (unrefillable) and require a form for ordering. Schedule III and IV drugs are available by prescription, may have five refills in 6 months, and may be ordered orally. Most Schedule V drugs are available over the counter.

†Taking drugs by injection can increase the risk of infection through needle contamination with staphylococci, HIV, hepatitis, and other organisms.

‡Associated with sexual assaults.

§Not available by prescription in the United States.

REPRODUCED FROM: National Institute on Drug Abuse. *Prescription Drug Abuse Chart.* 2011. Available at: http://www.drugabuse.gov/DrugPages/PrescripDrugsChart.html.

TABLE 12.4	Other Commonly Abused Drugs

Substance (by Category)	Examples of Commercial and/ or Street Names	U.S. DEA Schedule*/ How Administered†	Acute Effects/Health Risks
Tobacco			
Nicotine	Nicotine. Found in cigarettes, cigars, bidis, and smokeless tobacco; snuff, spit tobacco, chew	Not scheduled/ smoked, snorted, chewed	Increased blood pressure and heart rate/chronic lung disease; cardiovascular disease; stroke; cancers of the mouth, pharynx, larynx, esophagus, stomach, pancreas, cervix, kidney, bladder, and acute myeloid leukemia; adverse pregnancy outcomes; addiction.
Alcohol			
Alcohol (ethyl alcohol)	Ethyl alcohol. Found in liquor, beer, and wine	Not scheduled/ swallowed	In low doses, euphoria, mild stimulation, relaxation, lowered inhibitions; in higher doses, drowsiness, slurred speech, nausea, emotional volatility, loss of coordination, visual distortions, impaired memory, sexual dysfunction, loss of consciousness/increased risk of injuries, violence, fetal damage (in pregnant women); depression; neurologic deficits; hypertension; liver and heart disease; addiction; fatal overdose.
Cannabinoids			
Marijuana	Blunt, dope, ganja, grass, herb, joint, bud, Mary Jane, pot, reefer, green, trees, smoke, sinsemilla, skunk, weed	I/smoked, swallowed	Euphoria; relaxation; slowed reaction time; distorted sensory perception; impaired balance and coordination; increased heart rate and appetite; impaired learning, memory; anxiety; panic attacks; psychosis/cough, frequent respiratory infections; possible mental health decline; addiction.
Hashish	Boom, gangster, hash, hash oil, hemp	I/smoked, swallowed	
Opioids			
Heroin	Diacetylmorphine; smack, horse, brown sugar, dope, H, junk, skag, skunk, white horse, China white; cheese (with over-the-counter cold medicine and antihistamine)	I/injected, smoked, snorted	Euphoria; drowsiness; impaired coordination; dizziness; confusion; nausea; sedation; feeling of heaviness in the body; slowed or arrested breathing/ constipation; endocarditis; hepatitis; HIV; addiction; fatal overdose.
Opium	Laudanum, paregoric; big O, black stuff, block, gum, hop	II, III, V/ swallowed, smoked	

(Continues)

TABLE 12.4   Other Commonly Abused Drugs *(Continued)*

Substance (by Category)	Examples of Commercial and/ or Street Names	U.S. DEA Schedule*/ How Administered†	Acute Effects/Health Risks
Stimulants			
Cocaine	Cocaine hydrochloride; blow, bump, C, candy, Charlie, coke, crack, flake, rock, snow, toot	II/snorted, smoked, injected	Increased heart rate, blood pressure, body temperature, metabolism; feelings of exhilaration; increased energy, mental alertness; tremors; reduced appetite; irritability; anxiety; panic; paranoia; violent behavior; psychosis/ weight loss, insomnia; cardiac or cardiovascular complications; stroke; seizures; addiction.
Amphetamine	Biphetamine, Dexedrine; bennies, black beauties, crosses, hearts, LA turnaround, speed, truck drivers, uppers	II/swallowed, snorted, smoked, injected	
Methamphetamine	Desoxyn; meth, ice, crank, chalk, crystal, fire, glass, go fast, speed	II/swallowed, snorted, smoked, injected	Also: For cocaine: nasal damage from snorting. For methamphetamine: severe dental problems.
Club Drugs			
Methylenedioxy-methamphetamine (MDMA)	Methylenedioxy-methamphetamine, MDMA; ecstasy, Adam, clarity, Eve, lover's speed, peace, uppers	I/swallowed, snorted, injected	For MDMA: mild hallucinogenic effects; increased tactile sensitivity; empathic feelings; lowered inhibition; anxiety; chills; sweating; teeth clenching; muscle cramping/sleep disturbances; depression; impaired memory; hyperthermia; addiction.
Flunitrazepam‡	Rohypnol; forget-me pill, Mexican Valium, R2, roach, Roche, roofies, roofinol, rope, rophies	IV/swallowed, snorted	For flunitrazepam: sedation; muscle relaxation; confusion; memory loss; dizziness; impaired coordination/ addiction.
Gamma-hydroxybutyrate (GHB)‡	Gamma-hydroxybutyrate, GHB; G, Georgia home boy, grievous bodily harm, liquid ecstasy, soap, scoop, goop, liquid X	I/swallowed	For GHB: drowsiness; nausea; headache; disorientation; loss of coordination; memory loss/unconsciousness; seizures; coma.
Dissociative Drugs			
Ketamine	Ketalar SV: cat Valium, K, Special K, vitamin K	III/injected, snorted, smoked	Feelings of being separate from one's body and environment; impaired motor function/anxiety; tremors; numbness; memory loss; nausea.
Phencyclidine (PCP) and analogues	Phencyclidine, PCP; angel dust, boat, hog, love boat, peace pill	I, II/swallowed, smoked, injected	

TABLE 12.4   **Other Commonly Abused Drugs** *(Continued)*

Substance (by Category)	Examples of Commercial and/ or Street Names	U.S. DEA Schedule*/ How Administered†	Acute Effects/Health Risks
Dissociative Drugs *(continued)*			
Salvia divinorum	Salvia; shepherdess's herb, Maria Pastora, magic mint, Sally-D	Not scheduled/ chewed, swallowed, smoked	Also: For ketamine: analgesia; impaired memory; delirium; respiratory depression and arrest; death.
Dextromethorphan (DXM)	Dextromethorphan, DXM. Found in some cough and cold medications; robotripping, robo, triple C	Not scheduled/ swallowed	For PCP and analogues: analgesia; psychosis; aggression; violence; slurred speech; loss of coordination; hallucinations. For DXM: euphoria; slurred speech; confusion; dizziness; distorted visual perceptions.
Hallucinogens			
Lysergic acid diethylamide (LSD)	Lysergic acid diethylamide, LSD; acid, blotter, cubes, microdot yellow sunshine, blue heaven	I/swallowed, absorbed through mouth tissues	Altered states of perception and feeling; hallucinations; nausea. Also: For LSD and mescaline: increased body temperature, heart rate, blood pressure; loss of appetite; sweating; sleeplessness; numbness, dizziness, weakness, tremors; impulsive behavior; rapid shifts in emotion.
Mescaline	Mescaline; buttons, cactus, mesc, peyote	I/swallowed, smoked	
Psilocybin	Psilocybin; magic mushrooms, purple passion, shrooms, little smoke	I/swallowed	For LSD: flashbacks, hallucinogen persisting perception disorder. For psilocybin: nervousness; paranoia; panic.
Other Compounds			
Anabolic steroids	Anadrol, Oxandrin, Durabolin, Depo-Testosterone, Equipoise; roids, juice, gym candy, pumpers	III/injected, swallowed, applied to skin	For steroids: no intoxication effects/ hypertension; blood clotting and cholesterol changes; liver cysts; hostility and aggression; acne.

(Continues)

TABLE 12.4   **Other Commonly Abused Drugs** *(Continued)*

Substance (by Category)	Examples of Commercial and/ or Street Names	U.S. DEA Schedule*/ How Administered†	Acute Effects/Health Risks
Other Compounds			
Inhalants	Solvents (paint thinners, gasoline, glues), gases (butane, propane, aerosol propellants, nitrous oxide), nitrites (isoamyl, isobutyl, cyclohexyl); laughing gas, poppers, snappers, whippets	Not scheduled/ inhaled through nose or mouth	In adolescents: premature stoppage of growth. In males: prostate cancer, reduced sperm production, shrunken testicles, breast enlargement. In females: menstrual irregularities, development of beard and other masculine characteristics. For inhalants (varies by chemical): stimulation; loss of inhibition; headache; nausea or vomiting; slurred speech; loss of motor coordination; wheezing/cramps; muscle weakness; depression; memory impairment; damage to cardiovascular and nervous systems; unconsciousness; sudden death.

*Schedule I and II drugs have a high potential for abuse. They require greater storage security and have a quota on manufacturing, among other restrictions. Schedule I drugs are available for research only and have no approved medical use. Schedule II drugs are available only by prescription (unrefillable) and require a form for ordering. Schedule III and IV drugs are available by prescription, may have five refills in 6 months, and may be ordered orally. Some Schedule V drugs are available over the counter.

†Some of the health risks are directly related to the route of drug administration. For example, injection drug use can increase the risk of infection through needle contamination with staphylococci, HIV, hepatitis, and other organisms.

‡Associated with sexual assaults.

REPRODUCED FROM: National Institute on Drug Abuse. *Commonly Abused Drugs*. 2011. Available at: http://www.drugabuse.gov/DrugPages/DrugsofAbuse.html.

street names, and the health risks associated with their use. The abuse of these drugs leads to dependence on them and/or addiction to them.

Prescription Drug Misuse and Abuse

Although prescription drugs can be an ally in the fight against disease and illness, like all drugs they can result in serious side effects. Therefore, it is important that they be used as prescribed. Prescription drug *misuse* is when medications are used in a way other than prescribed, but not to cause an intentional "high." Sometimes, people misunderstand the directions for taking a drug, taking too little or too much. Sometimes they think they will get better faster if they take more. That is far from the truth, however. If more than the recommended amount of a drug is taken, it is more likely that potential side effects develop—some of which can even be life threatening.

Prescription drug *abuse* is the intentional use of a medication without a prescription (or in a way other than as prescribed) for the experience or feeling (the "high") it causes. The prescribed medications most commonly abused are listed in Table 12.3. They include pain relievers,

What I Need to Know

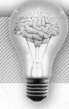

Risks of Commonly Misused or Abused Prescription Drugs

Prescription medication can be a vital adjunct to therapy and pain relief. However, it can also be misused and abused. The most commonly misused and abused prescription drugs are listed below, with associated risks of misuse or abuse.

Opioids (used to treat pain):

- *Addiction.* Prescription opioids act on the same receptors as heroin and therefore can be highly addictive. People who abuse them sometimes alter the route of administration (e.g., snorting or injecting vs. taking orally) to intensify the effect; some even report moving from prescription opioids to heroin.

- *Overdose.* Abuse of opioids, alone or in combination with alcohol or other drugs, can depress respiration and lead to death. Overdose is a major concern: The number of fatal poisonings involving prescription pain relievers has more than tripled since 1999.

- *Heightened HIV risk.* Injection of opioids increases the risk of HIV and other infectious diseases through use of unsterile or shared equipment.

Central nervous system depressants (used to treat anxiety and sleep problems):

- *Addiction and dangerous withdrawal symptoms.* These drugs are addictive and, in chronic users or abusers, discontinuing them absent a physician's guidance can bring about severe withdrawal symptoms, including seizures that can be life threatening.

- *Overdose.* High doses can cause severe respiratory depression. This risk increases when central nervous system depressants are combined with other medications or alcohol.

Stimulants (used to treat ADHD—attention deficit hyperactivity disorder—and narcolepsy):

- *Addiction and other health consequences.* These include psychosis, seizures, and cardiovascular complications.

REPRODUCED FROM: National Institute on Drug Abuse. *Prescription Drug Abuse: A Research Update from the National Institute on Drug Abuse.* 2011. Available at: http://www.drugabuse.gov/tib/prescription.html.

tranquilizers, stimulants, and sedatives (National Institute on Drug Abuse, 2011).

Drug Dependence and Addiction

Drug abuse can lead to drug dependence or addiction. **Drug dependence** is when a person needs a drug to function normally and abruptly stopping the drug leads to withdrawal symptoms (PubMed Health, 2010). **Drug addiction** is a chronic, relapsing brain disease characterized by compulsive drug-seeking behaviors and drug use despite harmful consequences. It is considered a brain disease because the addiction changes the brain's structure and how it works. Brain imaging studies from drug-addicted individuals show physical changes in areas of the brain that are critical to judgment, decision making, learning and memory, and behavior control (National Institute on Drug Abuse, 2010).

Dependence and addiction are not necessarily linked. A person may have a physical dependence on a substance without having an addiction. For example, certain blood pressure medications do not cause addiction but they can cause physical dependence. Other drugs, such as cocaine, cause addiction without leading to physical dependence.

Myths and Facts

What Is Known About Marijuana

MYTH	
Use of marijuana is pretty much harmless.	Marijuana increases heart rate by 20–100% shortly after smoking it; this effect can last up to 3 hours. Some heart attacks have been reported during marijuana use. Furthermore, marijuana intoxication can cause distorted perceptions, impaired coordination, difficulty with thinking and problem solving, and problems with learning and memory. Research has shown that in chronic users, marijuana's adverse impact on learning and memory can last for days or weeks after the acute effects of the drug wear off.
One of the positive aspects of marijuana use is that it does not produce addiction.	Research studies find that about 9% of users become addicted to marijuana; this number increases among those who start young (to about 17%) and among daily users (25–50%).
There are no withdrawal symptoms once someone stops using marijuana.	Long-term marijuana abusers trying to quit report withdrawal symptoms including irritability, sleeplessness, decreased appetite, anxiety, and drug craving; all of which can make it difficult to remain abstinent. These symptoms begin within about 1 day after drug cessation, peak at 2–3 days, and subside within 1–2 weeks after drug cessation.
Marijuana use is safer than smoking cigarettes because marijuana does not contain any carcinogens.	Numerous studies have shown marijuana smoke to contain carcinogens and to be an irritant to the lungs. In fact, marijuana smoke contains 50–70% more carcinogenic hydrocarbons than that contained in tobacco smoke. Marijuana users usually inhale more deeply and hold their breath longer than tobacco smokers do, which further increase the lungs' exposure to carcinogenic smoke.

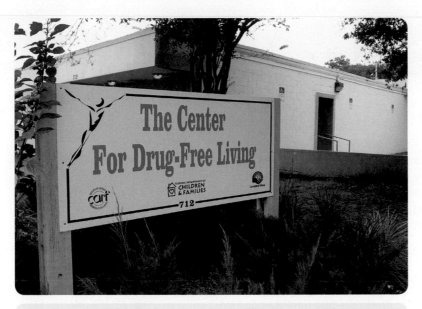

Treatment for drug abuse often requires a stay at a treatment facility to detoxify and to explore the reasons for the abuse and strategies to prevent its recurrence.

Why Are Drugs Abused in Spite of Known Health Risks?

Most abused drugs directly or indirectly target the brain's reward system by flooding the circuit with dopamine. Dopamine is a neurotransmitter present in regions of the brain that regulate movement, emotion, cognition, motivation, and feelings of pleasure. When some drugs of abuse are taken, they can release 2–10 times the amount of dopamine that natural rewards (such as eating and sex) release. In some cases, this occurs almost immediately (as when drugs are smoked or injected), and the effects can last much longer than those produced by natural rewards. The overstimulation of this system produces the euphoric effects sought by people who abuse drugs, and they repeat the abuse of these drugs to obtain repeatedly those pleasurable sensations.

Drug Tolerance

As a person continues to abuse drugs that cause surges of dopamine, the brain responds by producing less dopamine or by reducing the number of dopamine receptors in the reward circuit. The result is a lessening of dopamine's impact on the reward circuit, which reduces the abuser's ability to enjoy the drugs. This decrease compels the addicted person to increase his or her drug dosage in an attempt to bring the dopamine function back to normal. When larger amounts of the drug are required to achieve the same dopamine high, this is a sign of **drug tolerance**. Drug tolerance is usually part of addiction.

Treatment for Drug Abuse

Treatment of drug dependency involves stopping drug use either gradually or abruptly (detoxification), support, and staying drug free (abstinence). **Detoxification** is the withdrawal of an abused substance in a controlled environment. Sometimes a drug with a similar action is taken instead to reduce the side effects and risks of withdrawal. Detoxification can be done on an inpatient or outpatient basis. Given the degree of dependence, a residential treatment program in which the dependent person lives at the treatment facility may be required. Residential treatment programs monitor and address possible withdrawal symptoms and behaviors. These programs use behavior modification techniques, which are designed to get users to recognize their destructive behaviors.

Treatment programs include counseling, both individually for the person (and perhaps family) and in group settings. Drug abuse treatment programs have a long aftercare component that continues when the user is released from the medical facility. There is also a peer support component.

Drug dependence: when a person needs a drug to function normally and abruptly stopping the drug leads to withdrawal symptoms.

Drug addiction: a chronic, relapsing brain disease that is characterized by compulsive drug seeking and use despite harmful consequences.

Drug tolerance: needing a higher dose of a drug to attain the same effect.

Detoxification: the withdrawal of an abused substance in a controlled environment.

What I Need to Know
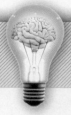

College Students and Substance Use

College students have a lot of experience with alcohol, tobacco, and other drugs. Even if they do not use these drugs, they know classmates and friends who do. However, they often estimate that more students use these drugs than actually do use them. That erroneous perception is likely to lead to the conclusion that the use of these drugs is not so bad if everyone else seems to be using them. The data in the table that follows are from a national study of the health behavior of college students.

Parameter	Male (%)	Female (%)
Percentage that drank more than two alcoholic drinks the last time they partied.	54	44
Perception of what percentage of students drank more than two alcoholic drinks the last time they partied.	85	87
During the last 2 weeks, the percentage that drank five or more drinks at one sitting.	42	27
Percentage that drove a car in the past 30 days after drinking.	18	14
Percentage that did something they regretted after drinking.	24	23
Percentage that smoked cigarettes in the past 30 days.	19	13
Percentage that used marijuana in the past 30 days.	17	11
Percentage that used cocaine in the past 30 days.	1	1
Percentage that used ecstasy (MDMA) in the past 30 days.	7	6
Percentage that used club drugs (GHB, ketamine, Rohypnol) in the past 30 days.	2	2

DATA FROM: American College Health Association. *American College Health Association–National College Health Assessment II: Reference Group Data Report Fall 2010*. Linthicum, MD: American College Health Association, 2011.

SUMMARY

The goal of this chapter is to provide you with the tools you need to make decisions regarding the use of alcohol, tobacco, and other drugs. To help you do that, a summary of important information included in this chapter is provided.

■ Alcohol affects many different parts of the brain including the cerebellum, limbic system, and the cerebral cortex. These brain changes explain the symptoms of alcohol abuse and intoxication.

■ One neurotransmitter—chemicals produced by the nervous system that convey information between nerve cells—susceptible to even small amounts of alcohol is called *glutamate*. Glutamate affects memory. Alcohol also causes an increased release of *serotonin*, another neurotransmitter, which helps regulate emotional expression, and *endorphins*, which are natural substances that may spark feelings of relaxation and euphoria as intoxication sets in.

■ Neurotransmitters adapt to create balance in the brain despite the presence of alcohol. These adaptations, however, have negative results such as building of alcohol tolerance, development of alcohol dependence, and alcohol withdrawal symptoms.

■ Different people react differently to alcohol. This is because of a variety of factors such as how much and how often one drinks, one's genetic background and family history of alcoholism, one's physical health, the size of the person, food in the stomach, and how quickly one drinks.

■ Strategies to overcome alcohol-related problems include keeping track of how much you drink, counting and measuring your drinks, setting goals, avoiding triggers to drinking, planning to handle urges to drink, and being ready to say NO when offered an alcoholic beverage.

■ A hangover is a combination of unpleasant physical and mental symptoms that occur after heavy alcohol drinking. Symptoms of hangover include fatigue, thirst, head and muscle aches, nausea, vomiting, stomach pain, dizziness, sensitivity to light and sound, decreased concentration, depression, anxiety, irritability, tremors, sweating, and increased blood pressure. There is no scientifically proven method of overcoming a hangover.

■ Binge drinking is a pattern of drinking of alcohol that brings BAC to 0.08 gram-percent or above. For a typical adult, this pattern corresponds to consumption of five or more drinks (male) or four or more drinks (female) in about 2 hours. Among other consequences, binge drinking is the major cause of alcohol poisoning.

■ Ingestion of toxic amounts of alcohol can lead to alcohol poisoning. Symptoms of alcohol poisoning include confusion, vomiting, seizures, slow and irregular breathing, blue-tinged or pale skin, low body temperature, and unconsciousness. Alcohol poisoning is a very serious condition that can result in death.

■ Fetal alcohol syndrome refers to growth, mental, and physical problems that may occur in a baby when a mother drinks alcohol during pregnancy. When a pregnant woman drinks alcohol, it easily passes across the placenta to the fetus. A pregnant woman who drinks any amount of alcohol is at risk, as no *safe* level of alcohol use during pregnancy has been established.

■ The adverse health effects from cigarette smoking account for an estimated 443,000 deaths, or nearly one of every five deaths, each year in the United States. More deaths are caused each year by tobacco use than by all deaths from HIV, illegal drug use, alcohol use, motor vehicle injuries, suicides, and murders combined.

■ Secondhand smoke is the combination of smoke from the burning end of a cigarette and the smoke breathed out by smokers. Secondhand smoke causes an estimated 46,000 premature deaths from heart disease each year in the United States among nonsmokers and an estimated 3,400 lung cancer deaths.

■ Tobacco use creates a dependence on nicotine. When a person quits smoking and nicotine is thereby withdrawn, anxiety, irritability, headache, hunger, and a craving for cigarettes or other sources of nicotine occur. These and other symptoms are called withdrawal symptoms.

- There are several strategies that have been found effective in helping people quit smoking. These include writing what you do not like about smoking and why you want to quit; enlisting support of family, friends, classmates, and coworkers; withdrawing gradually; avoiding smoking triggers; trying stop-smoking medications; managing stress; keeping busy; and rewarding not smoking.

- Prescription drug abuse is the intentional use of a medication without a prescription, in a way other than as prescribed, or for the experience or feeling it causes. The prescribed medications most commonly used inappropriately are pain relievers, tranquilizers, stimulants, and sedatives.

- The abuse of recreational drugs leads to dependence on them and/or addiction to them. *Drug dependence* is when a person needs a drug to function normally and abruptly stopping the drug leads to withdrawal symptoms. *Drug addiction* is the compulsive use of a substance despite its negative or dangerous effects.

- Most drugs of abuse directly or indirectly target the brain's reward system by flooding the circuit with the neurotransmitter dopamine. The overstimulation of this system produces the euphoric effects sought by people who abuse drugs, and they repeat the abuse of these drugs to obtain repeatedly those pleasurable sensations.

- As a person continues to abuse drugs, the brain recognizes this and produces less dopamine or reduces the number of dopamine receptors. The result is a lessening of dopamine's impact on the reward circuit, which reduces the abuser's ability to enjoy the drugs. A larger dose is then required to achieve the desired effect. This is known as *drug tolerance*.

REFERENCES

Centers for Disease Control and Prevention. Smoking-attributable mortality, years of potential life lost, and productivity losses—United States, 2000–2004. *Morbidity and Mortality Weekly Report* 57 (2008): 1226–1228.

Centers for Disease Control and Prevention. *Alcohol and Public Health. Fact Sheets: Binge Drinking.* 2010a. Available at: http://www.cdc.gov/alcohol/fact-sheets/binge-drinking.htm.

Centers for Disease Control and Prevention. *Fetal Alcohol Spectrum Disorders (FASDs).* 2010b. Available at: http://www.cdc.gov/ncbddd/fasd/facts.html.

Centers for Disease Control and Prevention. *Smoking and Tobacco Use: Health Effects of Cigarette Smoking.* 2011. Available at: http://www.cdc.gov/tobacco/data_statistics/fact_sheets/health_effects/effects_cig_smoking/index.htm.

Dawson, D. A., Grant, B. F., Stinson, F. S., and Chou, P. S. Another look at heavy episodic drinking and alcohol use disorders among college and noncollege youth. *Journal of Studies on Alcohol* 65(4) (2004): 477–488.

DrugAlcohol-rehab.com. *Famous Celebrity Addicts.* 2011. Available at: http://www.drugalcohol-rehab.com/famous-addicts.htm.

Mayo Clinic Staff. *Alcohol Poisoning: Symptoms.* 2010. Available at: http://www.mayoclinic.com/health/alcohol-poisoning/ds00861/dsection=symptoms

Mayo Foundation for Medical Education and Research. *Alcohol Poisoning: Symptoms.* 2010. Available at: http://www.mayoclinic.com/health/alcohol-poisoning/DS00861/DSECTION=symptoms.

Mayo Foundation for Medical Education and Research. *Quit Smoking: Proven Strategies to Help You Quit.* 2011. Available at: http://www.mayoclinic.com/health/quit-smoking/SK00056.

Medline Plus. *Nicotine Addiction and Withdrawal.* 2010. Available at: http://www.nlm.nih.gov/medlineplus/ency/article/000953.htm.

National Institute on Alcohol Abuse and Alcoholism. *Tips for Cutting Down on Drinking.* 2008. Available at: http://pubs.niaaa.nih.gov/publications/Tips/tips.htm.

National Institute on Alcohol Abuse and Alcoholism. *Beyond Hangovers: Understanding Alcohol's Impact on Your Health.* Bethesda, MD: National Institute on Alcohol Abuse and Alcoholism, 2011.

National Institute on Drug Abuse. *Drugs, Brains, and Behavior: The Science of Addiction.* Washington, DC: U.S. Department of Health and Human Services, 2010.

National Institute on Drug Abuse. *Prescription Drug Abuse: A Research Update from the National Institute on Drug Abuse.* 2011. Available at: http://www.drugabuse.gov/tib/prescription.html.

National Institutes of Health. Alcohol use and safe drinking. *MedlinePlus.* 2011. Available at: http://www.nlm.nih.gov/medlineplus/ency/article/001944.htm.

PubMed Health. *Fetal Alcohol Syndrome.* 2009. Available at: http://www.ncbi.nlm.nih.gov/pubmedhealth/PMH0001909/.

PubMed Health. *Drug Dependence.* 2010. Available at: http://www.ncbi.nlm.nih.gov/pubmedhealth/PMH0002490/.

Smokefree.gov. *Quit Guide: Quitting.* 2011. Available at: http://www.smokefree.gov/qg-quitting-quitday.aspx.

Timberlake, D. S., Hopfer, S. H. R., Rhee, S. H., Friedman, B. C., Haberstick, B. C., Lessem, J. M., and Hewitt, J. K. College attendance and its effects on drinking behaviors in a longitudinal study of adolescents. *Alcoholism: Clinical and Experimental Research* 31 (2007): 1020–1030.

Weschler, H. and Nelson, T. F. What we have learned from the Harvard School of Public Health College Alcohol Study: Focusing attention on college student alcohol consumption and the environmental conditions that promote it. *Journal of Studies on Alcohol and Drugs* 69 (2008): 481–490.

INTERNET RESOURCES

National Institute on Alcohol Abuse and Alcoholism
http://www.niaaa.nih.gov/Pages/default.aspx
National Institute on Drug Abuse
http://www.nida.nih.gov/nidahome.html
Substance Abuse and Mental Health Administration
http://www.samhsa.gov/

U.S. Food and Drug Administration
http://www.fda.gov/
Centers for Disease Control and Prevention
http://www.cdc.gov

Glossary

Abortion: the termination of a pregnancy; induced abortion is the purposeful termination of a pregnancy.

Adoption: a legal arrangement in which birth parents turn over responsibility of parenting the child to others, the adoptive parents.

Advice support: providing advice that will help a person make good decisions and improve that person's life.

Aerobic exercise: exercise in which the body can provide all of its need for oxygen, allowing the activity to be sustained and continuous.

Aggressiveness: a behavior whereby people get their entitlements but violate someone else's rights.

Alcohol poisoning: ingestion of a toxic amount of alcohol.

Anaerobic exercise: exercise that depletes oxygen over a short period of time—such as running a 100-yard dash or sprinting—and, therefore, cannot be sustained as long as aerobic exercise.

Angina: chest pain resulting from coronary arteries not being able to bring enough oxygen and nutrients to the heart muscle because they are partly blocked by plaque.

Anorexia nervosa: an eating disorder characterized by emaciation, a relentless pursuit of thinness, a distortion of body image, and intense fear of gaining weight.

Anxiety: an unrealistic fear accompanied by physiological arousal and avoidance or withdrawal behavior.

Arteries: large blood vessels that leave the heart to supply oxygen and nutrients to organs and tissues of the body.

Assertiveness: a behavior whereby people get their entitlements without violating anyone else's rights.

Atherosclerosis: when plaque narrows coronary blood vessels and makes them less flexible; also called hardening of the arteries.

Attachment anxiety: being dependent on one's partner to affirm one's worthiness of having his or her needs met. People with high attachment anxiety seem to be less psychologically willing or able to break up a relationship.

Attitude of gratitude: a focus on being grateful for what one has rather than bemoaning what one does not have.

Autoerotic behavior: sexually stimulating oneself with images or fantasies or by masturbating.

Binge drinking: a pattern of drinking of alcohol that brings blood alcohol concentration (BAC) to 0.08 grampercent or above; for a typical adult, this pattern corresponds to consumption of five or more drinks (male) or four or more drinks (female) in about 2 hours.

Blended families: separate families that unite as a result of remarriage, after divorce, or after the death of a spouse.

Body composition: the amount of body fat compared to other body components (called *lean body mass*).

Body image: the mental image we have of our physical appearance.

Body language: nonverbal physical reactions and positions of the body that relay information during communication.

Body mass index (BMI): a measure of body fat based on height and weight that is often used to define underweight, overweight, and obesity.

Bulimia nervosa: an eating disorder characterized by recurrent and frequent episodes of eating unusually large amounts of food (binge eating), followed by behavior that compensates for the binge, such as purging.

Cancer: uncontrolled growth of abnormal cells in the body (called *malignant* cells) that can result in disability or death.

Capillaries: small blood vessels that transport oxygen and nutrients from the arteries to all cells of the body and from body cells to veins.

Cardiorespiratory fitness: the efficiency and effectiveness of the heart and lungs to transport oxygen to cells throughout the body.

Case report: a type of study that provides a detailed report of the diagnosis, treatment, and follow-up of an individual patient or research subject.

Case series: a type of study that provides a detailed report of the diagnosis, treatment, and follow-up of several patients or research subjects.

Case-controlled study: a type of study that compares two groups of people, one with the disease or condition and another group that does not have the disease or condition.

Celibacy: a lifestyle of sexual abstinence.

Cervical cap: a rubber, plastic, or metal cap containing a spermicidal agent that covers the cervix; similar to, but smaller than, the diaphragm.

Cervix: where the uterus opens into the vagina.

Chaining: a behavior change strategy that considers the many obstacles to performing a behavior as links in a chain; decreasing the number of links makes the behavior easier to do and more likely to occur.

Cholesterol: a waxy, fat-like substance found in the membranes of cells in all parts of the body that is used to make hormones, bile acids, vitamin D, and other substances.

Circumcision: the surgical removal of the foreskin of the penis.

Clinical depression: a mood disorder in which feelings of sadness, loss, anger, or frustration interfere with everyday life for a long period of time.

Clinical significance: the clinical meaningfulness of the results of a study; that is, whether the results actually impact health in a real or meaningful way.

Clitoris: external female sex organ that holds the highest concentration of nerves in the female body; during sexual arousal, the clitoris becomes erect and engorged with blood, similar to the male penis.

Cognitive behavior therapy: a psychological treatment that helps people change the thoughts that support their unrealistic fear.

Cohabitation effect: the finding that couples who cohabit premaritally are at greater risk for marital distress and divorce.

Cohabitation: living with a romantic partner to whom one is not married.

Cohort study: a type of study that compares an outcome in groups of people who are mostly alike but differ on selected characteristics.

Communicable diseases: diseases that are transmitted from person to person or by contact with infected objects.

Complementary or alternative medicine (CAM): diverse medical and healthcare systems, practices, therapies, and products that are not currently considered to be part of conventional medicine.

Conception: when a sperm penetrates an egg; the beginning of a pregnancy.

Consequences: the stage on the stress model at which the overall results of stress are seen: there may be negative consequences (e.g., illnesses and diseases or impaired relationships) or positive consequences (e.g., improved grades or job performance).

Contraceptive pills: birth control method that involves taking a daily dose of hormones in pill form; the hormones, usually estrogen and progestin, prevent ovulation, and therefore no egg is available to be fertilized.

Contraceptive sponge: a sponge containing a spermicidal agent that is placed over the cervix to prevent live sperm from entering the uterus.

Control theory: an explanation for the way in which spirituality affects health: control can be *primary control* (activities designed to change the situation) or *secondary control* (activities designed to take charge of oneself).

Controlled clinical trial: a type of study in which an experimental group is given a treatment or engages in a health behavior and a control group is not given that treatment or does not engage in that behavior.

Conventional medicine: medicine as practiced by holders of MD or DO degrees and by allied health professionals, such as physical therapists, psychologists, and registered nurses.

Copay: fees needing to be paid when visiting a doctor, hospital, or emergency room.

Corpora cavernosa: a structure in the penis that fills with blood during sexual arousal resulting in penile erection.

Corpus spongiosum: a structure in the penis that fills with blood during sexual arousal resulting in penile erection.

Cowper's gland: small glands adjacent to the urethra that secrete small amounts of an alkaline fluid.

Date rape: rape that occurs between two people who date; this form can also occur in instances when the victim is unable to give consent because of intoxication or other altered states of consciousness.

Deductible: the amount of the covered expenses a patient must pay each year before the plan starts to reimburse the patient.

Dehydration: too little water/fluid in the body, which can cause nausea, diarrhea, and weakness.

Depo-Provera: birth control method that involves receiving an injection of progestin every 12 weeks to prevent ovulation.

DESC form: a method of making an assertive statement that involves Describing the situation, Expressing feelings, Specifying the desired change, and identifying the Consequences of making or not making the change.

Detoxification: the withdrawal of an abused substance in a controlled environment.

Diabetes: a group of diseases marked by high levels of blood glucose resulting from defects in insulin production, insulin action, or both.

Diaphragm: a shallow, rubber or synthetic rubber cap surrounding a flexible metal ring that covers the cervix to prevent sperm from entering the uterus.

Diaphragmatic breathing: using the diaphragm rather than the chest muscles to breathe.

Dietary fiber: known as roughage or bulk, it includes all parts of plant foods that your body cannot digest or absorb.

Distress: stress that leads to negative, or unwelcome, consequences.

Doctors of osteopathy (DOs): physicians who have received training in hands-on manual medicine and the body's musculoskeletal system.

Dopamine: a brain chemical that plays a crucial part in how we perceive pleasure. Many drugs of abuse act through the dopamine reward system. Problems with the dopamine reward system can lead to clinical depression and other mental illness.

Double-blind study: a type of study in which neither the researchers nor the subjects know who receives the treatment and who does not.

Double-blind, randomized, controlled clinical trial: a controlled clinical trial in which subjects are assigned randomly to treatment groups and neither researchers nor subjects know to which group subjects are assigned.

Drug addiction: a chronic, relapsing brain disease that is characterized by compulsive drug seeking and use despite harmful consequences.

Drug dependence: when a person needs a drug to function normally and abruptly stopping the drug leads to withdrawal symptoms.

Drug tolerance: needing a higher dose of a drug to attain the same effect.

Emergency contraception: a method of using oral contraceptives to prevent pregnancy after unprotected sex, commonly referred to as the morning-after pill.

Emotional arousal level: the stage on the stress model at which feelings arise, such as anger, nervousness, or fear.

Emotional health: being able to express emotions and feelings appropriately.

Emotional support: expressions of empathy, concern, caring, love, and trust that generally come from family and close friends.

Environmental planning: an anxiety-management technique that involves adjusting the surroundings to cause less anxiety.

Erotic love (eros): a passionate, all-enveloping love. When erotic lovers meet, the heart races and a fluttering in the stomach and a shortness of breath occur.

Esteem support: expressions of confidence or encouragement, affirmation of an individual's strengths, or just the knowledge that others believe in an individual in order for the individual to feel better about himself or herself.

Eustress: stress that leads to positive, or welcome, consequences.

External locus of control: the perception that events in your life are the result of fate, luck, chance, and significant others.

Fallopian tubes: tubes that connect the ovaries to the uterus. After being released from an ovary, an egg travels through a fallopian tube to the uterus. Fertilization usually takes place in the fallopian tube.

Female condom: a loose-fitting sheath made of polyurethane that is placed in the vagina to collect the ejaculate.

Fertility: the ability to conceive a child.

Fetal alcohol syndrome: growth, mental, and physical problems that may occur in a baby when a mother drinks alcohol during pregnancy.

Fight or flight: the preparedness of the body to fight or flee from a perceived threat.

Flexibility: the range of motion around a joint.

Force field analysis: a method of adopting desired behavior by maximizing forces that encourage the behavior and minimizing forces that oppose the behavior.

Forgiveness: a sincere intention not to seek revenge on or avoid the transgressor and to replace negative emotions such as resentment, hate, and anger with positive emotions such as compassion, empathy, and sympathy.

Genitalia: structures of the reproductive system, some of which are external and some internal.

Hangover: a combination of unpleasant physical and mental symptoms that occur after heavy alcohol drinking.

Health belief model: a health behavior change theory that includes the constructs of perceived susceptibility, perceived seriousness, perceived benefit, perceived barriers, cues to action, and self-efficacy.

Health maintenance organization (HMO): a health insurance plan that negotiates payments with specific doctors, hospitals, and clinics that are part of a network; members must receive all of their medical care from network providers, except in emergencies, for the reduced fees to be provided.

Health: composed of physical health, mental health, emotional health, social health, and spiritual health.

Homologous: developing from the same tissue.

HONcode: a symbol that health-related websites can display if certified valid by the Health on the Net Foundation.

Hospice: an organization that cares for dying patients by comforting them, administering pain medications, and that provides counseling and comfort for families of the patients.

Hyponatremia: drinking too much water resulting in low blood sodium levels, which can lead to nausea, disorientation, muscle weakness, coma, or death.

Imagery: a relaxation technique that requires thinking of a relaxing scene or event.

Indemnity plans: managed care plans in which there are no networks involved so patients can change doctors at any time and usually do not need a referral to see a specialist or to go for x-ray procedures or tests.

Informational support: providing information that will help a person make good decisions and improve that person's life.

Insulin: a hormone that is needed to convert sugar, starches, and other food into energy needed for daily life.

Internal locus of control: the perception that you are in control of most events in your life.

Intrauterine devices (IUDs): synthetic objects inserted by a medical provider into the uterus for the purpose of contraception.

Labia majora: two large folds of skin that protect the external genitalia in a female.

Labia minora: two folds of skin that lie within the labia majora.

Life situation level: the stage on the stress model at which a significant life event occurs to which one needs to adjust.

Lifestyle diseases: diseases caused by health behaviors that place one at risk of developing such conditions as coronary heart disease, stroke, and cancer.

Locus of control: your perception of the control you have over events in your life.

Loneliness: a psychological condition characterized by a deep sense of social isolation, emptiness, and worthlessness.

Ludic love (ludus): a playful, flirtatious love. It involves no long-term commitment and is basically for amusement. Ludic love is usually played with several partners at once.

Male condom: a latex, polyurethane, or lambskin sheath that covers the penis and collects semen thereby preventing it from entering the vagina.

Mammogram: an x-ray of the breast to detect lumps.

Manic love (mania): a combination of erotic and ludic love. A manic lover's needs for affection are insatiable. He or she is often racked with highs of irrational joy, lows of anxiety and depression, and bouts of extreme jealousy.

Medical doctors (MDs): physicians who have received training in 4-year medical schools and performed residencies in which they learned a specialty branch of medicine.

Medical self-care: those things individuals do to deal with minor illness and injuries at home; this includes preventing, detecting, and treating illness and disease.

Meditation: a relaxation technique that requires focusing on something repetitive (such as breathing) or unchanging (such as a spot on the wall).

Menarche: a female's first menstrual period; usually occurs between the ages of 11 and 14 years.

Mental health: a state of well-being in which the individual realizes his or her own abilities, can cope with the normal stresses of life, can work productively and fruitfully, and is able to make a contribution to his or her community.

Mental illness: alterations in thinking, emotions, or behaviors that produce distress and impaired functioning.

Mons pubis: the rounded, soft area above the pubic bone in a female.

Muscle dysmorphia: sometimes referred to as bigorexia or reverse anorexia, it is a preoccupation with muscle development.

Muscular endurance: the ability of the muscle to contract repeatedly or for a sustained period of time.

Muscular strength: the maximum force a muscle can contract.

SuperTracker: an online dietary and physical activity assessment tool that provides information on diet quality and physical activity status, provides weight management guidance, and helps you set goals to achieve long-lasting health and wellness.

National health objectives: objectives developed by the federal government every 10 years targeted at health issues.

Natural family planning: a method of birth control that involves abstaining from intercourse during the fertile period in the menstrual cycle.

Neurotransmitters: chemicals produced by the nervous system that convey information between nerve cells.

Nonassertiveness: a behavior whereby people give up their entitlements so as not to bother someone else.

Nutrition Facts label: appearing on the packaging of most foods, it contains product-specific information (serving size, calories, and nutrient information), Daily Values (DVs) for 2,000- and 2,500-calorie diets, and dietary information for important nutrients, including fats, sodium, and fiber.

Nuva Ring: birth control method that involves the insertion of a vaginal ring that releases a form of estrogen and progesterone.

Observational studies: studies in which researchers observe the medical conditions that occur in association with particular behaviors without interfering with those behaviors.

Ortho Evra: birth control method that involves wearing a patch on the skin that steadily releases estrogen and progesterone.

Outercourse: sexual activities that do not involve penetration, such as hugging, massage, caressing, and rubbing clothed bodies together.

Out-of-pocket limit: the maximum amount of money per year a patient would have to pay for healthcare.

Ovaries: the female organ that produces and stores eggs and from which an egg ruptures each menstrual cycle.

Ovulation: the rupturing of an ovum (egg) from an ovary, which occurs cyclically.

Ovum: an egg; one ruptures from an ovary each menstrual cycle.

Oxytocin: a hormone produced by the hypothalamus that makes people feel good, lowers the levels of stress hormones in the body, reduces blood pressure, improves mood, and increases tolerance for pain. Physical contact increases oxytocin levels.

Panic disorder: a psychological disorder characterized by panic attacks: sudden feelings of terror accompanied by a pounding heart, perspiration, weakness, faintness, or dizziness.

Pap smear: a screening test for cervical cancer that involves scraping tissue off the cervix and examining it.

Penis: the external male sex organ through which urine and semen are passed out of the body.

Perception level: the stage on the stress model at which a life situation is interpreted as a threat.

Physical fitness: having the energy to meet daily demands and unexpected challenges effectively and efficiently. It is composed of four components: cardiorespiratory fitness, muscular strength and endurance, flexibility, and body composition.

Physical health: having your physiology functioning well such as blood pressure within normal range, blood cholesterol within recommended limits, and sufficient muscular strength and endurance to meet life's demands.

Physiological arousal level: the stage on the stress model at which the body reacts physically to a stressor, such as with increased heart rate, blood pressure, and muscle tension.

Placebo theory: when people believe something (e.g., being affiliated with a religious or spiritual organization) will help them, they often report that it actually does help them.

Point of service (POS): a health insurance plan in which members can choose their own physician as long as that physician has previously agreed to provide services at a discounted fee.

Posttraumatic stress disorder: a condition that develops in some people who have experienced a traumatic or extreme psychological or physical event resulting in recurrent fears, flashbacks, and nightmares.

Poverty: defined by the federal government poverty guidelines based on income: in 2009, if a family of four had an income of less than $21,954, the federal guidelines defined the family as living in poverty.

Preferred provider organization (PPO): a health insurance plan that negotiates payments with specific doctors, hospitals, and clinics that are part of a network, but members can choose the physician they want to see instead of being solely restricted to the network providers.

Primary care doctors: provide medical care when needed, encourage health-related behavior and discourage risky behaviors to help patients remain healthy, and oversee and coordinate patients' health and medical care; the first point of contact, a sort of gatekeeper for the medical and health needs of patients.

Problem drinking: when alcohol causes trouble in relationships, in school, in social activities, or in how one thinks and feels.

Prostate gland: a gland that secretes an alkaline medium that neutralizes the acidity in the vagina.

Psychological health: the ability to express, think, and behave appropriately relative to one's emotions.

Psychoneuroimmunology: a field of science that studies the relationship between the health of the mind and the health of the body.

Randomized clinical trial: a study in which subjects are assigned to different groups by chance rather than purposefully.

Rape: forcible sexual intercourse.

Relative risk: how much a particular risk factor influences the risk of a particular outcome in a prospective study.

Relaxation response: physiological changes that occur in the body as a state of relaxation is achieved; for example, decreased heart rate, blood pressure, and muscle tension.

Religion: a social entity that involves beliefs, practices, and rituals related to the sacred—sacred defined as mystical or supernatural or God or, in Eastern religious traditions, the ultimate truth or reality.

Reps (repetitions): the number of lifts during each set.

Resistance skills: ways to resist pressure to engage in objectionable activities while still maintaining positive personal relationships.

RESPECT: a conflict resolution technique that **R**ecognizes a difference of opinion exists, **E**liminates thoughts about what you want, **S**cans and *listens* to what the other person is communicating in words and feelings, **P**araphrases the *words* and *feelings* of the other person, **E**xpresses what you want and your reasons, **C**ollects several alternative solutions, and **T**ries the best alternative solution.

Resting heart rate: how fast your heart beats when you are at rest.

RICE: self-treatment for injury that includes rest, ice, compression, and elevation of the injured body part.

Risk perception: the likelihood of a negative outcome as a result of a health behavior.

Safer sex: sexual behaviors performed in a way that offers some protection against contraction of sexually transmitted infections, such as using a condom and limiting the number of sexual partners.

Safer sex strategies: behaviors that decrease the chance of someone who is sexually active contracting a sexually transmitted infection or creating pregnancy; included are using a condom, limiting the number of sexual partners, and maintaining a monogamous sexual relationship.

Scrotum: a sac of skin containing the testes.

Secondhand smoke: the combination of smoke from the burning end of a cigarette and the smoke breathed out by smokers.

Self-esteem: how high a regard or opinion one has of oneself.

Self-forgiveness: the willingness to abandon self-resentment in the face of one's own acknowledged objective wrong while fostering compassion, generosity, and love toward oneself.

Self-talk: an anxiety-management technique that involves making reassuring statements to oneself to feel less anxious.

Semen: sperm and the secretions of the seminal vesicles, prostate gland, and Cowper's gland.

Seminal vesicles: two sacs that secrete a substance believed to activate the ability of sperm to move spontaneously.

Service learning: using the knowledge and skills learned in class to improve the lives of other people, thereby learning more oneself and feeling a sense of spirituality.

Sets: successive periods of lifting without rest.

Sexual abstinence: refraining from engaging in sexual activity; usually refers to vaginal intercourse.

Sexual harassment: unwelcome sexual advances, requests for sexual favors, and other verbal and physical conduct of a sexual nature that negatively affects an individual's school or work performance or creates an intimidating, hostile, or offensive learning or working environment.

Sexual orientation: one's erotic, romantic, and affectional attraction to the same sex, the opposite sex, or to both sexes.

Shyness: being afraid of people, especially people who for some reason are emotionally threatening.

Social health: interacting well with others and the environment; having satisfying relationships, close friends, and people in whom to confide.

Social learning theory: a health behavior change theory that includes the constructs of reciprocal determinism, behavioral capability, expectations, self-efficacy, observational learning, and reinforcement.

Social phobia: a severe form of shyness.

Social support theory: support provided by others; composed of emotional support, esteem support, tangible support, informational support, and advice support.

Spermicides: chemical agents that kill sperm; can be foams, creams, suppositories, films, or gels.

Spiritual health: having a clear view of meaning and purpose in life, connections with others and with nature, peacefulness, and comfort with life choices.

Spirituality: a feeling of connection to the world and others in it, which may or may not be conceptualized as religion.

Stages of change theory: a health behavior change theory that considers people to be at different stages of readiness for change.

Staging: determination of the extent of a cancer in the body based on the size of the tumor, whether lymph nodes contain cancer, and whether the cancer has spread from the original site to other parts of the body.

Statistical significance: the likelihood that a study's findings are a result of chance.

Storgic love (storge): a calm, companionate love. Storgic lovers are quietly affectionate and have goals of marriage and children for the relationship.

Stress: the combination of a life situation perceived as a threat and the resulting physiological and psychological arousal.

Stressor: a life situation that has the potential to elicit physical or psychological arousal.

Stress reaction: changes in the body that occur when a stressor is perceived as a threat; for example, increased heart rate, blood pressure, and muscle tension.

Stroke: when the brain is deprived of blood because of a blockage of the blood vessels supplying the brain or a rupture of those blood vessels.

Suicide: the purposeful taking of one's own life.

Systematic decision making: a method of making decisions that involves perceiving and defining the problem, brainstorming and evaluating ideas, and acting on an idea and reacting to the effects.

Systematic desensitization: an anxiety-management technique that involves working from a non-anxiety-provoking situation gradually toward doing the anxiety-provoking stimulus.

Tangible support: providing for tangible needs such as money, time, clothing, food, and the like.

Target heart rate: how fast the heart should beat during exercise to improve cardiorespiratory fitness.

Testes: structures that produce sperm and the male sex hormone testosterone.

Thought stopping: an anxiety-management technique that involves recognizing when anxious thoughts occur and purposefully thinking about something else.

Triglycerides: fatty substances in the blood and in food that lower HDL and are related to the development of coronary heart disease.

Urethra: a tube that runs through the penis providing a route for urine and semen to exit the body.

Uterus: a pear-shaped organ to which a fertilized egg attaches to grow and develop until birth.

Vagina: a hollow, tube-like structure that runs from the vaginal opening to the uterus.

Vas deferens: the tube through which sperm from the epididymis travel to the penis.

Veins: blood vessels that return blood to the heart after oxygen and nutrients are exchanged for carbon dioxide and waste products.

Wellness: having the components of health in the recommended amounts and in balance with each other.

Withdrawal: a method of birth control that requires removing the penis from the vagina just prior to ejaculation.

Zygote: a fertilized ovum.

Index

Index

Anxiety *(Cont.)*
   posttraumatic stress disorder and, 64
   prevalence rates for, 9*b*, 73*b*
   single-parent families and, 245
   symptoms of, 59
APA (American Psychological Association), 61, 75
Appetite, loss of, 57
Arteries, 152
Arthritis, 126
Asbestos, 160
Asian Americans
   diabetes and, 169
   food diet pyramid for, 216*b*
   stroke risk and, 158
Aspirin, 188
Assertiveness, 65–66
Association, statistical, 39*b*
Atheism, 105
Atherosclerosis, 153, 156, 232
Atkins diet, 213
Attachment anxiety, 234–235
Attitude of gratitude, 88, 89–90, 97*b*, 107

B

Basal metabolism, 209
Beauty pageants, 202
Bedside manner, 177
Behavioral capability, 47, 48
Behavioral change contract, 140
Behavioral change theory, 42–48
   explanation of behavior, 42, 43*f*
   health belief model, 45–46, 47*t*
   modification of behavior, 42–43, 43*f*
   myths and facts on, 44*b*
   physical fitness and, 138, 140
   social learning theory, 46–48, 48*t*
   stages of change theory, 43–45, 45*t*
   for stress management, 98*b*
   usefulness of, 42–43
   weight-loss strategies and, 211
Beta-blockers, 60
Bias, researcher, 37
Bigorexia, 224–225
Binge drinking, 17*b*
Binge eating, 224
Bipolar disorder, 73*b*
Blended families, 246–247
Blindness, 170
Blisters, 141, 142*t*
Blood pressure. *See* High blood pressure; Hypertension
BMI (body mass index), 202, 204–205
Body cathexis, 202
Body composition, 125

Body image, 200–204
   cultural influences on, 201–202
   myths and facts about, 203*b*
   self-esteem and, 202, 204
Body mass index (BMI), 202, 204–205
Booz Allen Hamilton, 112*b*
Borderline personality disorder, 74*b*
Brain aneurysms, 158
Breast cancer, 159, 162–163, 166*t*
Breast self-examination (BSE), 166*b*
Bulimia, 224
Bulk (dietary fiber), 206*b*
Burial instructions, 116

C

CAM. *See* Complementary or alternative medicine
Cancer, 159–169
   breast, 162–163
   cervical, 163
   colorectal, 160–161
   dietary fiber and, 206*b*
   discrimination linked to, 14
   endometrial, 163–164
   humor and, 69*b*
   lung, 160
   myths and facts about, 168*b*
   physical fitness and, 126
   prevalence rates for, 159, 159*f*
   prostate, 164
   relationships and, 232
   screening guidelines, 166–167*t*
   skin, 161–162
   spiritual health and, 106
   symptoms, 159–160
   testicular, 165–169
   tobacco use and, 8, 160
   types of, 160–169
Cannon, Walter, 82
Capillaries, 152
Carbohydrates, 156*b*, 205*t*
Cardiopulmonary resuscitation (CPR), 188
Cardiorespiratory fitness, 124, 131–132, 131*b*
Case-controlled studies, 37
Case reports, 37
Case series, 37
Cause-and-effect relationships, 39*b*
CBE (clinical breast examination), 166*b*
CBT. *See* Cognitive behavior therapy
Census Bureau, 240, 246
Center for Cognitive and Social Neuroscience at University of Chicago, 61
Centers for Disease Control and Prevention (CDC), 34, 106

Index

Index

Index

Index

Romantic relationships, 233–237
    breakups, 234–237
    hormones and, 236*b*
    types of love, 233–234
Rotter, Julian, 90
Roughage (dietary fiber), 206*b*
Roy Rogers Restaurants, 112*b*

S

Safer sex strategies, 10
Safety gear for physical activities, 141
SAMHSA (Substance Abuse and Mental Health Services
    Administration), 75
Saturated fats, 155, 210
Scheduling of physical exercise, 136–137, 136*t*
Schizophrenia, 74*b*
Screening guidelines
    for breast cancer, 163
    for cervical cancer, 163
    for diabetes, 169
    for preventive healthcare, 182*t*
    for prostate cancer, 164
Screening guidelines for cancer, 166–167*t*
Secondary control, 108
Second-hand smoke, 160
Sedentary lifestyle, 8–10. *See also* Physical fitness
Selective serotonin reuptake inhibitors (SSRIs), 60
Self-care, 186–191
    emergency conditions needing healthcare provider, 191
    Internet information for, 189–191, 190*b*
    resources for, 189
    skills for, 186, 188
    supplies and medications, 188–189
Self-confidence, 56
Self-directing behaviors, 108
Self-efficacy, 45, 46, 47, 48
Self-esteem
    body image and, 202, 204
    psychological health and, 56–57, 70*b*
    spiritual health and, 108
    suicide and, 71
Self-forgiveness, 110, 114
Self-talk, 59, 88, 90
Selye, Hans, 82
Sender of verbal communication, 66
Service learning, 111–112
Serving size, 221
Sets of weight-training exercises, 133
Seventh-day Adventists, 30, 107
Sexual assaults, 239
Sexual behavior
    among college students, 9*b*
    cervical cancer and, 163

health and, 10–11
    marriage and, 244*b*
Sexually transmitted infections (STIs), 11, 17*b*
Sexual violence, 237–240
Shared intimacy, 233
Shin splints, 141, 142*t*
Shock stage of grieving, 114, 115*t*
Shyness, 60–61
    management of, 61
    self-esteem and, 56
    symptoms of, 61
Significance, statistical vs. clinical, 36, 38–40, 39*b*
Single-parent families, 245–246
Skin cancer, 161–162
Sleep
    depression and, 57
    health effects of, 9*b*
    loneliness and, 61
    poverty and, 13
    suicide and, 71
Slim-Fast, 213
Smoking. *See* Tobacco use
Social health. *See also* Relationships
    defined, 4
    physical fitness benefits for, 126, 130
    spiritual health's effects on, 107
Social learning theory, 46–48, 48*t*
Socially avoidant behavior, 61
Social phobia, 60–61, 73*b*
Social policy
    health behaviors and, 31
    health impact of, 12–16
Social support theory, 107, 108–109
Socioeconomic class, 31. *See also* Poverty
Sodium, 210
Spinal manipulation, 185
Spiritual health, 103–121
    advice support and, 109
    biological effects on health, 106–107
    control theory and, 107–108, 112, 114
    death and dying and, 114–116
    defined, 4–5
    emotional support and, 108
    esteem support and, 108
    faith-based health programs, 113*b*
    forgiveness and, 5, 109–111, 114
    grieving process and, 114, 115*t*
    health effects of, 105–109
    hospice care and, 114–115
    informational support and, 109
    modern conceptions of, 105
    placebo theory and, 109
    psychological health affected by, 107

Photo Credits

Recurring Features

Myths and Facts: *Cloud* © hugolacasse/ShutterStock, Inc.; *Magnifying Glass* © Kraska/ShutterStock, Inc.; **What I Need to Know** © Andresr/ShutterStock, Inc.

Chapter 1

Opener © ema/ShutterStock, Inc.; **2** © Photodisc/Getty Images; **3** © Michal Kowalski/ShutterStock, Inc.; **4** *bottom* © auremar/ShutterStock, Inc.; *top* © CEFutcher/istockphoto.com; **7** © Shariff Che› Lah/Dreamstime.com; **11** *bottom* © Tyler Olson/ShutterStock, Inc.; *top* © AbleStock; **16** © mangostock/ShutterStock, Inc.; **18** *bottom* © Kurhan/ShutterStock, Inc.; *top left* © Samuel Borges/ShutterStock, Inc.; *top right* © stefanolunardi/ShutterStock, Inc.; **19** © J. Scott Applewhite/AP Images

Chapter 2

Opener © Blend Images/ShutterStock, Inc.; **29** *left* © Wallenrock/ShutterStock, Inc.; *right* © BananaStock/Thinkstock; **30** © Eyecandy Images/Thinkstock; **31** © Tom Carter/PhotoEdit; **32** © iStockPhoto/Thinkstock; **33** © Juriah Mosin/ShutterStock, Inc.; **36** © iStockphoto/Thinkstock; **39** © Subbotina Anna/ShutterStock, Inc.; **46** © Digital Vision/Thinkstock; **49** © Ilja Ma ík/ShutterStock, Inc.

Chapter 3

Opener © PT Images/ShutterStock, Inc.; **55** © CEFutcher/istockphoto.com; **57** © asiseeit/istockphoto.com; **58** © bowdenimages/istockphotos.com; **63** © Image Source/Alamy; **65** © Monkey Business/Thinkstock; **68** © Blueberries/istockphoto.com; **72** © ZUMA Wire Service/Alamy; **75** © PaulaConnelly/istockphoto.com

Chapter 4

Opener © auremar/ShutterStock, Inc.; **83** *bottom* © s_bukley/ShutterStock, Inc.; *top* © Dmitry Melnikov/ShutterStock, Inc.; **91** © Huntstock/Thinkstock; **92** © Phil Date/ShutterStock, Inc.; **95** © Blend Images/ShutterStock, Inc.; **96** © OLJ Studio/ShutterStock, Inc.; **97** © auremar/ShutterStock, Inc.

Chapter 5

Opener © Maxim Tupikov/ShutterStock, Inc.; **105** *bottom* © iStockphoto.com/Thinkstock; *top* © CEFutchcr/istockphoto.com; **106** © Brad Wilson/Photonica/Getty Images; **107** © David Coates/AP Images; **111** © Lisa F. Young/ShutterStock, Inc.; **113** © asiseeit/istockphoto.com; **115** © Stockbyte/Thinkstock

Chapter 6

Opener © Photodisc/Getty Images; **125** © Minerva Studio/ShutterStock, Inc.; **130** © Andresr/ShutterStock, Inc.; **134** *a* Courtesy of Mark Dutton; *b* © Alin Dragulin/Alamy; *c left, c right* © Juriah Mosin/Shutterstock, Inc.; *d* © S.P./ShutterStock, Inc.; *e bottom, e top, f* Courtesy of Mark Dutton; **135** *d bottom left* © Jones & Bartlett Learning; *d bottom right* © Artur Bogacki/Shutterstock, Inc.; *d center* Courtesy of Mark Dutton; **138** © Tetra Images/Alamy; **139** © Stephen Coburn/ShutterStock, Inc.; **140** © kizilkayaphotos/istockphoto.com

Chapter 7

Opener *center* © Yuri Arcurs/ShutterStock, Inc.; *left* © Dmitriy Shironosov/ShutterStock, Inc.; *right* © wavebreakmedia ltd/ShutterStock, Inc.; **153** © Monkey Business Images/ShutterStock, Inc.;

Photo Credits

154 © iStockphoto/Thinkstock; 155 © Creatas/ Thinkstock; 162 © Photodisc/Getty Images; 170 © Arkady/ShutterStock, Inc.

Chapter 8

Opener © Photodisc/Getty Images; 176 © deepblue-phtographer/ShutterStock, Inc.; 178 © iStockphoto/Thinkstock; 180 © Photodisc/ Getty Images; 183 © Keith Brofsky/Thinkstock; 186 © wavebreakmedia ltd/ShutterStock, Inc.; 188 © Dennis D. Potokar/Photo Researchers/Getty Images; 189 iPad Photo: © ra2 studio/ShutterStock, Inc.; inset: Courtesy of CDC; 191 © Curt Ziegler/ ShutterStock, Inc.

Chapter 9

Opener © Warren Goldswain/ShutterStock, Inc.; 201 © Anton Oparin/ShutterStock, Inc.; 204 © Serg64/ShutterStock, Inc.; 209 *right* © Flashon Studio/ ShutterStock, Inc.; *left* © Kraska/ShutterStock, Inc.; 213 © DNY59/istockphoto.com; 224 © Ron Chapple Studios/Dreamstime.com; 225 *bottom* © Losevsky Photo and Video/ShutterStock, Inc.; *top* © Darren Hubley/ShutterStock, Inc.

Chapter 10

Opener © Yuri Arcurs/ShutterStock, Inc.; 232 © Stephen Coburn/ShutterStock, Inc.; 233 © mangostock/istockphoto.com; 235 *bottom* © dogboxstudio/ShutterStock, Inc.; *top* © Galina Barskaya/ShutterStock, Inc.; 237 © Ingram Publishing/ Thinkstock; 238 © oliveromg/ShutterStock, Inc.; 245 © J. Henning Buchholz/ShutterShock, Inc.

Chapter 11

Opener © oliveromg/ShutterStock, Inc.; 267 © Don W. Fawcett/Photo Researchers; 270 *bottom* © Photodisc/ Getty Images; 272 *sponge* Courtesy of Allendale Pharmaceuticals, Inc. (http://www.allendalepharm .com); 273 © John T. Takai/ShutterStock, Inc.; 286 *bottom* Courtesy of Renelle Woodall/CDC; *top* Courtesy of Joe Miler and Jim Piedger/CDC; 287 *bottom* Courtesy of Dr. Thomas F. Sellers/Emory University/CDC; *center* © Wellcome Trust Library/ Custom Medical Stock Photo; *top* Courtesy of M. Rein, VD/CDC; 288 *bottom* © DermPics/Photo Researchers.; *center* © National Medical Slide Bank/ Custom Medical Stock Photo; *top* Courtesy of Joe Millar/CDC; 289 *bottom* © Photodisc/Getty Images; *center* Courtesy of Susan Lindsley/CDC; *top* Courtesy of Reed and Carnrick Pharmaceuticals/CDC

Chapter 12

Opener © LiquidLibrary; 300 © LPJ/ShutterStock, Inc.; 302 © Ingram Publishing/Thinkstock; 306 © iStockphoto/Thinkstock; 309 © Science Source/ Photo Researchers; 310 © Jupiterimages/Thinkstock; 311 © Richard Levine/Alamy; 323 © Chris Livingston/ Getty Images

Unless otherwise indicated, all photographs and illustrations are under copyright of Jones & Bartlett Learning, or have been provided by the author.